Yearbook of NEUROLOGY 2022

DISCLAIMER

All the abstracts included in this book have been paraphrased in accordance with standard norms. The comments listed beneath the abstracts solely reflect the views and opinions of the corresponding authors.

Yearbook of
NEUROLOGY
2022

Editors

Kalyan B Bhattacharya MD DM MAMS FIAN FRCP (Edin)
Adviser and Senior Consultant
Department of Neurology
Medica Superspecialty Hospital
and
Formerly Professor and Head
Department of Neurology
RG Kar Medical College
Kolkata, West Bengal, India

Gagandeep Singh MD DM (Neurology) FAMS FRCP (London) FIAN FICP
Professor and Head
Department of Neurology
Dayanand Medical College and Hospital
Ludhiana, Punjab, India
and
Honorary Senior Research Fellow
Department of Clinical and Experimental Epilepsy
Institute of Neurology, Queen Square
London, UK

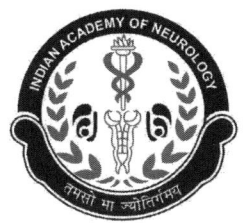

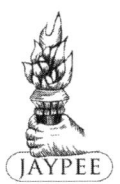

JAYPEE BROTHERS MEDICAL PUBLISHERS
The Health Sciences Publisher
New Delhi | London

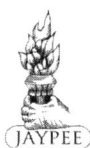 **Jaypee Brothers Medical Publishers (P) Ltd**

Headquarters
EMCA House
23/23-B, Ansari Road, Daryaganj
New Delhi 110 002, India
Landline: +91-11-23272143, +91-11-23272703
+91-11-23282021, +91-11-23245672
E-mail: jaypee@jaypeebrothers.com

Corporate Office
Jaypee Brothers Medical Publishers (P) Ltd.
4838/24, Ansari Road, Daryaganj
New Delhi 110 002, India
Phone: +91-11-43574357
Fax: +91-11-43574314
E-mail: jaypee@jaypeebrothers.com

Overseas Office
JP Medical Ltd.
83, Victoria Street, London
SW1H 0HW (UK)
Phone: +44-20 3170 8910
Fax: +44(0)20 3008 6180
E-mail: info@jpmedpub.com

Website: www.jaypeebrothers.com
Website: www.jaypeedigital.com

© 2023, Jaypee Brothers Medical Publishers

The views and opinions expressed in this book are solely those of the original contributor(s)/author(s) and do not necessarily represent those of editor(s) or publisher of the book.

All rights reserved by the author. No part of this publication may be reproduced, stored or transmitted in any form or by any means, electronic, mechanical, photocopying, recording or otherwise, without the prior permission in writing of the publishers.

All brand names and product names used in this book are trade names, service marks, trademarks or registered trademarks of their respective owners. The publisher is not associated with any product or vendor mentioned in this book.

Medical knowledge and practice change constantly. This book is designed to provide accurate, authoritative information about the subject matter in question. However, readers are advised to check the most current information available on procedures included and check information from the manufacturer of each product to be administered, to verify the recommended dose, formula, method and duration of administration, adverse effects and contraindications. It is the responsibility of the practitioner to take all appropriate safety precautions. Neither the publisher nor the author(s)/editor(s) assume any liability for any injury and/or damage to persons or property arising from or related to use of material in this book.

This book is sold on the understanding that the publisher is not engaged in providing professional medical services. If such advice or services are required, the services of a competent medical professional should be sought.

Every effort has been made where necessary to contact holders of copyright to obtain permission to reproduce copyright material. If any have been inadvertently overlooked, the publisher will be pleased to make the necessary arrangements at the first opportunity.

Inquiries for bulk sales may be solicited at: jaypee@jaypeebrothers.com

Yearbook of Neurology 2022/ Kalyan B Bhattacharya, Gagandeep Singh

First Edition: **2023**

ISBN: 978-93-5465-943-0

Printed at: Replika Press Pvt. Ltd.

CONTRIBUTORS

Editors

Kalyan B Bhattacharya MD DM MAMS FIAN FRCP (Edin)
Adviser and Senior Consultant
Department of Neurology
Medica Superspecialty Hospital
and
Formerly Professor and Head
Department of Neurology
RG Kar Medical College
Kolkata, West Bengal, India

Gagandeep Singh MD DM (Neurology) FAMS FRCP (London) FIAN FICP
Professor and Head
Department of Neurology
Dayanand Medical College and Hospital
Ludhiana, Punjab, India
and
Honorary Senior Research Fellow
Department of Clinical and Experimental Epilepsy
Institute of Neurology, Queen Square
London, UK

Section Editors

Achal Kumar Srivastava MD DM FRCP (London) FAAN FIAN FAMS FNASc
Professor
Department of Neurology
All India Institute of Medical Sciences
New Delhi, India

Atanu Biswas MD DM
Professor
Department of Neuromedicine
Bangur Institute of Neurosciences
IPGMER and SSKM Hospital
Kolkata, West Bengal, India

Bijoy Jose DM
Senior Resident
Department of Neurology
Amrita Institute of Medical Sciences
Kochi, Kerala, India

Debashish Chowdhury MD DM (Neurology)
Director Professor and Head
Department of Neurology
GB Pant Institute of Postgraduate Medical Education and Research
New Delhi, India

Faheem Arshad MD DM (Neurology)
Assistant Professor
Department of Neurology
National Institute of Mental Health and Neurosciences
Bengaluru, Karnataka, India

Hrishikesh Kumar MD DM (Neurology)
Vice Chairman
Movement Disorders Specialist
Institute of Neurosciences
Kolkata
Kolkata, West Bengal, India

Jino Vincent DM
Senior Resident
Department of Neurology,
Amrita Institute of Medical
Sciences
Kochi, Kerala, India

MV Padma Srivastava MD DM
FRCP (Edin) FAMS FNASc FIAN FNA
Professor and Head
Department of Neurology
Chief-Neurosciences Center
All India Institute of Medical
Sciences
New Delhi, India

Netravathi M DM (Neurology)
Professor
Department of Neurology
National Institute of Mental
Health and Neurosciences
(NIMHANS)
Bengaluru, Karnataka, India

Nirmal Surya MD DNB (Neuro)
FIAN MNAMS FRCP (London)
Chairman, Surya Neuro Center
Founder Trustee and Chairman
Epilepsy Foundation India
Mumbai, Maharashtra, India
President Indian Academy of
Neurology (IAN)
Member at Large, Presidium,
WFNR
President Indian Federation of
Neuro - Rehabilitation (IFNR)

Pramod Kumar Pal MD DNB DM
FIAN FRCP (Lon)
Professor
Department of Neurology
National Institute of Mental
Health and Neurosciences
Bengaluru, Karnataka, India

Prashanth LK MD DM (Neurology)
Consultant Neurologist and
Specialist
Parkinson's Disease and
Movement Disorders Clinic
Manipal Hospital, Miller's Road
Bengaluru, Karnataka, India

Pratap Sanchetee MD
(Medicine) DM (Neurology)
Consultant Neurologist
Sanchetee Neurology Research
Institute
Jodhpur, Rajasthan, India

Samhita Panda MD (Medicine)
DM (Neurology)
Additional Professor and Head
Department of Neurology
AIIMS Jodhpur
Jodhpur, Rajasthan, India

Sanjib Sinha MD DM FIAN FAMS
Professor and Head
Department of Neurology
National Institute of Mental
Health and Neurosciences
(NIMHANS)
Bengaluru, Karnataka, India

Satish V Khadilkar MD DM DNB
FIAN FICP FAMS FRCP (Lond)
Dean, Bombay Hospital
Institute of Medical Sciences
Mumbai, Maharashtra, India

Sudheeran Kannoth DM
Associate Professor
Neuroimmunology Laboratory
Department of Neurology
Amrita Institute of Medical
Sciences
Kochi, Kerala, India

Sunil Narayan MD DM DNB PhD
FIAN FRCP (UK) FEAN FAAN
Professor (Senior Scale)
Department of Neurology
Jawaharlal Institute of
Postgraduate Medical
Education and Research
(JIPMER), Dhanvantari Nagar,
Puducherry, India

Suvarna Alladi DM (Neurology)
Professor
Department of Neurology
National Institute of Mental
Health and Neurosciences
Bengaluru, Karnataka, India

Sudhir V Shah MD
DM (Neurology)
HOD and Professor
Department of Neurology
Smt NHL Municipal Medical
College and Sardar
Vallabhbhai Patel Institute of
Medical Sciences and
Research
Director of Neurosciences
Sterling Hospital
Ahmedabad, Gujarat, India

Tapas Kumar Banerjee MD
FRCP (London) FRCP (Edin) FAAN
FIAN
Medical Director and Chief
Consultant Neurologist
National Neurosciences Centre
Calcutta
Peerless Hospital Campus
Kolkata, West Bengal, India

Viswanathan LG DM (Neurology)
Assistant Professor
Department of Neurology
National Institute of Mental
Health and Neurosciences
(NIMHANS)
Bengaluru, Karnataka, India

Vivek Lal MD (Medicine) DM
(Neurology) FIAN FRCP (Edin)
Director, PGIMER
Professor and Head
Department of Neurology
Postgraduate Institute of
Medical Education and
Research (PGIMER)
Chandigarh, India

Associate Editors

Aastha Takkar Kapila MD (Medicine) DM (Neurology)
Associate Professor
Department of Neurology
Postgraduate Institute of Medical Education and Research (PGIMER)
Chandigarh, India

Adreesh Mukherjee MD DM (Neurology)
Assistant Professor
Bangur Institute of Neurology and Institute of Postgraduate Medical Education and Research
Kolkata, West Bengal, India

Ajith Cherian MD DM (Neurology)
Associate Professor
Department of Neurology
Sree Chitra Tirunal Institute of Medical Sciences and Technology
Thiruvananthapuram, Kerala, India

Akanksha Jain DM (Neurology)
Senior Resident 3rd year
Department of Neurology
Smt NHL Municipal Medical College
Ahmedabad, Gujarat, India

Amey Bhise DM (Neurology)
Senior Resident 2nd year
Department of Neurology
Smt NHL Municipal Medical College
Ahmedabad, Gujarat, India

Andelwar SL DM (Neurology)
Senior Resident 3rd year
Department of Neurology
Smt NHL Municipal Medical College
Ahmedabad, Gujarat, India

Ashish Kumar Duggal MD DM (Neurology)
Associate Professor
Department of Neurology
GB Pant Institute of Postgraduate Medical Education and Research
New Delhi, India

Ayush Agarwal MD DM DNB MNAMS
Assistant Professor
Department of Neurology
All India Institute of Medical Sciences
New Delhi, India

Divya KP MD DM (Neurology)
Assistant Professor
Department of Neurology
Sree Chitra Tirunal Institute of Medical Sciences and Technology
Thiruvananthapuram, Kerala, India

Divya M Radhakrishnan MD DM
Assistant Professor
Department of Neurology
All India Institute of Medical Sciences
New Delhi, India

Elavarasi A MD DM (Neurology)
Assistant Professor
Department of Neurology
All India Institute of Medical Sciences (AIIMS)
New Delhi, India

Gaurav Shah DM (Neurology)
Senior Resident 3rd year
Department of Neurology
Smt NHL Municipal Medical College
Ahmedabad, Gujarat, India

Heli Shah MD DM (Neurology)
Consultant Neurologist
Chaitanyam Neurology Clinic
Sterling Group of Hospitals
Jivraj Mehta Hospital
Ahmedabad, Gujarat, India

Hitav Someshwar BPTh MPTh (Neurophysiotherapy)
Junior Physiotherapist
Physiotherapy School and Centre
TNMC and BYL Nair Charitable Hospital
Mumbai, Maharashtra, India

Jacky Ganguly MD DM (Neurology)
Consultant Movement Disorders
Institute of Neurosciences
Kolkata, West Bengal, India

Jaslovleen Kaur MD DM (Neurology)
Fellow-Movement Disorders
National Neuroscience Institute
Singapore

Joydeep Biswas MD DNB (Neurology)
Consultant Neurologist
Ruby General Hospital
Kolkata, West Bengal, India

Kamalesh Chakravarty MD DM (Neurology)
Associate Professor
Department of Neurology
Postgraduate Institute of Medical Education and Research
Chandigarh, India

Contributors

Karthik Harishankar MD (Medicine)
Senior Resident
Department of Neurology
Postgraduate Institute of Medical Education and Research (PGIMER)
Chandigarh, India

Karthik Vinay Mahesh MD (Medicine) DM (Neurology)
Assistant Professor
Department of Neurology
Postgraduate Institute of Medical Education and Research (PGIMER)
Chandigarh, India

KP Vinayan MD DNB DM
Professor and Head
Department of Pediatric Neurology
Amrita Institute of Medical Sciences
Kochi, Kerala, India

Manjari Tripathi DM (Neurology) FNASc FRCP (Edin)
Professor and Unit Head
Department of Neurology
NIH Fellow (UCLA)
Neurosciences Centre
All India Institute of Medical Sciences
New Delhi, India

Mitesh Chandarana MD DM (Neurology)
Consultant Movement Disorders Specialist
Medisquare Superspeciality Hospital
Health1 Superspeciality Hospital
Ahmedabad, Gujarat, India

Raghunandan Nadig MD DNB
Professor
Department of Neurology
St John's Medical College Hospital
Bengaluru, Karnataka, India

Rakhil S Yadav MD DM (Neurology)
Consultant Neurologist
Suyog Neurology Center
Ahmedabad, Gujarat, India

Sandeep Kumar MD DM
Postdoctoral fellow
Cognitive Neurosciences
Department of Neurology
National Institute of Mental Health and Neurosciences
Bengaluru, Karnataka, India

Srinivas Raju MD DM (Neurology)
Consultant Neurologist
Manipal Hospital and Baptist Hospital
Bengaluru, Karnataka, India

Surbhi Mahajan MD (Medicine)
Senior Resident
Department of Neurology
Postgraduate Institute of Medical Education and Research (PGIMER)
Chandigarh, India

Suvorit Subhas Bhowmick MD DM (Neurology)
Consultant Movement Disorders Specialist
Movement Disorders Clinic
Vadodara Institute of Neurological Sciences
Vadodara, Gujarat, India

Thomas Mathew MD DM
Professor and Head
Department of Neurology
St John's Medical College Hospital
Bengaluru, Karnataka, India

Umangkumar Mukeshbhai Patel DM (Neurology)
Senior Resident 2nd year
Department of Neurology
Smt NHL Municipal Medical College
Ahmedabad, Gujarat, India

Zubin A Shah DM (Neurology)
Senior Resident 2nd year
Department of Neurology
Smt NHL Municipal Medical College
Ahmedabad, Gujarat, India

PREFACE

It is with great pleasure that we write the preface for the first edition of the *Yearbook of Neurology* in our country brought out under the aegis of the Indian Academy of Neurology.

The idea of bringing out such a compilation was conceived in January 2020 when the officials of the Indian Academy of Neurology approached and appointed me as the Editor-in-Chief for the book targeted to be published at the time of the annual conference in 2021. However, all hell broke loose within 2 months and we plunged into the disaster of the COVID-19 pandemic. Since everything went haywire and the publication houses were constrained to work with a substantially curtailed number of staff, the book could not be brought out. We tightened our belt and pledged sincerely to bring it out in 2022.

The book contains 16 chapters dedicated to different subspecialties in neurology. Each chapter is headed by one or two editors who are recognized experts in their chosen field and they with their associates have culled 10–12 publications from various peer-reviewed and indexed journals of international repute. The content of the papers has been condensed into abstracts in their own style and language, and the editors have written an expert commentary at the end as the key message, in keeping with what is the practice in the international volumes. There were occasional hiccoughs of various natures and therefore, we could not incorporate some chapters, despite our best intentions, as well as the contributors.

This is the maiden endeavor of the Indian Academy of Neurology to venture into such a project and it is hoped that it will be a regular project every year.

Yearbooks are generally meant for academicians, practicing consultants, and postdoctoral students with the aim of getting acquainted with the latest developments in the subjects and we sincerely hope that this book will serve that purpose.

We are thankful to the editors and their co-workers of the subsections for helping us to bring out the first volume of the book. We also extend our sincerest thanks to M/s Jaypee Brothers Medical Publishers (P) Ltd, New Delhi, India for kindly agreeing to publish the book and bringing it out on time.

We shall feel that our job is well done if it meets the requirements of the neurologists in our country.

Kalyan B Bhattacharya
Gagandeep Singh

CONTENTS

Section 1: Headaches
Section Editor: Debashish Chowdhury
Associate Editor: Ashish Kumar Duggal

1. A Clinical, Oculographic, and Vestibular Test Characteristics of Vestibular Migraine — 1
2. TOP-PRO Study: A Randomized Double-blind Controlled Trial of Topiramate versus Propranolol for Prevention of Chronic Migraine — 2
3. Randomized, Controlled Trial of Erenumab for the Prevention of Episodic Migraine in Patients from Asia, the Middle East, and Latin America: The EMPOWER Study — 3
4. If Headache has any Association with Hypertension, it is Negative. Evidence from a Population-based Study in Nepal — 5
5. Safety and Efficacy of Ubrogepant in Participants with Major Cardiovascular Risk Factors in Two Single-attack Phase 3 Randomized Trials: ACHIEVE I and II — 6
6. Randomized, Controlled Trial of Lasmiditan over Four Migraine Attacks: Findings from the CENTURION Study — 7
7. Characteristics and Outcomes of Patients with Cerebral Venous Sinus Thrombosis in SARS-CoV-2 Vaccine-induced Immune Thrombotic Thrombocytopenia — 9
8. Clinical Presentation, Investigation Findings, and Treatment Outcomes of Spontaneous Intracranial Hypotension Syndrome: A Systematic Review and Meta-analysis — 11
9. Calcitonin Gene-related Peptide Monoclonal Antibodies in Migraine: An Efficacy and Tolerability Comparison with Standard Prophylactic Drugs — 12
10. Clinical Features of New Daily Persistent Headache: A Retrospective Chart Review of 328 Cases — 13
11. An Internet-based Study on the Impact of COVID-19 Pandemic-related Lockdown on Migraine in India — 14
12. Characteristics and Natural Disease History of Persistent Idiopathic Facial Pain, Trigeminal Neuralgia, and Neuropathic Facial Pain — 16
13. Pediatric-onset Trigeminal Autonomic Cephalalgias: A Systematic Review and Meta-analysis — 18

14. Guidelines of the International Headache Society for Clinical Trials with Neuromodulation Devices for the Treatment of Migraine ... 19
15. Development and Validation of a Novel Patient-reported Outcome Measure in People with Episodic Migraine and Chronic Migraine: The Activity Impairment in Migraine Diary ... 21

Section 2: Neuroinfections
Section Editors: Pratap Sanchetee, Samhita Panda

1. Neurosyphilis, a True Chameleon of Neurology ... 25
2. Neurological Disorders Seen during Second Wave of SARS-CoV-2 Pandemic from Two Tertiary Care Centers in Central and Southern Kerala ... 26
3. Recurrent Neurocysticercosis: Not so Rare ... 28
4. 6-month Neurological and Psychiatric Outcomes in 236,379 Survivors of COVID-19: A Retrospective Cohort Study using Electronic Health Records ... 29
5. Severe Acute Respiratory Syndrome Coronavirus 2 Encephalitis is a Cytokine Release Syndrome: Evidences from Cerebrospinal Fluid Analyses ... 31
6. Determinants of Brain Swelling in Pediatric and Adult Cerebral Malaria ... 32
7. Presenting Symptoms of Leprosy at Diagnosis: Clinical Evidence from a Cross-sectional, Population-based Study ... 33
8. Association between High Proviral Load, Cognitive Impairment, and White Matter Brain Lesions in Human T-lymphotropic Virus Type 1-infected Individuals ... 35
9. Combined Testing of Cerebrospinal Fluid Interleukin-12 (p40) and Serum C-reactive Protein as a Possible Discriminator of Acute Bacterial Neuroinfections ... 37
10. Cycloserine and Linezolid for Tuberculosis Meningitis: Pharmacokinetic Evidence of Potential Usefulness ... 38

Section 3: Stroke
Section Editor: MV Padma Srivastava
Associate Editor: Ayush Agarwal

Important/Landmark Stroke Trials between June 2018 and February 2022

Thrombolysis

1. PRISMS: Effect of Alteplase versus Aspirin on Functional Outcome for Patients with Acute Ischemic Stroke and Minor Nondisabling Neurologic Deficits ... 41
2. EXTEND: Thrombolysis Guided by Perfusion Imaging up to 9 Hours after Onset of Stroke ... 42

3. Effect of Intravenous Tenecteplase Dose on Cerebral Reperfusion before Thrombectomy in Patients with Large Vessel Occlusion Ischemic Stroke: The EXTEND-IA TNK Part 2 Randomized Clinical Trial 43

Endovascular Treatment

1. BASILAR: Assessment of Endovascular Treatment for Acute Basilar Artery Occlusion via Nation-wide Prospective Registry 44
2. Aspiration Thrombectomy versus Stent Retriever Thrombectomy as First-line Approach for Large Vessel Occlusion (COMAPSS): A Multicenter, Randomized, Open-label, Blinded Outcome, Non-inferiority Trial 45
3. MR CLEAN-NO IV: A Randomized Trial of Intravenous Alteplase before Endovascular Treatment for Stroke 46
4. Safety and Efficacy of Aspirin, Unfractionated Heparin, Both, or Neither during Endovascular Stroke Treatment (MR CLEAN-MED): An Open-label, Multicentre, Randomized Controlled Trial 47
5. Safety and Efficacy of Intensive Blood Pressure Lowering after Successful Endovascular Therapy in Acute Ischaemic Stroke (BP-TARGET): A Multicentre, Open-label, Randomized Controlled Trial 48

Secondary Prevention

1. The Acute Stroke or Transient Ischemic Attack Treated with Ticagrelor and Aspirin for Prevention of Stroke and Death (THALES) Trial: Rationale and Design 49
2. The ESUS Trials: NAVIGATE ESUS 49
3. RESPECT ESUS 50
4. PRASTRO-II: Safety and Efficacy of Prasugrel in Elderly/Low Body Weight Japanese Patients with Ischemic Stroke: Randomized PRASTRO-II 51
5. Relationship of Spontaneous Microembolic Signals to Risk Stratifcation, Recurrence, Severity, and Mortality of Ischemic Stroke: A Prospective Study 52
6. Early Prolonged Ambulatory Cardiac Monitoring in Stroke (EPACS): An Open-label Randomized Controlled Trial 52

Neuroprotection

1. ESCAPE-NA1: Efficacy and Safety of Nerinitide for the Treatment of Acute Ischemic Stroke 53
2. Randomized, Controlled, Dose Escalation Trial of a Protease-activated Receptor-1 Agonist in Acute Ischemic Stroke: Final Results of the RHAPSODY Trial 54
3. A Multicentre, Randomized, Sham-controlled Trial on Remote Ischemic Conditioning in Patients with Acute Stroke (RESIST): Rationale and Study Design 55

Stroke Recovery

1. The SHINE Randomized Clinical Trial: Intensive versus Standard Treatment of Hyperglycemia and Functional Outcome in Patients with Acute Ischemic Stroke — 56
2. PROSCIS-B: Serum Anti-N-methyl-D-aspartate-receptor Antibodies and Long-term Clinical Outcome after Stroke — 57
3. RESTORE BRAIN Study — 58
4. Effects of Fluoxetine on Outcomes at 12 Months after Acute Stroke: Results from EFFECTS, a Randomized Controlled Trial — 58

Mobile Stroke Units

1. Prospective, Multicentre, Controlled Trial of Mobile Stroke Units — 59

Section 4: Epilepsy
Section Editor: Viswanathan LG, Sinha S

1. Epilepsy Outcome at Four Years in a Randomized Clinical Trial Comparing Oral Prednisolone and Intramuscular ACTH in West Syndrome — 61
2. Safety and Tolerability of Transdermal Cannabidiol Gel in Children with Developmental and Epileptic Encephalopathies: A Nonrandomized Controlled Trial — 62
3. Cost-effectiveness of Adrenocorticotropic Hormone versus Oral Steroids for Infantile Spasms — 64
4. The SANTÉ Study at 10 Years of Follow-up: Effectiveness, Safety, and Sudden Unexpected Death in Epilepsy — 65
5. Identifying Seizure Risk Factors: A Comparison of Sleep, Weather, and Temporal Features using a Bayesian Forecast — 67
6. The SANAD II Study of the Effectiveness and Cost-effectiveness of Valproate versus Levetiracetam for Newly Diagnosed Generalized and Unclassifiable Epilepsy: An Open-label, Non-inferiority, Multicenter, Phase 4, Randomized Controlled Trial — 68
7. Prevention of Epilepsy in Infants with Tuberous Sclerosis Complex in the EPISTOP Trial — 70
8. When Should a Brain MRI be Performed in Children with New-onset Seizures? Results of a Large Prospective Trial — 72
9. Improved Everyday Executive Functioning Following Profound Reduction in Seizure Frequency with Fenfluramine: Analysis from a Phase 3 Long-term Extension Study in Children/Young Adults with Dravet Syndrome — 73
10. Virtual Epilepsy Clinics: A Canadian Comprehensive Epilepsy Center Experience pre-COVID and during the COVID-19 Pandemic Period — 75

Section 5: Movement Disorders
Section Editors: Hrishikesh Kumar, Prashanth LK

Associate Editors: Adreesh Mukherjee, Ajith Cherian, Divya KP, Elavarasi A, Heli Shah, Jacky Ganguly, Jaslovleen Kaur, Mitesh Chandarana, Srinivas Raju, Suvorit Subhas Bhowmick

1.	Effects of Statins on Dopamine Loss and Prognosis in Parkinson's Disease	79
2.	Onset of Skin, Gut, and Genitourinary Prodromal Parkinson's Disease: A Study of 1.5 Million Veterans	80
3.	Safety and Efficacy of Mevidalen in Lewy Body Dementia: A Phase 2, Randomized, Placebo-controlled Trial	81
4.	Clinical Study of 668 Indian Subjects with Juvenile, Young, and Early Onset Parkinson's Disease	82
5.	Non-invasive Vagus Nerve Stimulation Improves Clinical and Molecular Biomarkers of Parkinson's Disease in Patients with Freezing of Gait	83
6.	Divergent Pallidal Pathways Underlying Distinct Parkinsonian Behavioral Deficits	84
7.	Detection of α-synuclein in CSF by RT-QuIC in Patients with Isolated Rapid-eye-movement Sleep Behavior Disorder: A Longitudinal Observational Study	85
8.	Predictors of Short-term Impulsive and Compulsive Behavior after Subthalamic Stimulation in Parkinson Disease	86
9.	Gene Therapy in Movement Disorders: A Systematic Review of Ongoing and Completed Clinical Trials	87
10.	Assessment of Botulinum Neurotoxin Injection for Dystonic Hand Tremor: A Randomized Clinical Trial	88

Section 6: Ataxia
Section Editors: Pramod Kumar Pal, Achal Kumar Srivastava

Associate Editor: Divya M Radhakrishnan

1.	SCA2 in the Indian Population: Unified Haplotype and Variable Phenotypic Patterns in a Large Case Series	90
2.	Cognitive Impairment in Spinocerebellar Ataxia Type 12	91
3.	Cognitive Impairment and its Neuroimaging Correlates in Spinocerebellar Ataxia 2	92
4.	Motor and Cognitive Outcomes of Cerebello-spinal Stimulation in Neurodegenerative Ataxia	94
5.	Quantitative Evaluation of Cerebellar Function in Multiple System Atrophy with Transcranial Magnetic Stimulation	95

6.	Nicotinamide Riboside Improves Ataxia Scores and Immunoglobulin Levels in Ataxia Telangiectasia	96
7.	Safety and Efficacy of Acetyl-DL-leucine in Certain Types of Cerebellar Ataxia: The ALCAT Randomized Clinical Crossover Trial	97
8.	Developments and Validation of a Patient-reported Outcome Measure of Ataxia	99
9.	Serum Neurofilament Light Chain as a Severity Marker for Spinocerebellar Ataxia	100
10.	Fampridine and Acetazolamide in EA2 and Related Familial EA: A Prospective Randomized Placebo-controlled Trial	102

Section 7: Dementia and Cognition
Section Editors: Suvarna Alladi, Atanu Biswas, Faheem Arshad
Associate Editor: S Sandeep Kumar

1.	Estimation of the Global Prevalence of Dementia in 2019 and Forecasted Prevalence in 2050: An Analysis for the Global Burden of Disease Study 2019	105
2.	Validation of ICMR Neurocognitive Toolbox for Dementia in the Linguistically Diverse Context of India	106
3.	Progression of Subjective Cognitive Decline to MCI or Dementia in Relation to Biomarkers for Alzheimer's Disease: A Meta-analysis	108
4.	Longitudinal Cognitive Changes in Genetic Frontotemporal Dementia within the GENFI Cohort	109
5.	Longitudinal Changes in Hearing and Visual Impairments and Risk of Dementia in Older Adults in the United States	110
6.	Sex Differences in the Genetic Architecture of Cognitive Resilience to Alzheimer's Disease	112
7.	Longitudinal Study of the Effect of a 5-year Exercise Intervention on Structural Brain Complexity in Older Adults. A Generation 100 Substudy	113
8.	Yoga Prevents Gray Matter Atrophy in Women at Risk for Alzheimer's Disease: A Randomized Controlled Trial	114
9.	Clinical Characteristics with Inflammation Profiling of Long COVID and Association with 1-year Recovery Following Hospitalization in the UK: A Prospective Observational Study	115
10.	Cognition, Behavior, and Caregiver Stress in Dementia during the COVID-19 Pandemic: An Indian Perspective	117
11.	A Randomized, Double-blind, Phase 2b Proof-of-concept Clinical Trial in Early Alzheimer's Disease with Lecanemab, an Anti-Aβ Protofibril Antibody	118

Section 8: Peripheral Neuropathy
Section Editor: Tapas Kumar Banerjee
Associate Editor: Joydeep Biswas

1. Characterization of Mononeuropathy of the Lateral Cutaneous Nerve of the Calf — 121
2. Mononeuritis Multiplex: An Unexpectedly Frequent Feature of Severe COVID-19 — 122
3. Efficacy of a Fixed Combination of Palmitoylethanolamide and Acetyl-l-carnitine in the Treatment of Neuropathies Secondary to Rheumatic Diseases — 123
4. Finger Drop Sign as a New Variant of Acute Motor Axonal Neuropathy — 125
5. Small Fiber Neuropathy in the Cornea of COVID-19 Patients Associated with the Generation of Ocular Surface Disease — 126
6. Antecedent Infections in Guillain–Barré Syndrome Patients from South India — 127
7. Motor Demyelinating Tibial Neuropathy in COVID-19 — 128
8. Calprotectin in Chronic Inflammatory Demyelinating Polyneuropathy and Variants: A Potential Novel Biomarker of Disease Activity — 129
9. Guillain–Barré Syndrome in Patients with SARS-CoV-2: A Multicentric Study from Maharashtra, India — 130
10. Epidermal Neurite Density in Skin Biopsies from Patients with Juvenile Fibromyalgia — 132

Section 9: Muscle Disorders
Section Editor: Satish Khadilkar
Associate Editor: Rakhil Yadav

1. Clinical Practice with Steroid Therapy for Duchenne Muscular Dystrophy: An Expert Survey in Asia and Oceania — 134
2. Deflazacort versus Prednisone/Prednisolone for Maintaining Motor Function and Delaying Loss of Ambulation: A Post-HOC Analysis from the ACT DMD Trial — 135
3. Management of Adrenal Insufficiency Risk after Long-term Systemic Glucocorticoid Therapy in Duchenne Muscular Dystrophy: Clinical Practice Recommendations — 136
4. AdipoRon, A New Therapeutic Prospect for Duchenne Muscular Dystrophy — 137
5. Phase 1 Study of Edasalonexent (CAT-1004), an Oral NF-κB Inhibitor, in Pediatric Patients with Duchenne Muscular Dystrophy — 139
6. Long-term Natural History Data in Duchenne Muscular Dystrophy Ambulant Patients with Mutations Amenable to Skip Exons 44, 45, 51, and 53 — 140

7. CRISPR Correction of Duchenne Muscular Dystrophy — 141
8. Emerging Strategies in the Treatment of Duchenne Muscular Dystrophy — 142
9. Cardiac Management of the Patient with Duchenne Muscular Dystrophy — 145
10. Respiratory Management of the Patient with Duchenne Muscular Dystrophy — 146
11. Making Sense of the Clinical Spectrum of Limb-girdle Muscular Dystrophies — 147
12. Plasmid-mediated Gene Therapy in Mouse Models of Limb-girdle Muscular Dystrophy — 149
13. The Limb-girdle Muscular Dystrophies: Is Treatment on the Horizon? — 150
14. The Effects of Resistance Exercise Training on Strength and Functional Tasks in Adults with Limb-girdle, Becker, and Facioscapulohumeral Dystrophies — 152
15. Genetic Determinants of Disease Severity in the Myotonic Dystrophy Type 1 OPTIMISTIC Cohort — 153
16. Efficacy and Safety of Dichlorphenamide for Primary Periodic Paralysis in Adolescents Compared with Adults — 154
17. The PRINTO Evidence-based Proposal for Glucocorticoids Tapering/Discontinuation in New Onset Juvenile Dermatomyositis Patients — 155
18. A Randomized, Double-blind, Placebo-controlled Trial of Infliximab in Refractory Polymyositis and Dermatomyositis — 157

Section 10: Sleep Medicine
Section Editor: Manjari Tripathi
Associate Editor: Kamalesh Chakravarty

1. High-risk Characteristics for Recurrent Cardiovascular Events among Patients with Obstructive Sleep Aponea in the SAVE Study — 160
2. Effects of Continuous Positive Airway Pressure on Depression and Anxiety Symptoms in Patients with Obstructive Sleep Apnoea: Results from the Sleep Apnoea Cardiovascular Endpoint Randomized Trial and Meta-analysis — 161
3. Sleep Duration and Risk of Cardiovascular Events: The SAVE Study — 162
4. Sleep Abnormalities and Polysomnographic Profile in Children with Drug-resistant Epilepsy — 164
5. Guidelines of the Indian Society for Sleep Research (ISSR) for Practice of Sleep Medicine during COVID-19 — 165
6. Cognitive and Behavioral Therapy for Insomnia Increases the Use of Continuous Positive Airway Pressure Therapy in Obstructive Sleep Apnea Participants with Comorbid Insomnia: A Randomized Clinical Trial — 166
7. Association of Obstructive Sleep Apnea and Cerebral Small Vessel Disease: A Systematic Review and Meta-analysis — 167

8. Long-term Efficacy and Safety of Phrenic Nerve Stimulation for the Treatment of Central Sleep Apnea	169
9. Multiple Treatment Comparison in Narcolepsy: A Network Meta-analysis	170
10. Clinical and Video-polysomnographic Analysis of Rapid Eye Movement Sleep Behavior Disorder and Other Sleep Disturbances in Dementia with Lewy Bodies	171
11. Insomnia with Objective Short Sleep Duration and Risk of Incident Cardiovascular Disease and All-cause Mortality: Sleep Heart Health Study	172
12. Sleep Disturbances and Sleep Disorders in Adults Living with Chronic Pain: A Meta-analysis	174
13. Long-term Effects of an Unguided Online Cognitive Behavioral Therapy for Chronic Insomnia	175
14. Effect of CPAP Treatment of Sleep Apnea on Clinical Prognosis after Ischemic Stroke: An Observational Study	176
15. Effectiveness of an Intensive Weight-loss Program for Severe OSA in Patients Undergoing CPAP Treatment: A Randomized Controlled Trial	177
16. Effects of a 12-week Yoga versus a 12-week Educational Film Intervention on Symptoms of Restless Legs Syndrome and Related Outcomes: An Exploratory Randomized Controlled Trial	179
17. Sleepiness and Sleepiness Perception in Patients with Parkinson's Disease: A Clinical and Electrophysiological Study	180
18. The Associations of Long-time Mobile Phone Use with Sleep Disturbances and Mental Distress in Technical College Students: A Prospective Cohort Study	181

Section 11: Neuro-ophthalmology
Section Editor: Vivek Lal

Associate Editors: Aastha Takkar Kapila, Karthik Vinay Mahesh, Surbhi Mahajan, Karthik Harisankar

1. Incidentally Detected MRI Signs of Increased Intracranial Pressure	185
2. Statistical Significance of Neuroimaging Signs in Idiopathic Intracranial Hypertension	186
3. More Guts than Brains	187
4. Papilledema – 'True' or 'Pseudo'!	188
5. Diplopia: Causes and Outcomes	189
6. Pregnancy and Neuromyelitis Optica Spectrum Disorder: Important Considerations	190
7. Newer Treatment Regimens in Neuromyelitis Optica-associated Optic Neuritis	191
8. The Epidemic of Idiopathic Intracranial Hypertension	192

9.	Diagnosing Idiopathic Intracranial Hypertension without Lumbar Puncture	194
10.	Optic Nerve Drusen and Pseudotumor Cerebri: Dual Pathology?	195

Section 12: Autoimmune Disorders
Section Editors: Bijoy Jose, Jino Vincent, Sudheeran Kannoth
Associate Editors: Thomas Mathew, Raghunandan Nadig

1.	Updated Diagnostic Criteria for Paraneoplastic Neurologic Syndromes	197
2.	Difference in the Source of Antiaquaporin-4-immunoglobulin G and Antimyelin Oligodendrocyte Glycoprotein-immunoglobulin G Antibodies in Cerebrospinal Fluid in Patients with Neuromyelitis Optica Spectrum Disorder	198
3.	Rituximab Treatment and Long-term Outcome of Patients with Autoimmune Encephalitis: Real-world Evidence from the GENERATE Registry	199
4.	Characterization of LRP4/Agrin Antibodies from a Patient with Myasthenia Gravis	200
5.	Autoimmune Encephalitis Resembling Dementia Syndromes	201
6.	Discontinuation of Immunosuppressive Therapy in Patients with Neuromyelitis Optica Spectrum Disorder with Aquaporin-4 Antibodies	202
7.	Overlapping Central and Peripheral Nervous System Syndromes in Myelin Oligodendrocyte Glycoprotein Antibody-associated Disorders	203
8.	Use and Safety of Immunotherapeutic Management of N-methyl-D-aspartate Receptor Antibody Encephalitis: A Meta-analysis	205
9.	Characterization of Extracranial Giant Cell Arteritis with Intracranial Involvement and its Rapidly Progressive Subtype	206
10.	Clinical Features and Risk of Relapse in Children and Adults with Myelin Oligodendrocyte Glycoprotein Antibody-associated Disease	207

Section 13: Rehabilitation
Section Editor: Nirmal Surya
Associate Editor: Hitav Someshwer

1.	Effect of Aquatic versus Land Motor Dual Task Training on Balance and Gait of Patients with Chronic Stroke: A Randomized Controlled Trial	209
2.	Early Mobilization and Quality of Life after Stroke: Findings from AVERT	210
3.	Botulinum Toxin and Occupational Therapy for Writer's Cramp	212
4.	A Newly Designed Intensive Caregiver Education Program Reduces Cognitive Impairment, Anxiety, and Depression in Patients with Acute Ischemic Stroke	214

5. Combining Virtual Reality Motor Rehabilitation with Cognitive Strategy Use in Chronic Stroke — 216

6. Virtual Reality Rehabilitation versus Conventional Physical Therapy for Improving Balance and Gait in Parkinson's Disease Patients: A Randomized Controlled Trial — 217

7. Urinary Symptoms in Patients with Parkinson's Disease and Progressive Supranuclear Palsy: Urodynamic Findings and Management of Bladder Dysfunction — 218

8. The Effects of Vestibular Rehabilitation on Dizziness and Balance Problems in Patients after Traumatic Brain Injury: A Randomized Controlled Trial — 220

9. Effects of High- and Low-frequency Repetitive Transcranial Magnetic Stimulation on Motor Recovery in Early Stroke Patients: Evidence from a Randomized Controlled Trial with Clinical, Neurophysiological and Functional Imaging Assessments — 222

10. A Randomized Control Trial Comparing the Effects of Motor Relearning Programme and Mirror Therapy for Improving Upper Limb Motor Functions in Stroke Patients — 224

11. The Use of Virtual Reality Rehabilitation for Individuals Post Stroke — 225

12. A Stimulus for Eating. The Use of Neuromuscular Transcutaneous Electrical Stimulation in Patients Affected by Severe Dysphagia after Subacute Stroke: A Pilot Randomized Controlled Trial — 227

13. The Effects of Aerobic Exercise on Sleep Quality Measures and Sleep-related Biomarkers in Individuals with Multiple Sclerosis: A Pilot Randomized Controlled Trial — 228

14. Task-based Mirror Therapy Enhances the Upper Limb Motor Function in Subacute Stroke Patients: A Randomized Control Trial — 230

15. Combined Cognitive-motor Rehabilitation in Virtual Reality Improves Motor Outcomes in Chronic Stroke: A Pilot Study — 232

16. Effects of Fluoxetine on Functional Outcomes after Acute Stroke (FOCUS): A Pragmatic, Double-blind, Randomized, Controlled Trial — 233

Section 14: Neurogenetics
Section Editor: Sunil Narayan
Associate Editor: KP Vinayan

Novel Therapies

1. Onasemnogene Abeparvovec Gene Therapy for Symptomatic Infantile-onset Spinal Muscular Atrophy in Patients with Two Copies of SMN2 (STR1VE): An Open-label, Single-arm, Multicentre, Phase 3 Trial — 236

2. Safety and Efficacy of Omaveloxolone in Friedreich Ataxia (MOXIe Study) — 237

3. Hematopoietic Stem- and Progenitor-cell Gene Therapy for Hurler Syndrome — 239
4. Treatment of Infantile-onset Spinal Muscular Atrophy with Nusinersen: Final Report of a Phase 2, Open-label, Multicentre, Dose-escalation Study — 240
5. A Major Successful Early Step towards Effective Vaccination for Arresting Progression of IDH1 Grade III Glioma – Phase I Human Trial — 242
6. Safety and Sustained 6 Years Effects of Treatment for Adult SMA Therapy – Phase I Trial — 243
7. Long-term (1 Year) Safety and Efficacy of High-dose Pyridoxine in IGD Deficiency Epilepsy — 244
8. Oral Prednisolone up to 1 mg/kg Orally Improved the Functional Status of Children with Congenital Fukuyama Myopathy (as for DMD) — 246
9. In Parkinson's Disease, Yearlong Administration of Sargramostim 3 μg/kg, Stopped UPDRS Progression, Decreased Numbers and Severity of Adverse Events and Restored Peripheral Immune Function Correlating with Increased Numbers and Function of Treg: Phase 1b Study — 247
10. Long 5.5-year Follow-up of Adeno-associated Vector-mediated Intracerebral Gene Therapy Encoding Human α-N-acetylglucosaminidase (rAAV2/5-hNAGLU) plus Immunotherapy in Sanfilippo B was Safe and Showed Sustained Enzyme Production — 248
11. European Pompe Consortium: In Classic Infantile Pompe Disease, High ERT Dosage of 40 mg/kg/week (Alglucosidase α had Significantly Improved Survival when Compared with Patients Treated with the Standard Recommended ERT Dosage of 20 mg/kg Every Other Week. Recommend Dosage Reconsideration — 249
12. In NF1, No Evidence of Neurotoxicity on 1 Year of Treatment with an MEKi and a Potential Clinical Signal of Cognitive Improvement, Supporting Future Research of Mitogen Activated Protein Kinase Inhibitor (MEKi) as a Cognitive Intervention — 251

Symptomatic Therapy

1. Prevention of Epilepsy in Infants with Tuberous Sclerosis Complex in the EPISTOP Trial — 252
2. Pharmacogenetic Predictors of Cannabidiol Response and Tolerability in Treatment-resistant Epilepsy — 253

Pharmacogenomics

1. Association between COMT Methylation and Response to Treatment in Children with ADHD — 254
2. Integrative Network-based Analysis Reveals Gene Networks and Novel Drug Repositioning Candidates for Alzheimer's Disease — 255

Genetic Markers

1. KCNT1-related Epilepsies and Epileptic Encephalopathies: Phenotypic and Mutational Spectrum — 256
2. APOE Genotype Contributes to the Heterogeneity in Rate of Clinical Progression in AD — 258
3. Adult GBA Variants, Parkinsonism is Linked to a more Aggressive Motor Disease Course over 7 Years from Diagnosis in Patients. Recruiting only GBA Carriers can Reduce Trial Size by up to 65% Compared to a Trial Recruiting all Patients with PD — 259
4. 1,250 plus Finnish Ageing Clinical Trial on Multidomain Interventions Facilitated LTL Maintenance among Subgroups of Older People and LTL (Telomere Length) Maintenance was Associated with more Pronounced Cognitive Intervention Benefits — 261
5. Most known CSF Biomarkers of Parkinsonism Predict Cognitive Decline in PD during Follow-up but only α-syn help Dissociate it from Healthy Controls — 262
6. CMT: UK CMT 6-year and US Follow-up Cohorts and Two Mouse Models—NfL Light Chain not a Helpful Biomarker to Assess Response to Therapy in Clinical Trials — 263
7. Increased Copy Number of APP is Sufficient to Cause AD and CAA, with likely Earlier Onset in Case of Triplication Compared with Duplication — 264
8. PME is One of the Best Genetically Defined Epilepsy Syndrome with Diagnostic Yield >80%. Using NGS Technology, Pathogenic Variants were Detected in both Established PME Genes and in Genes not Previously Associated with PME but Other Developmental Encephalopathies — 265

Natural History and Clinical Tools

1. First Long-term (2-year) Systematic Study in Progression of FSHD – Slow Progress but Considerable Unpleasant Soft Symptoms — 267
2. Ongoing Study Designed to Understand Natural History of Specific Congenital Muscular Dystrophy as an Essential Step for Reaching Trials Readiness — 268
3. Bayesian Models Adequately Predict the Natural Evolution of Congenital (Centronuclear) Myopathy and Facilitate a Sufficiently Powerful Trial Design — 269
4. Identification of Stage-dependent Progression Rates Provide Reliable Outcome Measures to Monitor Disease Progression, in all Trial Designs in Friedreich's Ataxia — 271
5. In GNE Myopathy 3-year Natural History Study, Insight into the Appropriate Tools to Detect Clinically Meaningful Changes for Future Interventional Trials — 272
6. 30-year Follow-up Study in 350 Patients of NF Type 2 to Guide Clinical Trial Design — 273
7. RESCUE and REVERSE LHON Studies: LHON Progresses Rapidly in the First Months Following Onset during the Subacute Phase, Followed by Relative Stabilization during the Dynamic Phase — 275

8. Different Rates of Progression of Disease in Subgroups of Patients with Different Deletions Amenable to Exon Skipping Therapy in Duchenne Muscular Dystrophy ... 276

9. Delphi-method Consensus-derived Canadian Outcome Measurement Toolkit Claimed to Improve Monitoring and Assessment of Adult SMA Patients ... 277

10. AI-based Model from Data of Two Largest Cohort Imaging Studies in HD TRACK-HD PREDICT-HD and Structural MRI Changes Together Predict Huntington Disease Progress ... 278

Genetic Screening

1. WISCOSIN Newborn Screening for SMA: 1/10000 Prevalence; both Timely SMN2 Information and SMN1 and SMN2 Confirmation as Parts of the Algorithm Facilitated Timely Clinical Follow-up, Family Counseling, and Treatment Planning ... 279

Prevalence Studies

1. The IPaNeMA Study: Using Clinical, CPK and GAA Fluorometric Method, Late-onset Pompe Prevalence in Academic, Tertiary Neuromuscular Practices in the United States and Canada is Estimated to be 1%, with an Equal Prevalence Rate of Pseudodeficiency Alleles ... 280

2. CADASIL Defining Cysteine Altering Stroke Associated NOTCH3 Variants Common in Korean Population, Around 10/1000 Compared to Rare 2–5/1, 00,000 Prevalence in West ... 281

Section 15: Demyelination
Section Editor: Netravathi M

1. Disease-modifying Therapies in Relapsing-remitting Multiple Sclerosis: A Systematic Review and Network Meta-analysis ... 284

2. Multiple Sclerosis, Disease-modifying Therapies and COVID-19: A Systematic Review on Immune Response and Vaccination Recommendations ... 285

3. Prodromal Emesis in Myelin Oligodendrocyte Glycoprotein-antibody-associated Disorder ... 286

4. A Comparison of the Effects of Rituximab versus Other Immunotherapies for Myelin Oligodendrocyte Glycoprotein Immunoglobulin G-associated Central Nervous System Demyelination: A Meta-analysis ... 287

5. Treatment of Myelin Oligodendrocyte Glycoprotein Immunoglobulin G-associated Disease in Paediatric Patients: A Systematic Review ... 288

6. Distinct Patterns of Magnetic Resonance Imaging Lesions in Myelin Oligodendrocyte Glycoprotein-antibody Disease and Aquaporin-4 Neuromyelitis Optica Spectrum Disorder: A Systematic Review and Meta-analysis ... 289

7. Brain Magnetic Resonance Imaging Activity during the Year before
   Pregnancy can Predict Postpartum Clinical Relapses — 290

8. A Randomized Study of Natalizumab Dosing Regimens for
   Relapsing-remitting Multiple Sclerosis — 291

9. Treatment Escalation versus Immediate Initiation of Highly Effective
   Treatment for Patients with Relapsing-remitting Multiple Sclerosis: Data from
   2 Different National Strategies — 292

Section 16: Social Aspects of Neurology
Section Editor: Sudhir Shah

Associate Editors: Akanksha Jain, Zubin A Shah, Amey Bhise, Gaurav Shah, Umangkumar M Patel, Andelwar SL

1. American Academy of Neurology Position Statement: Ethical Issues in
   Clinical Research in Neurology — 293

2. Ethical Issues in the Care of People with Dementia — 295

3. Disabling Stroke in Persons already with a Disability: Ethical Dimensions
   and Directives — 296

4. Driving and Epilepsy: Ethical, Legal, and Healthcare Policy Challenges — 297

5. Patients' Views on the Ethical Challenges of Early Parkinson Disease Detection — 298

6. Ethical Considerations in Chronic Brain Injury — 299

7. Ethical Principles in Patient-centered Medical Care to Support Quality of
   Life in Amyotrophic Lateral Sclerosis — 300

8. Ethical, Palliative, and Policy Considerations in Disorders of Consciousness — 302

9. Neuroethics of Neuromodulation: An Update — 303

10. The COVID-19 Pandemic and the Ethical Duties of the Neurologist — 304

11. The Ethics of Motivational Neuro-doping in Sport: Praiseworthiness
    and Prizeworthiness — 305

12. Challenges and Ethical Issues in the Course of Palliative Care Management
    for People Living with Advanced Neurologic Diseases — 306

13. Reflections on Ethics and Humanity in Pediatric Neurology: The Value of
    Recognizing Ethical Issues in Common Clinical Practice — 308

14. Drugs, Genes, and Screens: The Ethics of Preventing and Treating Spinal
    Muscular Atrophy — 310

15. Understanding and Addressing Gender Equity for Women in Neurology — 311

Index — 315

Section 1: Headaches

Section Editor: Debashish Chowdhury

Associate Editor: Ashish Kumar Duggal

ARTICLE 1

A Clinical, Oculographic, and Vestibular Test Characteristics of Vestibular Migraine

Young AS, Nham B, Bradshaw AP, Calic Z, Pogson JM, D'Souza M, et al. Clinical, oculographic, and vestibular test characteristics of vestibular migraine. *Cephalalgia.* 2021;41(10):1039-52.

Abstract

Young et al. described the clinical features and vestibular tests in patients with vestibular migraine (VM). Amongst 101 adult patients who presented with recurrent spontaneous and/or positional vertigo, 27 patients were diagnosed with VM and 74 patients were diagnosed as probable VM on the basis of 2012 Barany Society criteria. Ictal and interictal video oculography (VOG), caloric and video head impulse tests (vHITs), vestibular-evoked myogenic potentials (VEMP), and audiometry were performed. Patients underwent home VOG or ictal VOG in the emergency department (ED) when they presented with acute vestibular event and rotatory vertigo. Videos were analyzed for nystagmus after the return of each patient device by authors who were blinded to the patient's final diagnosis. Additionally, patients presenting with acute vestibular syndrome (AVS) underwent vHIT and magnetic resonance imaging; caloric testing and audiometry were performed on all patients with prolonged spontaneous vertigo lasting >10 minutes and positional testing on all patients presenting with episodic positional vertigo (EPV). Common presenting symptoms were headache (81.2%), spinning vertigo (72.3%), Mal de debarquement (58.4%), and motion sensitivity (30.7%). Authors found that VM presented as AVS, episodic spontaneous vertigo (ESV), and EPV. Most patients with VM show normal interictal test results, including symmetrical hearing thresholds and normal caloric, vHIT, and VEMP results. Low-velocity spontaneous ictal nystagmus (horizontal, vertical, or torsional) was present in 71.3% of patients and was significantly enhanced in the supine and lateral positions, which may explain the large subset of patients who report significant positional vertigo in the absence of benign paroxysmal positional vertigo.

COMMENT

This article by Young et al. describes the clinical features and vestibular tests in patients with vestibular migraine (VM). VM refers to episodic vertigo or vestibular symptoms attributed to migraine. Proposed mechanisms of VM are: reciprocal connections between the vestibular nuclei and the trigeminal nucleus caudalis, migraine-induced ischemia of the inner ear, and enhanced perceptual sensitivity to head tilting movements.[1-3] By definition, the vestibular symptoms are of moderate or severe intensity and last from 5 minutes to 72 hours. This study found that patients with VM may present as acute vestibular syndrome (AVS), episodic spontaneous vertigo (ESV), and episodic positional vertigo (EPV). An important differential diagnosis of VM is Ménière's disease, but the normal audiovestibular test results even in the presence of subjective auditory symptoms may be helpful in differentiating the two conditions.[4]

ARTICLE 2

TOP-PRO Study: A Randomized Double-blind Controlled Trial of Topiramate versus Propranolol for Prevention of Chronic Migraine

Chowdhury D, Bansal L, Duggal A, Datta D, Mundra A, Krishnan A, et al. TOP-PRO study: A randomized double-blind controlled trial of topiramate versus propranolol for prevention of chronic migraine.
Cephalalgia. 2022;42(4-5):396-408.

Abstract

This study was a double-blind randomized controlled trial (RCT) aimed to assess the efficacy (noninferior efficacy) and tolerability of propranolol compared with topiramate for the preventive treatment of chronic migraine (CM). Patients with CM, aged between 18 and 65 years, and not on any preventive treatment were allocated randomly to receive topiramate (100 mg/day) or propranolol (160 mg/day). Mean change in migraine days per month at the end of 24 weeks was the primary efficacy outcome for the study. Secondary outcomes were mean change in headache days per month at the end of 24 weeks; 50% reduction in headache days compared to baseline; mean change in antimigraine therapy days, average visual analog scale score, and Headache Impact Test-6 (HIT-6) scores. The study enrolled 175 patients, of these, 95 (topiramate group: 46 and propranolol group: 49) patients completed the trial. The mean change in migraine days was −7.3 [standard deviation (SD) 1.1] days for propranolol and −5.3 (SD 1.2) days for topiramate. The findings revealed that propranolol was noninferior and nonsuperior as compared with topiramate in the prevention of headaches [point estimate of −1.99 with a 95% confidence interval (CI) of −5.23 to 1.25 days]. Similarly, secondary outcomes were similar in both the propranolol and topiramate groups. There was no significant difference in adverse events between the two groups 32/93 in the topiramate group and 30/82 in the propranolol group. The most common adverse event reported was paresthesias in both groups. Notably, no patients in the propranolol group discontinued due to adverse events as compared to four (4.3%) in the topiramate group. Although propranolol performed better compared to topiramate across all the outcome parameters in numerical terms, the difference was not statistically significant. Overall the authors concluded that this RCT provided evidence that propranolol is noninferior to topiramate and has better tolerability.

COMMENT

There are very few treatment options for the preventive management of chronic migraine (CM) with topiramate being the only oral agent that is approved for the prevention of CM. Two pivotal randomized controlled trials (RCTs) by Silberstein et al. and Diener et al. found that topiramate had good efficacy at a dose of 100 mg/day when compared to placebo although treatment-emergent adverse events were high.[5,6] Though propranolol is approved for use as a prophylactic agent in episodic migraine, evidence for use of propranolol in CM is limited.[7-9] This study used a robust protocol that included standardized outcome measures as suggested by the International Headache Society (IHS) for conducting an RCT in CM.[10] This study was marred by an inability to reach the target sample size and high rate of dropouts due to the unprecedented COVID-19 pandemic and lockdown. This study found no significant differences in terms of efficacy and adverse events between the topiramate and propranolol when used as a preventive treatment for CM and provides good quality evidence of noninferiority of propranolol over topiramate for the preventive treatment of CM which can be a useful treatment option in countries with limited healthcare resources.

ARTICLE 3

Randomized, Controlled Trial of Erenumab for the Prevention of Episodic Migraine in Patients from Asia, the Middle East, and Latin America: The EMPOWER Study

Wang SJ, Roxas AA Jr, Saravia B, Kim BK, Chowdhury D, Riachi N, et al. Randomised, controlled trial of erenumab for the prevention of episodic migraine in patients from Asia, the Middle East, and Latin America: The EMPOWER study. *Cephalalgia. 2021;41(13):1285-97.*

Abstract

EMPOWER was a double-blind, randomized, phase 3 study aimed to evaluate the safety and efficacy of Erenumab in adults with episodic migraines. The study included participants from Asia, the Middle East, and Latin America. Randomized patients (n = 900) received monthly subcutaneous injections of placebo, Erenumab 70 mg, or Erenumab 140 mg (3:3:2) for 3 months. Primary endpoint was a change from baseline in monthly migraine days at month 3. Secondary endpoints included a reduction of ≥50%, ≥75%, and 100% in monthly migraine days, a change in monthly acute migraine-specific medication treatment days and patient-reported outcomes [Headache Impact Test-6 (HIT-6), modified MIDAS, MPFID, EuroQOL, or EQ-5D-5L], and safety assessment. At month 3, change from baseline in monthly migraine days (primary endpoint) was −3.1, −4.2, and −4.8 days for placebo, Erenumab 70 mg, and Erenumab 140 mg, respectively. Statistically significant difference was observed for Erenumab versus placebo [$p = 0.002$ (70 mg) vs. $p < 0.001$ (140 mg)]. The study findings revealed that Erenumab was well-tolerated. In addition, the proportions of patients reporting at least one adverse event and serious adverse events were similar between groups. Treatment emergent adverse events were reported in 36.7% of the patients who received placebo, 34.9% of the patients who received Erenumab 70 mg, and 34.4% of the patients who received Erenumab 140 mg. However, none of the patients treated with Erenumab had any adverse events resulting in discontinuation of the treatment. This study validates the preexisting data from previous worldwide Erenumab studies indicating that at doses of 70 and 140 mg, Erenumab is a safe and well-tolerated treatment for various ethnicities underrepresented previously in earlier Erenumab trials.

COMMENT

Monoclonal antibodies targeting the calcitonin gene-related peptide pathway, involved in the pathogenesis of migraine, and represent a new paradigm of preventive migraine therapies. Erenumab is a fully human monoclonal antibody that selectively blocks the canonical calcitonin gene-related peptide receptor, involved in the pathogenesis of migraine.[11] This is the first study of Erenumab conducted in patients with episodic migraine from Asia (81.2%), the Middle East, and Latin America (18.8%). The results are consistent with previous studies of Erenumab versus placebo in patients with episodic migraine. STRIVE study, which was a pivotal phase 3 trial had demonstrated that Erenumab 70 and 140 mg showed a relative change of −1.4 and −1.9 migraine days per month over the final 3 months of the 6-month double-blind treatment phase, respectively as compared to placebo.[12] Although EMPOWER does not demonstrate long-term efficacy and safety of Erenumab, several open-label extension studies of up to 5 years duration have proven that Erenumab is safe and effective.[13] However, recent data suggest that constipation and hypertension may be important adverse events that can be seen with Erenumab.

ARTICLE 4

If Headache has any Association with Hypertension, it is Negative. Evidence from a Population-based Study in Nepal

Manandhar K, Risal A, Koju R, Linde M, Steiner TJ. If headache has any association with hypertension, it is negative. Evidence from a population-based study in Nepal.
Cephalalgia. 2021;41(13):1310-7.

Abstract

This cross-sectional nationwide study conducted in Nepal evaluated any positive association between hypertension (HTN) and headache disorders. Trained health workers conducted face-to-face structured interviews, during unannounced home visits, with a representative sample of the Nepalese adult population (18–65 years). They applied standard diagnostic criteria for headache disorders [Headache-Attributed Restriction, Disability, Social Handicap and Impaired Participation (HARDSHIP) modular structured questionnaire developed by Lifting The Burden (LTB) for population-based studies] and measured blood pressure digitally. HTN was defined as systolic pressure ≥ 140 mm Hg and/or diastolic ≥ 90 mm Hg. Of the total 2,100 participants (59.0% female, mean age 36.4 ± 12.8 years), 317 (15.1%) had HTN (41.0% female), and 1,794 (85.4%) had headache. Of the 1,794 participants with headaches 728 had migraine, 863 had tension-type headache, and 161 had headache on ≥15 days/month. All headache collectively was less prevalent among HTN cases (78.9%) than noncases (86.6%, $p = 0.001$). Participants with HTN appeared less likely to have any headache and each type of headache, although the difference was significant only for any headache ($p = 0.001$). The findings of this study contrast with those of several that have found mostly positive associations between HTN and headache prevalence. The authors conclude that there is no evidence that HTN (even untreated) is a significant cause of headache. So, headache disorders and HTN are unrelated entities requiring distinct policies for prevention, control, and management.

COMMENT

There is a common persistent belief, commonly expressed that hypertension (HTN) is an important cause of headaches. Several population-based epidemiological studies have found no correlation or negative correlation between headaches and HTN.[14-17] This study provides evidence that headache disorders and HTN are unrelated entities requiring distinct policies for prevention, control, and management. So, it can be concluded that mild (140-159/90-99 mm Hg) or moderate (160-179/100-109 mm Hg) chronic arterial HTN does not appear to cause headache, though acute rise in systolic (to ≥180 mm Hg) and/or diastolic (to ≥120 mm Hg) blood pressure can cause headache and is coded as 10.3 Headache attributed to arterial HTN by the International Classification of Headache Disorders, 3rd edition criteria (ICHD-3) classification.

ARTICLE 5

Safety and Efficacy of Ubrogepant in Participants with Major Cardiovascular Risk Factors in Two Single-attack Phase 3 Randomized Trials: ACHIEVE I and II

Hutchinson S, Silberstein SD, Blumenfeld AM, Lipton RB, Lu K, Yu SY, et al. Safety and efficacy of ubrogepant in participants with major cardiovascular risk factors in two single-attack phase 3 randomized trials: ACHIEVE I and II. *Cephalalgia. 2021;41(9):979-90.*

Abstract

ACHIEVE I and II were multicenter, double-blind, single-attack, phase 3 trials in adults with migraine, with or without aura that evaluated the safety and efficacy of ubrogepant for acute treatment of migraine across cardiovascular (CV) disease risk categories. Participants were randomized 1:1:1 to placebo or ubrogepant (50 or 100 mg in ACHIEVE I; 25 or 50 mg in ACHIEVE II), to treat one migraine attack of moderate or severe headache pain intensity. Exclusion criteria were individuals with clinically significant CV or cerebrovascular disease (per the investigator's opinion), with recent CV/cerebrovascular events, as well as those with clinically uncontrolled hypertension [defined by sitting systolic blood pressure (BP) > 160 mm Hg or sitting diastolic BP > 100 mm Hg at visit 1 or 2]. At baseline, participants were classified into one of three CV risk categories (high, moderate, and low) using an algorithm based on the National Cholesterol Education Program [(NCEP); National Institutes of Health, 2001] and Framingham risk factors along with the presence of CV heart disease or other forms of vascular disease, as well as diabetes. A fourth category with no risk factors was also created to separate participants in the low-risk group. Because of the small sample size, participants in the moderate and high-risk groups were clubbed together for analytical purposes. The primary endpoints were pain freedom and absence of most bothersome symptom 2 hours after the initial dose, and level of functional disability at 1, 2, 4, and 8 hours after the dose of ubrogepant. Secondary efficacy endpoints included pain relief at 2 hours, sustained pain relief from 2 to 24 hours with no administration of either rescue medication or second dose of trial medication, sustained pain freedom from 2 to 24 hours with no administration of either rescue medication or second dose of trial medication, absence of photophobia, phonophobia, and nausea at 2 hours. Ubrogepant 50 mg and placebo treatment groups from the individual trials were pooled for analysis. A total of 3,358 participants were randomized into the ACHIEVE I and ACHIEVE II trials [intent-to-treat (ITT) population]. Approximately 11% of participants in the overall safety population (*n* = 2,901) were categorized as moderate/high risk (*n* = 311), 32% as low risk (*n* = 920), and 58% as no CV risk factors (*n* = 1,670). The proportion of participants reporting an adverse event (AE) was generally consistent across CV risk categories. Commonly reported treatment-emergent adverse events (TEAEs) included nausea, dry mouth, and somnolence (all <5%). There were no AEs leading to participant discontinuation. Cardiac-related AEs (e.g., palpitations, flutter, etc.) were low and similar between ubrogepant and placebo (0.1%) and treatment (0.3%) groups. One participant in the ubrogepant 50 mg group experienced a serious adverse event (SAE) in the cardiac disorder system organ class, pericardial effusion, which was deemed to be not treatment-related. The efficacy of ubrogepant 50 mg versus placebo was comparable across CV risk categories for the coprimary efficacy endpoints. This post-hoc analysis thus shows that ubrogepant is safe, tolerable, and efficacious across the three categories of CV disease risk status studied [no risk factors, low risk (<2 major risk factors), and moderate to high risk (≥2 major risk factors)].

COMMENT

Triptans are the most effective and migraine-specific, acute therapeutic agent available to date. The associated cardiovascular (CV) adverse events (AE) associated with make their use challenging in people who have or are at risk for CV disease. These patients with CV disease are more likely to receive opioids or barbiturates for treatment or may receive less specific and efficacious acute treatments with poor migraine control with the attendant risk of developing chronic migraine.[18] Ubrogepant is a recently Food and Drug Administration (FDA)-approved, oral calcitonin gene-related peptide (CGRP) receptor antagonist (gepant) developed for the acute treatment of migraine, which does not have the vasoconstrictor properties of triptans. The efficacy and safety of Ubrogepant in management of acute migraine overcome the unmet need for acute treatment options for migraine with improved benefit-risk profiles. Since individuals with clinically significant CV or cerebrovascular disease and uncontrolled hypertension were excluded from this study, the results cannot be generalized to this group of the population, and long-term studies may be needed before the use of gepants can be advocated in patients with clinically significant CV and cerebrovascular disease.

ARTICLE 6

Randomized, Controlled Trial of Lasmiditan over Four Migraine Attacks: Findings from the CENTURION Study

Ashina M, Reuter U, Smith T, Krikke-Workel J, Klise SR, Bragg S, et al. Randomized, controlled trial of lasmiditan over four migraine attacks: Findings from the CENTURION study.
Cephalalgia. 2021;41(3):294-304.

Abstract

Lasmiditan is a selective serotonin 1F (5-HT1F) receptor agonist (ditan), approved by the Food and Drug Administration (FDA) for the acute treatment of migraine, with or without aura, in adults, the CENTURION study was a multicenter, double-blind phase 3 study, designed to assess the efficacy of and consistency of response to lasmiditan in the acute treatment of migraine across four attacks. Patients were randomized 1:1:1 to one of three treatment groups—lasmiditan 200 mg, lasmiditan 100 mg, or a control group that received placebo for three attacks and lasmiditan 50 mg for either the third or fourth attack. The primary endpoints were pain freedom at 2 hours (first attack) and pain freedom at 2 hours in ≥2/3 attacks. Secondary endpoints included pain relief, sustained pain freedom, and disability freedom. Although patients with known cardiovascular risk factors or disease were included, those with a history of hemorrhagic stroke were excluded. Patients on migraine preventive therapies were eligible provided they were stable for 3 months prior to screening. The trial also included a subpopulation of patients with an insufficient response to triptans—an inconsistent response to their most recent triptan, those who were taking a triptan and had a poor/very poor migraine Treatment Optimization Questionnaire (mTOQ-6) score, or had discontinued their most recent triptan for efficacy or tolerability reasons or due to contraindications. The migraine attacks were to be treated within 4 hours, provided the headache was at least moderate severity. Primary endpoints were the percentage of patients who were pain-free at 2-hour post-dose during the first attack and the percentage of patients who were pain-free at 2-hour post-dose in at least two of three attacks (consistency of response). Additional secondary endpoints included the percentage of patients who were migraine-associated most bothersome symptom (MBS) free at 2 hours, who used rescue medication in the 2–24-hour period, who reported being "much better" or "very much better" as measured using the Patient Global Impression of Change (PGIC) at 2 and 24 hours, and who were pain-free at 2 hours but reported recurrence within 24 or 48 hours. A total of 1,613 patients were randomized, of which 1,471 had first attack efficacy data and 1,049 provided sufficient data to assess consistency. Lasmiditan at either dose was superior to placebo for pain freedom at 2 hours, with therapeutic gains of 17.4% and 20.9% for lasmiditan at 100 and 200 mg, respectively. Lasmiditan had an early onset of action for both doses, and the effect of lasmiditan on pain freedom was greatest between 4 and 6 hours post-dose. In triptan nonresponders, lasmiditan was superior to placebo for 2-hour pain freedom. The response of lasmiditan was consistent with lasmiditan being superior to placebo for pain freedom at 2 hours in ≥2 of 3 attacks, as well as pain relief at 2 hours in ≥2 out of 3 attacks. A total of 22 patients (1.5%) reported one or more serious adverse events, with a similar incidence across treatment groups. The most common treatment-emergent adverse events (TEAEs) with lasmiditan were dizziness, paresthesia, fatigue, and nausea; these were generally mild or moderate in severity. The trial confirms that lasmiditan is an efficacious acute treatment for migraine with a consistent response across multiple migraine attacks and is also associated with central nervous system (CNS) adverse events that are generally mild or moderate in severity.

COMMENT

Lasmiditan is a selective serotonin 1F (5-HT1F) receptor agonist that lacks vasoconstrictor activity and therefore can be used for patients with relative contraindications to triptans due to cardiovascular risk factors.[19] In two previous studies—SAMURAI and SPARTAN, lasmiditan demonstrated statistically significant superiority versus placebo in the proportion of patients who were pain-free as well as the proportion of patients who were free of their migraine-associated most bothersome symptom (MBS) at 2-hour post-dose.[20,21] The most common adverse event associated with lasmiditan is dizziness, other relatively frequent adverse events are paresthesia, somnolence, fatigue, and nausea. Lasmiditan thus provides another acute treatment option for the management of acute migraine in patients with vascular risk factors.

ARTICLE 7

Characteristics and Outcomes of Patients with Cerebral Venous Sinus Thrombosis in SARS-CoV-2 Vaccine-induced Immune Thrombotic Thrombocytopenia

Sánchez van Kammen M, Aguiar de Sousa D, Poli S, Cordonnier C, Heldner MR, van de Munckhof A, et al. Characteristics and outcomes of patients with cerebral venous sinus thrombosis in SARS-CoV-2 vaccine-induced immune thrombotic thrombocytopenia.
JAMA Neurol. 2021;78(11):1314-23.

Abstract

This was a cohort study that used data from an international registry of consecutive patients with cerebral venous sinus thrombosis (CVST) within 28 days of SARS-CoV-2 vaccination from 81 hospitals in 19 countries of 116 patients with CVST after SARS-CoV-2 vaccination. The data were compared with data of patients with CVST between 2015 and 2018 derived from an existing international registry. The patients were thus divided into three groups: (1) CVST in the setting of SARS-CoV-2 vaccine-induced immune thrombotic thrombocytopenia, (2) CVST after SARS-CoV-2 vaccination not fulfilling criteria for thrombotic thrombocytopenic syndrome (TTS), and (3) CVST unrelated to SARS-CoV-2 vaccination. Patients with CVST after SARS-CoV-2 vaccination were classified as having TTS if they met all of the following criteria: (1) confirmed thrombosis, (2) new-onset thrombocytopenia, and (3) no known recent exposure to heparin. Of 123 reported patients with CVST after SARS-CoV-2 vaccination, 7 were excluded (duplicate report—3; symptom onset before vaccination—2; symptom onset 28 days after vaccination). Of the 116 patients with postvaccination CVST—96 patients (82.8%) were vaccinated with ChAdOx1 nCov-19, 16 (13.8%) with BNT162b2 (Pfizer/BioNTech), 2 (1.7%) with CoronaVac (Sinovac), 1 (0.9%) with Ad26.COV2.S (Janssen/Johnson & Johnson), and 1 (0.9%) with mRNA-1273 (Moderna). Amongst the 116 patients with CVST—78 (67.2%) met the Brighton criteria for TTS. The pre-COVID-19 control group consisted of 207 patients. Of the 78 patients with TTS after SARS-CoV-2 vaccination, 76 (97%) had received ChAdOx1 nCov-19 (Oxford–AstraZeneca), 1 (1%) had received Ad26.COV2.S, and 1 (1%) had received BNT162b2. One patient developed CVST–TTS after the second ChAdOx1 nCov-19 vaccination. The median time from vaccination to CVST symptom onset was 9 (7–10) days in the CVST with TTS group as compared to 7 days in the CVST without TTS group. The median platelet count in the TTS group was 45 (25–71) × 10³/μL. Out of 69 patients in whom PF4 antibodies were measured, they were positive in 91% of patients. In the sole TTS patient after Pfizer BNT162b2 vaccine, the PF4 antibodies were negative, thrombocytopenia was mild, and an alternative explanation for TTS was found. In the TTS group, seven patients (9%) presented with petechiae, two (3%) with purpura, and four (5%) with mucosal bleeding. Anticoagulation with heparin was more commonly used in the non-TTS group (84%) as compared to nonheparin anticoagulants in the TTS group (47%). Immunomodulation therapy in the form of intravenous immunoglobulins was used in 60% of patients with TTS. In-hospital mortality was significantly higher in the TTS group (47%) as compared to non-TTS group (5%) and the control cerebral venous thrombosis (CVT) group (3.9%). The mortality rate in patients with CVST–TTS treated with intravenous immunoglobulins was 28 and 41% among patients receiving heparin as the first anticoagulant treatment. The in-hospital mortality rate of patients with CVST–TTS before March 19, 2021, when the scientific community first became aware of this new syndrome was 61 and 42% after March 2021.

COMMENT

Cerebral venous sinus thrombosis (CVST) is an important adverse effect associated with after SARS-CoV-2 vaccination. This study gives useful insight into the prognosis of CVST and CVST with thrombotic thrombocytopenic syndrome (TTS) after COVID-19 vaccinations. Vaccine-induced immune thrombotic thrombocytopenia (VITT) is caused by antibodies that recognize platelet factor 4 (PF4, also called CXCL4) bound to platelets. The adenoviral vector-based vaccines—ChAdOx1 nCoV-19 (AstraZeneca, University of Oxford, and Serum Institute of India) and Ad26.COV2.S (Janssen; Johnson & Johnson) are the vaccines mainly implicated in this syndrome. Cerebral venous thrombosis (CVT) after COVID vaccination can occur in isolation or in association with TTS. Therapeutic anticoagulation is one of the primary treatments for VITT and should be used even in cases with associated central nervous system (CNS) hemorrhage. A direct oral anticoagulant (DOAC) is usually preferred, other choices are Fondaparinux or parenteral direct thrombin inhibitor (argatroban or bivalirudin). There is no consensus on the duration of anticoagulation, but it is reasonable to continue anticoagulation for 3 months after normalization of the platelet count, as long as no further thrombosis occurs. High-dose intravenous immunoglobulin (IVIG) is recommended along with anticoagulation, as a means of interrupting VITT antibody-induced platelet activation. Therapeutic plasma exchange can be tried in refractory cases, while platelet transfusions should be minimized.

ARTICLE 8

Clinical Presentation, Investigation Findings, and Treatment Outcomes of Spontaneous Intracranial Hypotension Syndrome: A Systematic Review and Meta-analysis

D'Antona L, Jaime Merchan MA, Vassiliou A, Watkins LD, Davagnanam I, Toma AK, et al. Clinical presentation, investigation findings, and treatment outcomes of spontaneous intracranial hypotension syndrome: A systematic review and meta-analysis.
JAMA Neurol. 2021;78(3):329-37.

Abstract

This preferred reporting items for systematic reviews and meta-analyses (PRISMA) reporting guideline-compliant systematic review and meta-analysis of the literature on spontaneous intracranial hypotension (SIH) provides a summary of the evidence on SIH. Three databases (PubMed/MEDLINE, Embase, and Cochrane) were searched from inception to April 30, 2020, and original studies in the English language reporting 10 or more patients with SIH were selected by consensus. SIH is diagnosed when a headache has developed spontaneously and in temporal relation to a cerebrospinal fluid (CSF) leak (evident on imaging) and/or CSF hypotension (lumbar puncture opening pressure < 60 mm CSF). The predetermined main outcomes were the pooled estimate proportions of symptoms of SIH, imaging findings (brain and spinal imaging), and treatment outcomes [conservative, epidural blood patches (EBPs), and surgical]. The mean age of patients was 42.5 years [95% confidence interval (CI) 41.1–43.9] with a range of 2–88 years. Various risk factors for SIH identified in these studies included—connective tissue disorders, spinal pathologies (i.e., osteophytes, disc prolapse, and discogenic microspurs), and bariatric surgery. The most common symptoms were orthostatic headache [92% (95% CI 87–96%)], nausea [54% (95% CI 46–62%)], and neck pain/stiffness [43% (95% CI 32–53%)]. The most common abnormality identified on brain magnetic resonance imaging (MRI) was diffuse pachymeningeal enhancement identified in 73% of patients, while MRI was normal in 19% of patients. Other MRI abnormalities identified in various studies were subdural collections seen in 35%, brain sagging in 43%, signs of venous engorgement in 57%, and pituitary gland enlargement in 38% of cases. Spinal neuroimaging identified extradural CSF in 48–76% of patients. Digital subtraction myelography and MR myelography with the unconventional use of intrathecal gadolinium had the highest sensitivity for identifying the exact leak site (100 and 75.5%, respectively). The most common leak location was the thoracic spine (41%); followed by the cervicothoracic junction (25%), the cervical spine (14%), and the lumbar spine (12%); while multiple leaks were identified in 24% of cases. Lumbar puncture opening pressures were low in 67% of cases, normal in 32%, and high (>200 mmH$_2$O) in 3% of cases. Conservative treatment was effective in 28% while EBP was successful in 64% of cases. Large EBPs (>20 mL) had better success rates than small EBPs. The epidural patches were usually well tolerated with transient symptoms such as palpitation, nausea, and headache being reported. The results of this study suggest that the absence of orthostatic headache, normal imaging findings, or normal lumbar puncture opening pressures do not exclude a diagnosis of SIH. Treatment with EBPs could be attempted early, even if the exact leak location is unknown since this is a safe and effective procedure.

COMMENT

Spontaneous intracranial hypotension (SIH) is a clinical condition characterized by debilitating postural headaches secondary to spontaneous spinal cerebrospinal fluid (CSF) leak and/or CSF hypotension.[22] Although the most common pattern of headache is orthostatic headache a substantial proportion of patients (~10%) may have other types of headaches including—chronic daily headaches, which may replace the orthostatic headache,[23] paradoxical headache, worse with recumbency and better with the upright position[24] and diurnal headache characterized by onset late in the day.[25] Magnetic resonance imaging (MRI) brain with contrast is an essential diagnostic investigation and diffuse pachymeningeal enhancement is the most common finding seen in 75% of cases. Attempts should be made to localize the site of CSF leak which is most commonly seen in the thoracic spine, but this may not always be possible. Notably in this meta-analysis, the success rate of targeted epidural blood patch (EBP) (70%) was similar to nontargeted EBP (69%). Therefore, early treatment with a large EBP (~20 mL) may be an effective treatment option even if the site of leak is not identified.

ARTICLE 9

Calcitonin Gene-related Peptide Monoclonal Antibodies in Migraine: An Efficacy and Tolerability Comparison with Standard Prophylactic Drugs

Vandervorst F, Van Deun L, Van Dycke A, Paemeleire K, Reuter U, Schoenen J, et al. CGRP monoclonal antibodies in migraine: An efficacy and tolerability comparison with standard prophylactic drugs.
J Headache Pain. 2021;22(1):128.

Abstract

This study compares the oral prophylactic agents for episodic and chronic migraine (CM) with level A evidence—propranolol 80–160 mg, metoprolol 100–200 mg, topiramate 100 mg for episodic migraine (EM), and 50–200 mg for CM, valproate 250–1500 mg, candesartan 8–16 mg, amitriptyline 25 mg, and Onabotulinumtoxin A at the injection sites and dosing according to the PREEMPT trials with calcitonin gene-related peptide (CGRP) monoclonal antibodies (mAbs) with regards to efficacy and tolerability. Only trials in adults with a randomized (parallel-group or cross-over) double-blinded placebo-controlled design studying the efficacy of an agent in monotherapy, of which the full article was available in English, with at least 10 patients in each treatment arm and reporting of the administered dosages were considered. Outcome measures studies were mean reduction of monthly migraine days (MMDs). Results from all four CGRP mAb were lumped, considering their comparable mechanism of action and the fact that so far no clear difference in efficacy appears from clinical trials although no head-to-head trials have been performed. The average reductions in MMD for CGRP mAb versus placebo in EM and CM, were respectively 1.9 and 2.2 days. The reduction in MMD versus placebo was 0.9 days for candesartan, 1.2 days for EM, and 1.8 days for CM with topiramate; 1.7 days for valproate; 1.1 days for amitriptyline; 0.9 days for beta-blockers (pooled for both propranolol and metoprolol), and 2.0 days for Onabotulinumtoxin A. In both EM and CM, the highest MMD reduction was found for the CGRP mAb. The highest dropout rates compared to placebo were seen in patients treated with amitriptyline, valproate, or topiramate. CGRP mAb have an efficacy that is at least comparable to the efficacy of the currently used preventive drugs. The true clinical efficacy of CGRP mAb might even be higher since overall, a high placebo response was reached in most of the trials probably related to their more invasive route of administration. The limitations of this study are enormous variation in trial design, large differences in both the number of patients treated with the preventive agent and the number of trials performed, and a huge variation in the methodological quality of included studies.

COMMENT

Monoclonal antibodies (mAbs) are an exciting new treatment option for prophylaxis of episodic and chronic migraine (CM). The overall efficacy of these agents is similar to the other agents available such as candesartan, amitriptyline, topiramate, and Onabotulinumtoxin A. The number needed to treat ranges from 5 to 9 for various mAbs which is similar to topiramate (4) and Onabotulinumtoxin A (9).[26] What makes mAbs an attractive proposition is their excellent safety profile and tolerability. The likelihood to help versus harm ratio is lower for mAbs as compared to conventional agents. This review reenforces the fact that mAbs are safe and efficacious option for prophylaxis of migraine.

ARTICLE 10

Clinical Features of New Daily Persistent Headache: A Retrospective Chart Review of 328 Cases

Evans RW, Turner DP. Clinical features of new daily persistent headache: A retrospective chart review of 328 cases. *Headache. 2021;61(10):1529-38.*

Abstract

This study is a retrospective chart review of clinical features of patients with a provisional diagnosis of new daily persistent headache (NDPH) from September 1, 2011 through February

28, 2020 (8.5 years). Out of 328 patients who met the International Classification of Headache Disorders, 3rd edition criteria; 65.5% were females. NDPH constituted 6.6% of the total 5,001 cases of headache seen at the center over 8.5 years and was the second most common diagnosis after migraine. The mean age of onset was 40.3 years (range 12–87 years). The median [25th, 75th] duration of NDPH at initial consultation was 0.7 [0.3, 2.0] year. The headache was side locked unilateral in 8.5% of cases and had a thunderclap onset in 3.6% of cases. The migrainous phenotype was more common (79.3%) than the tension-type headache phenotype (20.7%). Precipitating factors were the following: stressful life events, 67/328 (20.4%); upper respiratory infection or flu-like illness, 33/328 (10.1%); and extracranial surgery, 5/328 (1.5%). The authors concluded that NDPH is typical of moderate-to-severe intensity often with migraine features without obvious seasonal or other cyclical variation and most cases are refractory.

COMMENT

This retrospective chart review describes the clinical features of new daily persistent headache (NDPH) in a cohort of 328 patients. NDPH is a chronic daily headache that begins one day and typically does not remit, many patients (80%) can recall the exact date or circumstances in which the headache starts.[27] The phenotype of NDPH frequently resembles migraine or, less often, tension-type headache. It is a rare disorder with a prevalence of 0.1% among Spanish adults and a prevalence of 0.03% amongst adults of age 30–44 years in Norway.[28,29] Diagnosis of NDPH requires the exclusion of secondary causes of headache even in the presence of a normal neurological examination. Some of the most important secondary causes, which are a differential of NDPH include—cerebral venous sinus thrombosis, headache due to spontaneous spinal cerebrospinal fluid leak, idiopathic intracranial hypertension (IIH), and giant cell arteritis.

ARTICLE 11

An Internet-based Study on the Impact of COVID-19 Pandemic-related Lockdown on Migraine in India

Chowdhury D, Krishnan A, Duggal A, Datta D, Mundra A, Deorari V, et al. An internet-based study on the impact of COVID-19 pandemic-related lockdown on migraine in India.
Acta Neurol Scand. 2021;144(6):706-16

Abstract

This study assessed the impact of lockdown during the COVID-19 pandemic on migraine patients in India on disease activity, healthcare accessibility, and quality of life (QoL). A web-based structured questionnaire was used to assess the impact of lockdown and COVID-19 on previous physician-diagnosed migraine patients or those fulfilling any two of three clinical features (limitation of activities for >1 day, associated nausea or vomiting, and photophobia or phonophobia). The primary outcome measure was the impact of the COVID-19 pandemic and lockdown on qualitative changes in attack frequency, headache days/last month, headache attack duration, and severity. Secondary outcome measure included QoL during the past 1 month that was compared between participants with and without migraine. A total of 4,078 persons completed the full survey out of which 984 (24.1%) had migraine. A majority (51.3%) of migraineurs reported worsening of their headaches in terms of increased attack frequency (95.6%), increased headache days (95%), increased attack duration (89.9%), and increased headache severity (88.1%). The worsening of headache was attributed to anxiety due to the pandemic (79.7%), inability or difficulty to access health care (48.4%) and migraine medicines (48.9%), and financial worries (60.9%). Among the migraineurs, only 278 (28.25%) had access to a doctor for their headache. Migraine affected QoL in 61.4% of migraineurs. The determinants of poor QoL by univariate analysis were female sex, married status, those who were employed, those with a monthly headache frequency of ≥15 days (prelockdown), those who were using a preventive medication, those who reported worsening of their migraine, and those who had difficulty or did not have access to doctors and medications during the lockdown. Those employed in essential COVID-19 duties had good QoL. This survey thus demonstrates that the COVID-19 pandemic and lockdown affected Indian migraine patients adversely with resultant poor QoL.

COMMENT

Migraine and other primary headaches are chronic neurological conditions that can be very disabling and have a significant impact on the quality of life (QoL). Patients with chronic headaches often require long-term treatment (including injectable therapies) and regular consultations with their healthcare providers. They are more vulnerable to variations in their habits and may have difficulties in adapting to various stressors which can worsen their headache. COVID-19 and the ensuing lockdown was a life-changing event that had a profound impact on the mental health of people with a resultant increase in many psychiatric disorders. During the early period of the pandemic and the lockdown in various parts of the world, there was a heightened level of psychosocial stress because of social isolation, anxiety because of the pandemic and fear of financial instability, inability to go out for exercise and recreation could lead to worsening of headache in migraineurs. Social isolation and vulnerability in subjects suffering from chronic diseases such as migraine may lead to inefficient psychological adjustment and have a negative impact on symptom perception leading to worsening of symptoms. In addition, the inability to access health care because of lockdown or conversion of the healthcare facility to dedicated COVID centers and difficulty in getting transport to the healthcare facility could have caused poor medication compliance and worsening of headache symptoms or medication overuse. On the other hand, amelioration of some of the stressors like every day travel to work, spending more time with family, and flexibility of planning and scheduling work from home (especially for persons living in cities) might have contributed to an improvement in the severity and frequency of migraine. Thus, the impact of COVID on migraine can be variable depending on the population studied and the social and medical support available in the population. Parodi and colleagues, in a study from Italy, reported fewer headache attacks, lesser pain, and moderate levels of depression in patients during the 2-month quarantine.[29] This is in contrast to this study and some other studies from Kuwait, where Al-Hashel et al. found that majority of their respondents had worsening of migraine during the pandemic.[30] This means that the pandemic and lockdown had a variable effect on headache frequency and severity which probably depends on the socioeconomic factors and access to healthcare.[31] Access to healthcare and headache specialists was severely impaired during the pandemic. Chowdhury et al. reported that only 28% of their respondents were able to access their doctors through personal visits. The pandemic and lockdown gave an opportunity to use telemedicine as a mode of healthcare access. Most of the studies have found that patients were satisfied with telemedicine. Chowdhury et al. found that 86% of their respondents were mostly satisfied with a telemedicine consultation. The pandemic and lockdown has thus given us opportunities for using telemedicine as an effective and patient-centered option even during the postpandemic period.

ARTICLE 12

Characteristics and Natural Disease History of Persistent Idiopathic Facial Pain, Trigeminal Neuralgia, and Neuropathic Facial Pain

Ziegeler C, Brauns G, May A. Characteristics and natural disease history of persistent idiopathic facial pain, trigeminal neuralgia, and neuropathic facial pain.
Headache. 2021;61(9):1441-51.

Abstract

This was a longitudinal prospective study that used a questionnaire filled by the patients and physicians to characterize key features and clinical development of common nondental facial pain syndromes such as persistent idiopathic facial pain (PIFP), trigeminal neuralgia (TN), and neuropathic facial pain (NEUROP). Later a telephone interview was conducted with the same patients in 2020 to assess their natural disease history. A total of 411 patients with chronic facial pain were included in the study with 150 patients with PIFP, 111 patients with TN, and 86 patients with NEUROP. The mean age of all patients with facial pain ($n = 411$) at the time of their first consultation was 51.9 (±15.3) years with a range from 11 to 91 years. Almost all patients (99.3%) with facial pain had primarily consulted a dentist for their pain syndrome and had underwent dental interventions in healthy teeth with the intention to treat the pain, most commonly in PIFP (83%). Acute medications were generally ineffective in patients with PIFP. Tricyclic antidepressants and calcium channel blockers (gabapentin, pregabalin) were used most often in patients with PIFP, with an efficacy rate of 13.5% for tricyclic antidepressants and 30% for gabapentin. Patients with TN had tried a preventative medication in 84.7% (94/111) of the cases and showed comparatively higher efficacy rates (50–60%) of the most commonly used medication classes. The authors also found that despite a high economic impact with significant personal expenses, most patients could not treat their pain adequately. The authors concluded that although treatment of TN seems to be effective in most patients, patients with PIFP, and NEUROP report poor effectiveness even when following guideline therapy suggestions.

COMMENT

Facial pain is defined as "pain below the orbitomeatal line, anterior to the pinnae, and above the neck."[22] Facial pain is widely prevalent in the community and may affect up to 25% of the population, with almost 11% of patients suffering from chronic facial pain.[32] Trigeminal neuralgia (TN) is the most common cranial neuralgia. Its prevalence is estimated to be between 5 and 29 per 100,000 person years.[33] TN classically manifests as paroxysmal stereotyped attacks of intense sharp electric shock-like sensation or stabbing pain in the distribution of one or more divisions of the trigeminal nerve. The pain responds to carbamazepine and oxcarbazepine at least in the initial stages, though later pain may become refractory and continuous causing diagnostic confusion. Facial pain in the distribution of one or more branches of cranial nerve V (CNV) can be a result of a disorder associated with neural damage—neuropathic facial pain. The primary pain is usually continuous or near continuous and is commonly described as burning, squeezing, or likened to pins and needles. There may be associated superimposed paroxysms, but they are not the predominant pain type.[34] Treatment with amitriptyline, gabapentin, pregabalin, and topical lidocaine may be beneficial in some cases, particularly those associated with herpes zoster infection but post-traumatic trigeminal neuropathic pain may not respond to these agents with significant social and economic impact. PIFP on the other hand is a chronic daily persistent facial pain that occurs in the absence of any clinical neurological deficit or preceding causative event. The pain is poorly localized and does not follow the distribution of a peripheral nerve. Treatment is primarily cognitive-behavioral therapy supplemented by tricyclic antidepressants and serotonin-norepinephrine reuptake inhibitors.[35] Facial pain is a common disorder that may present to neurologists and effective treatment often requires a multidisciplinary approach.

ARTICLE 13

Pediatric-onset Trigeminal Autonomic Cephalalgias: A Systematic Review and Meta-analysis

Ghosh A, Silva E, Burish MJ. Pediatric-onset trigeminal autonomic cephalalgias: A systematic review and meta-analysis. *Cephalalgia.* 2021;41(13):1382-95.

Abstract

This study was a systematic review and meta-analysis that extracted articles discussing cases of trigeminal autonomic cephalalgias (TACs) with age of onset 18 years or younger using PRISMA guidelines. Data extracted included age of onset, sex, and International Classification of Headache Disorders, 3rd edition criteria (ICHD-3) for TACs (including pain location, duration, frequency, autonomic features, restlessness) and some migraine criteria (photophobia, phonophobia, and nausea). Out of 1,788 studies that were extracted, 86 studies met the inclusion criteria (studies that reported any TAC and any study that mentioned either onset of age 18 years or younger or any epidemiological report). Most of the studies (56) examined cluster headaches. The final dataset included patients from 24 countries and five continents (excluding Africa and Antarctica). Cluster headache had an onset as young as 1-year-old with many preadolescent patients. Pediatric-onset cluster headache patients ($n = 124$) had pain in all typical locations, with a full range of durations (15–180 minutes), but a lower frequency (between every other day and six per day, official criterion is between every other day and eight per day). Pediatric cluster headache was most commonly associated with lacrimation in 81%, followed by restlessness in 63%, conjunctival injection in 61%, nasal congestion in 57%, ptosis in 52%, rhinorrhea in 45%, facial sweating in 16%, miosis in 14%, and eyelid edema in 3%. The sex ratio in pediatric-onset cluster headache patients was 1.8, which is much less than the sex ratio in adult population. Pediatric-onset paroxysmal hemicrania was found in 11 patients across six studies, with a range of onset between 2 and 14-year-old. Pediatric-onset SUNCT (short-lasting unilateral neuralgiform headache with conjunctival injection and tearing) was found in six patients across six studies, with a range of onset between 2 and 17-year-old. Pediatric-onset SUNA (short-lasting unilateral neuralgiform headache attacks with cranial autonomic symptoms) was found for three patients across three studies, with a range of onset between 1 and 18-year-old. Pediatric-onset hemicrania continua were found in two patients across two studies, ages 8 and 12 years. The systematic review found that TACs can start early in life, with the youngest documented cases at 1-year-old for cluster headache and SUNA, 2-year-old for paroxysmal hemicrania and SUNCT, and 6-year-old for hemicrania continua. Overall the authors conclude that the full range of each ICHD-3 criterion is appropriate for pediatric-onset cluster headache patients, but additional information is needed for the other TACs.

COMMENT

Trigeminal autonomic cephalalgia (TAC) is a group of five primary headache disorders that share features of the unilateral location and ipsilateral facial autonomic features such as conjunctival injection, nasal congestion, and ptosis. TACs typically begin in adulthood and are exceptionally rare in preteens.[36] This article provides a detailed overview of the clinical features of pediatric TACs and finds that the International Classification of Headache Disorders, 3rd edition criteria (ICHD-3) for diagnosis of TACs can be applied with similar precision in the pediatric population. It is important to remember that TACs can be seen in patients as young as 1 year. However, secondary causes must always be ruled out in pediatric cases, before classifying them as primary headaches.

ARTICLE 14

Guidelines of the International Headache Society for Clinical Trials with Neuromodulation Devices for the Treatment of Migraine

Tassorelli C, Diener HC, Silberstein SD, Dodick DW, Goadsby PJ, Jensen RH, et al. Guidelines of the International Headache Society for clinical trials with neuromodulation devices for the treatment of migraine.
Cephalalgia. 2021;41(11-12):1135-51.

Abstract

An international group of headache scientists and clinicians with expertise in neuromodulation evaluated clinical trials involving neuromodulation devices that have been published since 2000 published the guidelines for clinical trials with neuromodulation devices for the treatment of migraine. A neuromodulation device is defined as any medical device that modulates the activity of the brain, the spinal cord, or peripheral nerves by means of electricity, magnetic fields, or other device-mediated modalities to either inhibit or facilitate neural impulses to achieve a clinical benefit for patients. Eligible subjects should be less than 50 years of age and fulfill the diagnostic criteria for migraine in the most recent version of the International Classification of Headache Disorders (ICHD). Subjects with episodic migraine (EM) may be included in trials for acute or preventive treatment of migraine. Subjects with a history of secondary headaches including medication overuse headaches [those in whom the underlying headache is not migraine and do not fulfill the criteria for chronic migraine (CM)] should be excluded. Patients with current use of opioids for >2 days/month, botulinum toxin injections or calcitonin gene-related peptide inhibitors in the past 6 months should be excluded from the studies. Although subjects with CM and acute medication overuse are eligible for inclusion in these studies, it should be clearly indicated which subjects are with and without medication overuse. The duration of migraine should be at least 12 months in adults and at least 6 months in children and adolescents. Whenever possible sex differences in treatment response using prespecified or post-hoc analyses should be analyzed. For pivotal trials, an adequately powered, the multicenter study should be performed to demonstrate consistent tolerability and efficacy of an investigational device. The committee recommends that although blinding represents a significant challenge due to an active signal, but strategies to enhance and preserve blinding should be used whenever possible. Pivotal comparative studies should preferably utilize parallel-group design. Combined double-blind trials that evaluate the efficacy of a device in the acute and preventive treatment of migraine are possible once the device has proved to be effective in both indications separately. Randomized controlled trials should follow the principles of intention to treat, wherever possible. *For trial assessing the preventive efficacy of a device*: A minimum 28-day prospective baseline period and a 12-week double-blind treatment period is recommended. *For trial assessing the acute efficacy of a device*: A minimum 28-day prospective baseline period is recommended followed by a double-blind period of 4 weeks for one attack, and 6–8 weeks in trials evaluating the consistency of response across multiple attacks. The International Headache Society (IHS) recommends postapproval product registries (i.e., prospective open-label observational studies) to evaluate the use of newly cleared devices in clinical practice. For implanted devices, a long-term follow-up (several months to years) is recommended. These recommendations for the assessment of neuromodulation devices in the acute and preventive treatment of migraine will facilitate research and help to clarify their optimal role in clinical practice.

COMMENT

This article fulfills the unmet need for a standardized approach and guidelines for research in neuromodulation devices in headache medicine. Previous studies have used varying methodologies and endpoints, making it difficult to compare the results. Use of these guidelines will help in future research of neuromodulation devices for the treatment of migraine.

ARTICLE 15

Development and Validation of a Novel Patient-reported Outcome Measure in People with Episodic Migraine and Chronic Migraine: The Activity Impairment in Migraine Diary

Lipton RB, Gandhi P, Stokes J, Cala ML, Evans CJ, Knoble, et al. Development and validation of a novel patient-reported outcome measure in people with episodic migraine and chronic migraine: The Activity Impairment in Migraine Diary *Headache. 2022;62(1):89-105.*

Abstract

The activity impairment in migraine diary (AIM-D) is a patient-related outcome tool that was created from concepts that emerged during qualitative interviews with five clinicians experienced in treating migraine and concept elicitation (CE) interviews with 40 adults with episodic migraine (EM) or chronic migraine (CM). The AIM-D was psychometrically evaluated using data from 316 adults with EM or CM who participated in a 13-week prospective observational study. Concepts relevant for the AIM-D were identified through telephone interviews with five clinicians experienced in treating migraine and face-to-face interviews with adults with EM or CM. Subsequently, concepts emerged from in-person advisory meetings with a panel of clinical experts and experts in clinical outcome assessment research were used to develop and refine the AIM-D. To minimize recall bias, the AIM-D was developed as a 24-hour daily diary. Concepts were selected for inclusion based on their importance and relevance to patients and the extent to which they were aligned with the target measurement concepts. The AIM-D was debriefed in three waves of cognitive interviews with adults with EM or CM; wherein participants were asked to provide feedback on the instructions, items, and response options and suggest any changes they would make. Subsequently, content analysis and psychometric evaluation were done in a longitudinal observational study over 13 weeks including a 1-week baseline period, conducted at 28 clinical sites in the United States. Participants completed patient-reported outcome (PRO) assessments at home using an eDiary and at the clinical site using an eTablet. AIM-D had a headache and a nonheadache version. Each AIM-D item asks respondents to rate the level of difficulty on a six-point rating scale ranging from (0) "Not difficult at all" to (5) "I could not do it at all", with instructions to answer each question based on the level of difficulty experienced "in the past 24 hours for the nonheadache version." For the headache version respondents were instructed to specifically consider the period "during (their) headache." To test the psychometric properties of the AIM-D, participants completed additional PRO assessments using the eDiary or eTablet including—a daily headache diary, EuroQOL 5 Dimensions 5 Levels (EQ-5D-5L), FIMQ, Headache Impact Test-6 (HIT-6), PROs Measurement Information System (PROMIS) Pain Interference – Short Form 6a, PROMIS Pain Intensity Numeric Rating Scale (NRS), MSQ v2.1, and MIDAS. Participants also completed the patient global impression-severity (PGI-S), a single-item measure that assesses the overall severity of migraine symptoms over the previous 7 days. Only one item (item no 6 related to walking) had a floor effect. Item–item correlations on a randomly drawn headache day ranged from 0.65 to 0.93 and item–total correlations ranged from 0.85 to 0.9. Internal consistency reliability was high with Cronbach's alpha on a randomly drawn headache day of 9.7. Test–retest reliability was also good with intraclass correlation coefficients (ICCs) for AIM-D domain scores and total scores were >0.60 for participants with no change in PGI-S between baseline and week 2. The AIM-D demonstrated construct validity with activity level, headache days, activity limitations, number of migraine days, PGI-S scores, PROMIS pain interference total score, FIMQ total score, HIT-6 total score, and MSQ domain scores. The AIM-D showed evidence of being responsive to changes in migraine frequency and severity. Thus, the AIM-D is a content valid and psychometrically sound measure of activity impairment with migraine with a potential to evaluate patient outcomes in routine clinical practice.

COMMENT

Measuring the burden of migraine and the benefits of treatment relies on the use of patient-reported outcome (PRO) measures. Some common measures for outcomes that have been used in various research models are Migraine Disability Assessment (MIDAS),[11] Headache Impact Test-6 (HIT-6),[12] and Work Productivity and Activity Impairment (WPAI) questionnaire.[37-39] One PRO measure that has recently been used is the Migraine Specific Quality of Life Questionnaire, version 2.1 Role Function-Restrictive (MSQ v2.1 RFR) domain and Migraine Physical Function Impact Diary (MPFID).[40] The MSQ v2.1 has a 4-week recall period and is subject to recall bias. The activity impairment in migraine diary (AIM-D) is another PRO that was developed and evaluated following Food and Drug Administration (FDA) guidance as a measure for assessing activity impairment, with items and response options that are relevant for patients with episodic migraine (EM) or chronic migraine (CM).[41] AIM-D captures meaningful physical and cognitive impacts not captured by the MSQ v2.1, such as difficulty walking and difficulty thinking clearly, and assesses severity rather than frequency of impacts. Content of AIM-D is similar to MPFID, but despite their overlap, these two measure different aspects of migraine burden.

REFERENCES (Headaches)

1. Furman JM, Marcus DA, Balaban CD. Migrainous vertigo: development of a pathogenetic model and structured diagnostic interview. Curr Opin Neurol. 2003;16(1):5-13.
2. Lewis RF, Priesol AJ, Nicoucar K, Lim K, Merfeld DM. Dynamic tilt thresholds are reduced in vestibular migraine. J Vestib Res. 2011;21(6):323-30.
3. Lee H, Lopez I, Ishiyama A, Baloh RW. Can migraine damage the inner ear? Arch Neurol. 2000;57(11):1631-4.
4. Teggi R, Colombo B, Albera R, Libonati GA, Balzanelli C, Caletrio AB, et al. Clinical features, familial history, and migraine precursors in patients with definite vestibular migraine: The VM-Phenotypes projects. Headache. 2018;58:534-44.
5. Silberstein SD, Lipton RB, Dodick DW, Freitag FG, Ramadan N, Mathew N, et al. Efficacy and safety of topiramate for the treatment of chronic migraine: a randomized, double-blind, placebo-controlled trial. Headache. 2007;47:170-80.
6. Diener HC, Bussone G, Van Oene JC, Lahaye M, Schwalen S, Goadsby PJ, et al. Topiramate reduces headache days in chronic migraine: a randomized, double-blind, placebo-controlled study. Cephalalgia. 2007;27:814-23.

7. Stensrud P, Sjaastad O. Comparative trial of Tenormin (atenolol) and Inderal (propranolol) in migraine. Headache. 1980;20:204-7.
8. Palferman TG, Gibberd FB, Simmonds JP. Prophylactic propranolol in the treatment of headache. Br J Clin Prac. 1983;37:28-9.
9. Domingues RB, da Silva ALP, Domingues SA, Aquino CCH, Kuster GW. A double-blind randomized controlled trial of low doses of propranolol, nortriptyline, and the combination of propranolol and nortriptyline for the preventive treatment of migraine. Arq Neuropsiquiatr. 2009;67:973-7.
10. Tassorelli C, Diener HC, Dodick DW, Silberstein SD, Lipton RB, Ashina M, et al. Guidelines of the International Headache Society for controlled trials of preventive treatment of chronic migraine in adults. Cephalalgia. 2018;38:815-32.
11. Shi L, Lehto SG, Zhu DXD, Sun H, Zhang J, Smith BP, et al. Pharmacologic characterization of AMG 334, a potent and selective human monoclonal antibody against the calcitonin gene-related peptide receptor. J Pharmacol Exp Ther. 2016;356:223-31.
12. Goadsby PJ, Reuter U, Hallstrom Y, Broessner G, Bonner JH, Zhang F, et al. A controlled trial of erenumab for episodic migraine. N Engl J Med. 2017;377:2123-32.
13. Ashina M, Goadsby PJ, Reuter U, Silberstein S, Dodick D, Rippon GA, et al. Long-term safety and tolerability of erenumab: three-plus year results from a five-year open-label extension study in episodic migraine. Cephalalgia. 2019;39:1455-64.
14. He M, Yu S, Liu R, Yang X, Zhao G, Qiao X, et al. Elevated blood pressure and headache disorders in China—associations, under-treatment and implications for public health. J Headache Pain. 2015;16:86.
15. Abramson JH, Hopp C, Epstein LM. Migraine and non-migrainous headaches. A community survey in Jerusalem. J Epidemiol Commun Health. 1980;34:188-93.
16. Fagernaes CF, Heuch I, Zwart JA, Winsvold BS, Linde M, Hagen K, et al. Blood pressure as a risk factor for headache and migraine: a prospective population-based study. Eur J Neurol. 2015;22:156-62.
17. Hagen K, Stovner LJ, Vatten L, Holmen J, Zwart JA, Bovim G. Blood pressure and risk of headache: a prospective study of 22 685 adults in Norway. J Neurol Neurosurg Psychiat. 2002;72:463-6.
18. Lipton RB, Buse DC, Friedman BW, Feder L, Adams AM, Fanning KM, et al. Characterizing opioid use in a US population with migraine: Results from the CaMEO study. Neurology. 2020;95(5):e457-68.
19. Oswald JC, Schuster NM. Lasmiditan for the treatment of acute migraine: a review and potential role in clinical practice. J Pain Res. 2018;11:2221-7.
20. Kuca B, Silberstein SD, Wietecha L, Berg PH, Dozier G, Lipton RB; COL MIG-301 Study Group. Lasmiditan is an effective acute treatment for migraine: A phase 3 randomized study. Neurology. 2018;91(24):e2222-32.
21. Goadsby PJ, Wietecha LA, Dennehy EB, Kuca B, Case MG, Aurora SK, et al. Phase 3 randomized, placebo-controlled, double-blind study of lasmiditan for acute treatment of migraine. Brain. 2019;142:1894-904.
22. Headache Classification Committee of the International Headache Society (IHS) The International Classification of Headache Disorders, 3rd edition. Cephalalgia. 2018;38(1):1-211.
23. Häni L, Fung C, Jesse CM, Ulrich CT, Miesbach T, Cipriani DR, et al. Insights into the natural history of spontaneous intracranial hypotension from infusion testing. Neurology. 2020;95(3):e247-55.
24. Mokri B, Aksamit AJ, Atkinson JL. Paradoxical postural headaches in cerebrospinal fluid leaks. Cephalalgia. 2004;24(10):883-7.
25. Leep Hunderfund AN, Mokri B. Second-half-of-the-day headache as a manifestation of spontaneous CSF leak. J Neurol. 2012;259(2):306-10.
26. Drellia K, Kokoti L, Deligianni CI, Papadopoulos D, Mitsikostas DD. Anti-CGRP monoclonal antibodies for migraine prevention: A systematic review and likelihood to help or harm analysis. Cephalalgia. 2021;41(7):851-64.
27. Li D, Rozen TD. The clinical characteristics of new daily persistent headache. Cephalalgia. 2002;22(1):66-9.
28. Castillo J, Muñoz P, Guitera V, Pascual J. Kaplan Award 1998. Epidemiology of chronic daily headache in the general population. Headache. 1999;39(3):190-6.
29. Grande RB, Aaseth K, Lundqvist C, Russell MB. Prevalence of new daily persistent headache in the general population. The Akershus study of chronic headache. Cephalalgia. 2009;29(11):1149-55.
30. Parodi IC, Poeta MG, Assini A, Schirinzi E, Del Sette P. Impact of quarantine due to COVID infection on migraine: a survey in Genova, Italy. Neurol Sci. 2020;41(8):2025-7.
31. Al-Hashel JY, Abokalawa F, Alenzi M, Alroughani R, Ahmed SF. Coronavirus disease-19 and headache; impact on pre-existing and characteristics of de novo: a cross-sectional study. J Headache Pain. 2021;22(1):97.
32. Benolie IR, Birman N, Eliav E, Sharav Y. The international classification of headache disorders: accurate diagnosis of orofacial pain? Cephalalgia. 2008;28:752-62.
33. MacDonald BK, Cockerell OC, Sander JW, Shorvon SD. The incidence and lifetime prevalence of neurological disorders in a prospective community-based study in the UK. Brain. 2000;123(Pt 4):665-76.
34. Smith JH, Cutrer FM. Numbness matters: a clinical review of trigeminal neuropathy. Cephalalgia. 2011;31(10):1131-44.
35. Benoliel R, Gaul C. Persistent idiopathic facial pain. Cephalalgia. 2017;37(7):680-91.
36. Özge A, Faedda N, Abu-Arafeh I, Gelfand AA, Goadsby PJ, Cuvellier JC, et al. Experts' opinion about the primary headache diagnostic criteria of the ICHD-3rd edition beta in children and adolescents. J Headache Pain. 2017;18:109.

37. Stewart WF, Lipton RB, Kolodner K, Liberman J, Sawyer J. Reliability of the migraine disability assessment score in a population-based sample of headache sufferers. Cephalalgia. 1999;19(2):107-14.
38. Kosinski M, Bayliss MS, Bjorner JB, Ware JE Jr, Garber WH, Batenhorst A, et al. A six-item short-form survey for measuring headache impact: the HIT-6. Qual Life Res. 2003;12:963-74.
39. Reilly MC, Zbrozek AS, Dukes EM. The validity and reproducibility of a work productivity and activity impairment instrument. Pharmacoeconomics. 1993;4:353-65.
40. Hareendran A, Mannix S, Skalicky A, et al. Development and exploration of the content validity of a patient-reported outcome measure to evaluate the impact of migraine-the migraine physical function impact diary (MPFID). Health Qual Life Outcomes. 2017;15(1):224.
41. Food and Drug Administration. (2018). Discussion document for patient-focused drug development. Methods to identify what is important to patients and select, develop or modify fit-for-purpose clinical outcome assessments. [online] Available from https://www.fda.gov/drugs/news-events-human-drugs/patient-focused-drug-development-guidance-methods-identify-what-important-patients-and-select [Last accessed September, 2022].

Section 2: Neuroinfections

Section Editors: Pratap Sanchetee, Samhita Panda

ARTICLE 1

Neurosyphilis, a True Chameleon of Neurology

Pujari SS, Kulkarni RV, Duberkar D, Nirhale S, Nadgir D, Dhonde P, et al. Neurosyphilis, a true chameleon of neurology. Ann Indian Acad Neurol. 2021;24(4):566-72.

Abstract

Background: Nowadays, neurosyphilis (NS) is a rare occurrence. Antibiotic use has altered the characteristics of many manifestations, which are heterogeneous. Even with pertinent clinical and radiological findings, a differential diagnosis of NS is not frequently considered because it mimics a number of common neurological diseases.

Objectives: To assess the signs and symptoms of NS in present era and the diagnostic process.

Method: A total of 10 patients with NS were recruited and their data was analyzed. The demographic information, clinical characteristics, investigations, the steps used to arrive at a diagnosis, management, and results were all noted.

Results: Six individuals in our cohort had cognitive decline/encephalopathy, one had cerebellar ataxia, one had myelitis, and one had meningitis with cranial nerve palsies. These were the manifestations of NS. In one instance, the existence of an Argyll Robertson pupil aided in the diagnosis. In contrast to the six patients for whom treponemal tests were sought as part of the routine workup for dementia/ataxia, two patients had treponemal tests ordered only after other etiologies had been considered.

Conclusion: Degenerative, vascular, nutritional, autoimmune, or prion diseases are sometimes confused for NS dementia and behavioral abnormalities. Myelitis mimics demyelination or nutritional myelopathy, and meningitis is similar to infectious (tubercular), granulomatous (sarcoidosis, Wegener's), collagen vascular disease, and neoplastic meningitis (B12 deficiency). Cerebellar ataxia is a rare complication of NS. Consider NS as one of the uncommon causes of these symptoms, and effective outcomes are achieved when NS is treated quickly.

Keywords: Meningitis, Myelitis asymptomatic neurosyphilis, Dementia, Meningitis, Myelitis, Cerebellar ataxia

COMMENT

This article highlights an underestimated etiological differential when dealing with varied neurological presentations. The classical patterns and severity of presentation of neurosyphilis have changed in recent decades. Neurosyphilis can present as subtle mimics of neurological disorders affecting different parts of the neuraxis with acute, subacute, or chronic evolution. It can masquerade as dementia, cognitive impairment, extrapyramidal deficits, ataxia, seizures, strokes, myelopathy, cranial neuropathies, or even asymptomatic neurosyphilis. It is important to know that no clinical or radiological feature is specific to neurosyphilis. The presence of peripheral skin lesions, Argyll Robertson pupils, cerebrospinal fluid (CSF) pleocytosis with raised proteins, and CSF venereal disease research laboratory (VDRL)/ treponema pallidum hemagglutination assay (TPHA) tests guide to diagnose neurosyphilis. Hence, investigations should be tailored to maximize the yield to decrease the time to treatment initiation.

Key Messages

- Neurosyphilis should be considered in situations with atypical neurological presentations or as in typical syndromes like dementia, myelopathy, and strokes.
- A high index of suspicion will increase the yield of this eminently treatable disorder if detected early.

ARTICLE 2

Neurological Disorders Seen during Second Wave of SARS-CoV-2 Pandemic from Two Tertiary Care Centers in Central and Southern Kerala

George M, Baby N, Azad A, Rajan A, Radhakrishnan SK. Neurological disorders seen during second wave of SARS-CoV-2 pandemic from two tertiary care centers in central and Southern Kerala.
Ann Indian Acad Neurol. 2021;24(6):917-26.

Abstract

Background and objective: SARS-CoV-2 infections are characterized by predominant respiratory symptoms. Neurological involvement has so far only occasionally been mentioned in anecdotal reports from India. There have also been reports of adverse effects following COVID-19 immunization. We list the neurological signs and symptoms that were observed during the second wave in connection with either the COVID-19 infection or the vaccine.

Methods: This retrospective investigation covered sequential COVID-19 patient admissions to two tertiary healthcare facilities in Kerala from 1 March, 2021 to 31 May, 2021. The term "COVID-19-associated neurological disorders (CAND)" refers to neurological symptoms that appear 2 weeks before or 30 days after a positive status of antigen or reverse transcription-polymerase chain reaction (RT-PCR), and the term "postvaccinal neurological disorders (PVND)" refers to neurological symptoms that appear within 1 month of receiving the COVID-19 vaccination.

Results: There were 1,270 COVID-19 admissions recorded during the study period. A total of 42 individuals (3.3%) with neurological symptoms were detected; 35 of these patients had CAND symptoms, and 7 had PVND symptoms. Stroke was most prevalent (50%) and was followed by seizures and diseases of the peripheral nervous system (14.2% each). Additionally, infections related to COVID-19 (9.5%) and encephalitis/demyelination (11.9%) were observed.

Conclusion: The SARS-CoV-2 epidemic has seen the emergence of CAND and PVND. The association of some of them may be accidental, but it is important to note because it is yet unknown how COVID-19 affects different organ systems. Additionally, this might be beneficial for upcoming research that designs management choices.

Keywords: COVID-associated neurological disorders, Neurological disorders, COVID-19 vaccination, COVID-19 infection, Postvaccinal neurological disorders

COMMENT

The SARS-CoV-2 is a catastrophic event since the influenza pandemic of 1918. The factors implicated in the causation of the second wave are a complex interaction of mutant strains with changing immune status in the host and complacency on the part of the public and authorities. Enhanced transmission and rapid depletion of antibodies are major issues. Experimental studies have confirmed a considerable impact on the nervous system in the short as well as in the long run. This article, in spite of limitations, highlight increased neurological involvement along the entire neuraxis. Immunization, a major weapon in our armamentarium, is also loaded with critical neurological consequences. This study has convincingly documented this fact. Our experience with SARS-CoV-2 and consequent neurological involvement is still in its infancy. We are going to witness a large number of neurological sequelae such as stroke and demyelinating disorders related to SARS-CoV-2 in the future.[1,2]

Key Message

Clinicians must be vigilant of COVID-19 in all unexplained presentations and a registry should be maintained at the institutional and national level to document it.

ARTICLE 3

Recurrent Neurocysticercosis: Not so Rare

Kaur KP, Garg A, Sebastian LJD, Bhatia R, Singh MB, Srivastava A, Tripathi M, et al. Recurrent neurocysticercosis: Not so rare.
Neurol India. 2021;69(2):385-91.

Abstract

Background: In individuals with neurocysticercosis (NCC) in India, solitary cysticercus granuloma (SCG) manifesting as a single ring-enhancing lesion (SREL) is the most common imaging result. The majority of SCGs dissolve with or without calcifications during follow-up. Rare reports of recurrent SCG have been documented.

Objectives: The purpose of our study is to evaluate the incidence of recurrent SCG in a cohort of SCG patients and to propose the hypothesis.

Material and methods: A total of 278 SCG patients who met the NCC criteria were included in this retrospective analysis. We examined their magnetic resonance imaging (MRI) results and medical records.

Results: With a median follow-up of 14.23 months, 15.6% of patients developed recurrent NCC (range: 0.24–113.3). Out of 15 patients with recurrent NCC, 10 patients previously had imaging resolution or partial regression of the lesion followed by the appearance of new SCG in the same location, 3 patients had a change in the morphology of the lesion from a solitary discrete ring-enhancing lesion (REL) to a solitary conglomerate REL as a result of the development of new cysticercus granuloma next to the old lesion, patients had recurrent lesions next to the previous lesion. After the regressing of the original SCGs, two patients had new SCGs in various sites.

Conclusion: Solitary cysticercus granuloma recurrence is more likely to happen at the location of initial infection in NCC, where it is not unusual. It should not be confused with neurotuberculosis or other granulomatous infections that persist over time.

Keywords: Solitary cysticercus granuloma (SCG), Single ring-enhancing lesions, Neurocysticercosis, Enlarging NCC, Recurrent NCC, Conglomerate ring-enhancing lesions

COMMENT

Disappearing and reappearing lesions seen on computed tomography (CT) or magnetic resonance imaging (MRI) scan of the brain is a quite recent phenomenon. They have been described largely in patients with epilepsy and are mostly related to cysticercosis. It must be appreciated that such resolutions are essentially radiological or imaging resolutions and not necessarily biological or histological resolutions.[3] Recurrences have been noticed either at the original site or at a different site(s). This could be related to either aggravation of a dormant cyst or reinfection from persistent taeniasis or food handlers. Breakdown of the blood–brain barrier following a seizure has also been advanced in some of the symptomatic patients. Recurrence in these patients is with a solitary lesion rather than with multiple lesions suggesting unique interaction between host immunity and parasite-dependent factors.

> **Key Messages**
> - With liberal use of CT and MRI during follow-up, we will be witnessing a larger number of patients having reappearing lesions with or without concomitant clinical recovery in patients with SCG.
> - These patients must be treated on a conservative line with good follow-up rather than rushing to invasive procedures for the confirmation of diagnosis.

ARTICLE 4

6-month Neurological and Psychiatric Outcomes in 236,379 Survivors of COVID-19: A Retrospective Cohort Study using Electronic Health Records

Taquet M, Geddes JR, Husain M, Luciano S, Harrison PJ. 6-month neurological and psychiatric outcomes in 236 379 survivors of COVID-19: A retrospective cohort study using electronic health records.
Lancet Psychiatry. 2021;8(5):416-27.

Abstract

Background: More data are needed to assess the neurological and psychiatric sequel of COVID-19.

Methods: For this retrospective cohort study and time-to-event analysis, we used data from the electronic health records. Primary cohort comprised COVID-19 patients older than 10 years, and compared it with patients with influenza and other respiratory tract infections. We estimated the incidence of various neurological and psychiatric outcomes in the 6 months after the COVID-19 diagnosis. Using a Cox model, we compared incidences with those in patients with influenza or other respiratory tract infections.

Findings: The estimated incidence of a neurological or psychiatric diagnosis in the subsequent 6 months among 236,379 COVID-19 patients was 33.62% [95% confidence interval (CI) 33.17–34.07], with 12.84% (12.36–13.33) receiving their initial such diagnosis. The estimated incidence of a diagnosis was 46.42% (44.78–48.09) for patients admitted to an intensive therapy unit and 25.79% (23.50–28.25) for a first diagnosis. For each of the specific diagnoses associated with the study outcomes, the COVID-19 cohort as a whole had estimated incidences of 0.56% (0.50–0.63) for cerebral hemorrhage, 2.10% (1.97–2.23) for ischemic stroke, 0.11% (0.08–0.14) for parkinsonism,

0.67% (0.59–0.75) for dementia, 17.39% (17.04–17.74) for anxiety disorder, and 1.40% (1.30–1.51) for psychotic disorder. The majority of diagnostic categories were more frequent in COVID-19 patients than in patients with influenza [hazard ratio (HR) 1.44; 95% CI 1.40–1.47, for any diagnosis; 1.78, 1.68–1.89, for any first diagnosis] and in patients with other respiratory tract infections (1.16, 1.14–1.17, for any diagnosis; 1.32, 1.27–1.36, for any first diagnosis).

Interpretation: The 6 months following COVID-19 infection have been accompanied by significant neurological and psychiatric morbidity. Patients with severe COVID-19 risks exhibited greater risk factors.

Keywords: COVID-19, Psychiatric, Neurological, Dementia, Stroke, Anxiety, Mood disorders, Delirium

COMMENT

Considered initially to be a respiratory illness, COVID-19 is a multisystemic disease that has a large toll on nervous, gastrointestinal, hepatic, and genitourinary systems. It can cause or precipitate a spectrum of neurological and psychiatric disorders during the acute and postacute stages. Our understanding of the pathogenesis of neuropsychiatric involvement is evolving and various biological and psychosocial factors need to be researched. This study is one of the large epidemiological analyses based on electronic health records. Major risk factors are disease severity, duration of symptoms, and female gender. Exacerbation of preexisting illnesses has been noted commonly with seizures and psychiatric disorders. Considering the huge toll of neuropsychiatric morbidity with COVID-19, medical services and social care systems should be geared accordingly. Studies with longer follow-ups are needed to document late sequels.

Key Message

The literature on the long-term consequences of COVID-19 is emerging. Robust and high-quality longitudinal studies delineating neuropsychiatric complications and their relationship to neuroimaging and inflammatory biomarkers are needed.

ARTICLE 5

Severe Acute Respiratory Syndrome Coronavirus 2 Encephalitis is a Cytokine Release Syndrome: Evidences from Cerebrospinal Fluid Analyses

Pilotto A, Masciocchi S, Volonghi I, De Giuli V, Caprioli F, Mariotto S, et al. Severe acute respiratory syndrome coronavirus 2 (SARS-CoV-2) encephalitis is a cytokine release syndrome: Evidences from cerebrospinal fluid analyses. *Clin Infect Dis.* 2021;73(9):e3019-26.

Abstract

Background: Recent research showed that cytokine release syndrome, endothelial activation, blood–brain barrier disruption, and immune-mediated processes are all involved in the neurological symptoms of severe acute respiratory syndrome coronavirus 2 (SARS-CoV-2). The cerebrospinal fluid (CSF) correlates of SARS-CoV-2 encephalitis have very seldom been thoroughly studied.

Methods: A comprehensive panel of CSF neuronal (NfL, T-tau), glial (GFAP, TREM2, YKL-40), and inflammatory biomarkers [interleukin (IL)-1β, L-6, Il-8, tumor necrosis factor alpha (TNF-α), CXCL-13 and β2-microglobulin] was performed on patients with polymerase chain reaction (PCR)-confirmed SARS-CoV-2 infection and encephalitis (COV-Enc), encephalitis without SARS-CoV-2 infection (ENC).

Results: The study had 18 healthy controls (HC), 21 ENC, and 13 COV-Enc participants. In COV-Enc patients, CSF showed elevated IL-8 levels independently of the existence of pleocytosis/hyperproteinorrachia but was negative for SARS-CoV-2 real-time PCR. Patients with COV-Enc demonstrated elevated levels of IL-6, TNF-α, β2-microglobulin, and glial markers (GFAP, sTREM-2, and YKL-40) comparable to ENC, but normal CXCL13 levels. NfL and Tau, neuronal markers, were aberrant only in severe cases.

Conclusion: Glial activation and neuroinflammatory indicators were strongly linked to SARS-CoV-2-related encephalitis, but neuronal markers were only elevated in severe cases. The pattern of CSF abnormalities revealed that the primary inflammatory mechanism of SARS-CoV-2 associated encephalitis was cytokine-release syndrome.

Keywords: COVID-19, SARS-CoV-2, Encephalitis, Cytokine storm syndrome; Immune effector cell-associated neurotoxicity syndrome (ICANS)

COMMENT

The pathogenesis of SARS-CoV-2-associated central nervous system (CNS) disease is complex and cannot be explained by a sole mechanism. The neurotropism of the SARS-CoV-2 virus is selective and is not able to explain generalized involvement such as encephalitis. Dysregulated systemic inflammatory responses, hypoxia, and autoimmune responses have been advanced to explain widespread involvement. Cytokine release syndrome (CRS) is a potentially fatal complication of various infections including the SARS-CoV-2 virus. The majority of studies evaluated blood and other peripheral markers to support this hypothesis. The present study has analyzed an extensive panel of cerebrospinal fluid (CSF) neuronal, glial, and biomarkers of inflammatory responses and neuronal injuries to support CRS as an underlying mechanism of SARS-CoV-2-related encephalitis. This and many such studies will pave the way to devise better therapeutic strategies and use them as therapeutic and prognostic markers.

> **Key Message**
>
> Emerging evidence indicates that apart from neurotropism and neuroinvasiveness, neuroimmune dysfunction with the SARS-CoV-2 virus is a major determinant in patients with encephalitis.

ARTICLE 6

Determinants of Brain Swelling in Pediatric and Adult Cerebral Malaria

Sahu PK, Duffy FJ, Dankwa S, Vishnyakova M, Majhi M, Pirpamer L, et al. Determinants of brain swelling in pediatric and adult cerebral malaria.
JCI Insight. 2021;6(18):e145823.

Abstract

Both adults and children can get cerebral malaria (CM), although children are more likely to experience severe brain swelling. We did blood profiling and brain magnetic resonance imaging (MRI) on a cohort of pediatric and adult patients with CM in Rourkela, India, and compared them with an African pediatric CM cohort in Malawi to look at characteristics linked to brain swelling in malaria. We found that CM at both sites was associated with greater plasma *Plasmodium falciparum* histidine rich protein 2 (PfHRP2) levels and enhanced var transcripts that encode for binding to endothelial protein C receptor (EPCR). Due to overall lower parasite var transcript levels in this age group and more severe thrombocytopenia in Rourkela adults, machine learning models trained on the African pediatric cohort could classify brain swelling in Indian children with CM cases but performed less well for adult classification. Subdividing the CM patients into different groups demonstrated increased parasite biomass associated with severe thrombocytopenia and more Group A-EPCR var transcripts in mild thrombocytopenia. Despite age disparities in brain swelling, these data show that greater parasite biomass and a fraction of Group A-EPCR binding variants are shared characteristics in children and adult CM cases.

Keywords: Tuberculosis, Cerebrospinal fluid, Pharmacokinetics, Pharmacology, Meningitis

COMMENT

Cerebral malaria, in spite of adequate medical management, has high mortality to the tune of 20%. This study aims to unfold the molecular mechanism of CM by comparing two sets of populations, i.e., (1) African population with high disease transmission and higher immunity where severe malaria primarily affects children and (2) Indian population with low transmission and lower immunity where children and adults are equally affected. The biological mechanisms for severe malaria involve parasite virulence, and host's immunological and genetic factors. While cerebral edema is a prominent feature in children, adults with severe malaria are associated more with multiorgan failure and thrombocytopenia. This study has confirmed that high parasite biomass, as indicated by higher plasma levels of PfHRP2, is a good indicator of CM in both adult and pediatric populations. However, elevated var transcripts that encode EPCR are seen in pediatric CM only.

Key Messages

- The pathogenesis and clinical presentation of severe malaria differ depending on the immune status of a person.
- Delineation of the molecular mechanisms for severe malaria will pave the way for understanding varied clinical presentations and devising specific therapeutic modalities.

ARTICLE 7

Presenting Symptoms of Leprosy at Diagnosis: Clinical Evidence from a Cross-sectional, Population-based Study

Chen X, Zha S, Shui TJ. Presenting symptoms of leprosy at diagnosis: clinical evidence from a cross-sectional, population-based study.
PLoS Negl Trop Dis. 2021;15(11):e0009913.

Abstract

Background: Leprosy has a wide range of clinical symptoms across the dermatologic and neurological spectrum, making diagnosis difficult.

Objectives: To examine associations between common presenting symptoms of leprosy and stage at diagnosis.

Methods: In this cross-sectional study, we analyzed population-level data from the Leprosy Management Information System (LEPMIS) in Yunnan, China from 2010–2020 and enrolled patients with newly detected leprosy.

Results: The data of 2,125 newly detected leprosy patients, with 5,000 symptoms, were analyzed. Numbness (828/5,000; 16.56%), erythema (802/5,000; 16.04%), painless nor pruritic skin lesions (651/5,000; 13.02%), eyebrow hair loss (467/5,000; 9.34%), and tubercles (442/5,000; 8.84%) were the common symptoms. Symptoms related to skin (1,935/2,533; 76.39%) and leprosy reaction (279/297, 93.94%) were mainly existed in multibacillary (MB) group while symptoms related to disability (263/316, 83.49%), clinical features (38/56, 69.09%), and facial features (19/23, 82.61%) were predominantly present in the delayed diagnostic group. Despite low proportions, formic sensation (99/5,000; 1.98%), pain (92/5,000; 1.84%), pruritus (56/5,000; 1.12%), finger contracture (109/5,000; 2.18%), muscle atrophy (71/5,000; 1.42%), and motor dysfunction (18/5,000; 0.36%) were reported during the diagnosis of leprosy. The proportions of skin, skin and nerve, and nerve symptoms as initial symptoms were 33.25, 44.95, and 21.80% and as only symptoms were 28.66, 57.81, and 13.91%, respectively. In those with physical disability, nerve symptoms were the most frequent (57.65 and 65.36% for the initial and only symptoms, respectively). In the delayed diagnosis group, nerve symptoms were the most frequent symptoms (15.73 and 17.25%) and were associated with the longest diagnostic intervals [mean ± standard deviation (SD): 38.88 ± 46.02 and 40.35 ± 49.36 months for initial and only symptoms, respectively].

Conclusion: Leprosy awareness in the community would increase with a better understanding of the nature of the presenting symptoms and the creation of symptom awareness initiatives. We should work to raise awareness of nerve symptoms because they were linked to a larger percentage of physical disability and a longer diagnosis lag.

Keywords: Leprosy, Multibacillary, Paucibacillary, Disability, Diagnostic interval

COMMENT

Although leprosy elimination programs have been decentralized and integrated into the general health system in India, it continues to affect patients. However, there has been a changing pattern in clinical presentation in the recent past. This study, a decade long population level data analysis, throws light on these trends. Leprosy remains a disease primarily affecting the superficial peripheral nervous system and skin with rarer afflictions of the upper respiratory tract mucosa, bone, testes, and eyes. Multibacillary forms of leprosy predominate with its major manifestations restricted to skin and associated leprosy reactions.[4] On the contrary, a higher frequency of symptom signatures of nerve involvement is noted in paucibacillary forms. Delayed diagnosis and grade-2 disability in the form of motor weakness, finger contractures, and muscle atrophy are observed in the paucibacillary group. In order to target reduction in the grade-2 disability, the focus should shift to early identification of nerve involvement which at times may be challenging.

> **Key Messages**
> - Leprosy elimination programs should employ focused strategies to decrease grade-1 and -2 disabilities.
> - This can be achieved by earlier detection of paucibacillary forms and their associated nerve ± skin involvement.

ARTICLE 8

Association between High Proviral Load, Cognitive Impairment, and White Matter Brain Lesions in Human T-lymphotropic Virus Type 1-infected Individuals

Kalil RS, Vasconcellos I, Rosadas C, Cony A, Lima DP, Gonçalves CCA, et al. Association between high proviral load, cognitive impairment, and white matter brain lesions in HTLV-1-infected individuals.
J Neurovirol. 2021;27(6):810-9.

Abstract

Background: In human T-lymphotropic virus type 1 (HTLV-1)-infected people, there is still no obvious connection between high proviral load (PVL) in peripheral blood mononuclear cells (PBMCs), cognitive dysfunction, and white matter brain lesions.

Methods: In this cross-sectional study, all individuals fulfilling the following criteria were included: Between 18 and 65 years of age, >4 years of formal education, and completed neuropsychological evaluation and HTLV-1 serology. Infected individuals underwent brain conventional magnetic resonance imaging (MRI) and PVL quantitative polymerase chain reaction (qPCR). Statistical analysis was adjusted in the models by age and education.

Results: The study included 62 participants: 22 asymptomatic carriers (mean age 43.4 ± 13.1 years old), 22 patients with HTLV-1-associated myelopathy/tropical spastic paraparesis (HAM/TSP) (mean age 51.5 ± 8.7 years old), and 18 uninfected controls (mean age 52.3 ± 11.1 years old). Cognitive deficit was observed in all groups. Patients with HAM/TSP showed higher neurocognitive deviation in attention and motor skills, higher frequency (84%) of brain white matter lesions, and higher PVL median (range) 8.45 (0.5–71.4) copies/100 PBMC. Brain white matter lesion was associated with verbal memory deficit in HTLV-1-infected individuals (HAM/TSP and asymptomatic carriers) ($p = 0.026$). In addition, there was a correlation between higher PVL and neurocognitive dysfunction score (processing speed of visuomotor information and visuoconstructive praxis) in HTLV-1-infected patients.

Conclusion: The study demonstrated an association between HTLV-1 infection, neurocognitive disorder, and white matter brain lesions on MRI as well as a correlation with higher HTLV-1 PVL, suggesting that the central nervous system involvement by HTLV-1 is not restricted to the spinal cord but involves the whole neuroaxis. HTLV-1-infected individuals should be tested for cognitive impairment.

Keywords: Cognitive impairment, HTLV-1, HTLV-1-associated myelopathy, Magnetic resonance imaging, Tropical spastic paraparesis

COMMENT

Human T-lymphotropic virus type 1 (HTLV-1)-associated myelopathy/tropical spastic paraparesis (HAM/TSP) is a relatively neglected entity occurring in <4% of those infected. Few earlier studies have shown that white matter (WM) lesions in HTLV-I-infected individuals suggest potential early central nervous system inflammation but without correlation with cognitive impairment.[5] Other studies have shown the presence of cognitive impairment linked to heightened inflammatory markers in HAM/TSP. This study may be considered an extension of the knowledge from these studies which further expands the phenotype of HAM/TSP and HTLV-1-infected yet apparently asymptomatic individuals. HTLV-1-infected persons inclusive of both HAM/TSP and asymptomatic individuals were found to have a high frequency of cognitive deficits with associated brain magnetic resonance imaging (MRI) WM lesions. This also correlated with high proviral load suggesting subclinical involvement of the subcortical tracts involved in information processing.

Key Messages

- HTLV-1-associated infections should now be recognized to have involvement of the neuraxis beyond the spinal cord.
- Detailed assessment of cognitive functions along with inflammatory markers and proviral load may help guide an early institution of treatment in apparently asymptomatic subjects.

ARTICLE 9

Combined Testing of Cerebrospinal Fluid Interleukin-12 (p40) and Serum C-reactive Protein as a Possible Discriminator of Acute Bacterial Neuroinfections

Kalchev Y, Petkova T, Raycheva R, Argirova P, Stoycheva M, Murdjeva M. Combined testing of cerebrospinal fluid IL-12 (p40) and serum C-reactive protein as a possible discriminator of acute bacterial neuroinfections.
Cytokine. 2021;140:155423.

Abstract

Introduction: Meningitis is the most prevalent of the life-threatening illnesses of the central nervous system (CNS). While bacterial pathogens are linked to increased mortality rates and long-lasting neurological sequelae, viral infections are typically self-limiting illnesses.

Objectives: We aimed to study the role of interleukin (IL)-6, IL-8, IL-10, IL-12 (p40), tumor necrosis factor alpha (TNF-α) cytokines, classical cerebrospinal fluid (CSF) parameters, and serum C-reactive protein levels (CRP) for discriminating bacterial from viral CNS infections.

Material and methods: Eighty patients were enrolled in this prospective study at St George University Hospital in Plovdiv who had clinical signs and abnormal CSF test results indicative of a neuroinfection. The latex-agglutination test, multiplex polymerase chain reaction (PCR), and common techniques like direct microscopy, culturing, and identification were all used for the microbiological analysis. Enzyme-linked immunosorbent assay (ELISA) was used to measure the levels of cytokines. The patients' medical records were used to gather CRP and CSF data.

Results: Cerebrospinal IL-12 (p40) had the strongest discriminating power among the cytokines, (AUC = 0.925; p = 0.000). The greatest indicator of bacterial neuroinfection was CSF protein levels (AUC = 0.973; p = 0.000). As a standalone biomarker, serum CRP was predicted to have an AUC of 0.943. When blood CRP and CSF IL-12 (p40) are combined, the discriminatory power can be enhanced up to 0.995 (p = 0.000), with an ideal cutoff value of 144 (sensitivity 100%, specificity 90.9%).

Conclusion: The combination of CSF IL-12 (p40) and serum CRP testing yields the best diagnostic results.

Keywords: C-reactive protein, IL-12 (p40), Meningitis, Cerebrospinal fluid, Neuroinfection

COMMENT

Neuroinfections such as meningitis are characterized by the activation of an inflammatory cascade mediated by various cytokines, chemokines, and other pro- and anti-inflammatory mediators. The intrinsic ability of the blood–brain barrier and loss of its integrity during the infective process along with local activation of the endothelial cells, resting microglia, astrocytes, and meningeal macrophages lead to changes in these markers in the CSF. Neuroscientists and neurophysicians dealing with neuroinfections are interested in tests that can discriminate between bacterial and viral infections with a high degree of certainty. The authors found interleukin (IL)-6 and IL-8 to be nondiscriminatory. On the other hand, CSF IL-12 (p40) and protein, and combination with serum C-reactive protein increased the probability of bacterial meningitis. This could potentially help guide early antibiotic therapy.

Key Messages

- The search for strong markers of CNS bacterial infections has taken us from basic CSF biochemistry and microbiological investigations to the effect on inflammatory markers.
- IL-12 may be a potential stand-alone marker with high specificity and sensitivity which can also be used in combination with CSF protein and serum CRP.

ARTICLE 10

Cycloserine and Linezolid for Tuberculosis Meningitis: Pharmacokinetic Evidence of Potential Usefulness

Kempker RR, Smith AGC, Avaliani T, Gujabidze M, Bakuradze T, Sabanadze S, et al. Cycloserine and linezolid for tuberculosis meningitis: Pharmacokinetic evidence of potential usefulness.
Clin Infect Dis. 2022;75(4):682-9.

Abstract

Background: In order to effectively treat tuberculosis meningitis (TBM), antituberculosis medications must be able to pass the blood–brain barrier and reach the central nervous system. By giving information on how antituberculosis medications that have recently been developed and those that have been repurposed can enter the cerebrospinal fluid (CSF), we aimed to close a significant knowledge gap.

Methods: In Tbilisi, Georgia, from January 2019 to January 2020, we carried out a clinical pharmacology study on patients receiving TBM treatment. While the patients were in the hospital, serial serum and CSF samples were taken. To capture early and late CSF penetration, CSF was obtained from regular lumbar punctures that were timed alternatingly between 2 and 6 hours.

Results: A total of 17 TBM patients (8 with proven disease) were included; all took linezolid, with a subgroup also getting cycloserine (5), clofazimine (5), delamanid (4), and bedaquiline (2). Bedaquiline (12), clofazimine (24), and delamanid (19) were all detected at levels below the limit of detection in all CSF assays. At 2 and 6 hours, the median CSF concentrations of cycloserine were 15.90 and 15.10 g/mL, respectively, with adjusted CSF/serum ratios of 0.52 and 0.66.

Linezolid concentrations in the CSF were 0.90 and 3.14 g/mL at 2 and 6 hours, with corresponding adjusted CSF/serum ratios of 0.25 and 0.59. Rifampin coadministration had no effect on the level of linezolid in the CSF serum.

Conclusion: Linezolid and cycloserine may be useful medications for treating TBM based on their moderate-to-high CSF penetration, however bedaquiline, delamanid, and clofazimine's efficacy is unclear given their low CSF penetration.

Keywords: Cerebrospinal fluid, Pharmacology, Pharmacokinetics, Meningitis, Tuberculosis

COMMENT

Mortality from TBM is considerably high and substantially increases for drug resistant forms.[6] The World Health Organization (WHO) consolidated guidelines on tuberculosis (TB) have clearly promoted the use of new and repurposed drugs for treatment of TB, especially for drug resistant TB. However, treatment of tubercular meningitis has always been fraught with controversies regarding the duration and regimen of antitubercular drugs, more so in the presence of multidrug-resistant (MDR) TBM. This is important as most recommendations have been largely extensions to studies on pulmonary TB. The main issue of drug effectiveness in TBM is the need to have good penetration of the blood–brain barrier and therapeutic CSF levels. The authors have evaluated to the effectiveness of linezolid, cycloserine, clofazimine, bedaquiline, and delamanid in TBM. Linezolid, which has previously been found to benefit MDR-TBM, was again ratified as achieving good CSF penetration along with cycloserine unlike the others usually given in MDR regimens. This study showing around 50% CSF penetration for linezolid further makes it an attractive addition to existing TBM regimens.

Key Messages

- *Therapeutic regimens for TBM and drug-resistant TBM should evolve from direct assessments in these patient groups.*
- *Linezolid and cycloserine have good pharmacokinetic data to support their use in MDR-TBM compared to other newer drugs.*

REFERENCES (Neuroinfections)

1. Kulkarni R, Misra UK, Meshram C, Kochar D, Modi M, Vishnu VY, et al. Epidemic of mucormycosis in COVID-19 pandemic: A position paper. Ann Indian Acad Neurol. 2022;25:7-10.
2. Kulkarni R, Pujari S, Gupta D, Advani S, Soni A, Duberkar D; MAN Collaborative Study Group. Rhino-orbito-cerebral mycosis and COVID-19: From bad to worse? Ann Indian Acad Neurol. 2022;25:68-75.
3. Sanchetee PC, Dhamija RM, Sabharwal RK, Krishna NR. Appearance of subcutaneous cysticercosis: An unusual reaction with praziquantel. Neurol India. 1989;37:171-4.
4. Govindasamy K, John AS, Lal V, Arif M, Solomon RM, Ghosal J, et al. A comparison of three types of targeted, community-based methods aimed at promoting early detection of new leprosy cases in rural parts of three endemic states in India. PLoS One. 2021;16(12):e0261219.
5. Morgan DJ, Caskey MF, Abbehusen C, Oliveira-Filho J, Araujo C, Porto AF, et al. Brain magnetic resonance imaging white matter lesions are frequent in HTLV-I carriers and do not discriminate from HAM/TSP. AIDS Res Hum Retroviruses. 2007;23(12):1499-504.
6. Seddon JA, Tugume L, Solomons R, Prasad K, Bahr NC; Tuberculous Meningitis International Research Consortium. The current global situation for tuberculous meningitis: epidemiology, diagnostics, treatment and outcomes. Wellcome Open Res. 2019;4:167.

Section 3: Stroke

Section Editor: MV Padma Srivastava

Associate Editor: Ayush Agarwal

Important/Landmark Stroke Trials between June 2018 and February 2022

THROMBOLYSIS

ARTICLE 1

PRISMS: Effect of Alteplase versus Aspirin on Functional Outcome for Patients with Acute Ischemic Stroke and Minor Nondisabling Neurologic Deficits

Khatri P, Kleindorfer DO, Devlin T, Sawyer RN Jr, Starr M, Mejilla J, et al. Effect of alteplase vs aspirin on functional outcome for patients with acute ischemic stroke and minor nondisabling neurologic deficits.
JAMA. 2018;320(2):156-66.

Abstract

Randomized, double-blinded, placebo-controlled, multicenter clinical trial designed to evaluate the efficacy and safety of alteplase in individuals with nondisabling deficits and National Institutes of Health Stroke Scale (NIHSS) between 0 and 5. Patients were randomized to receive either intravenous (IV) alteplase [recombinant tissue plasminogen activator (rTPA)] (0.9 mg/kg) with oral placebo or oral aspirin (325 mg) with IV placebo and primary outcome was the percentage of patients with favorable clinical outcome at 90 days defined as modified Rankin Scale (mRS) 0–1.

122 patients (78.2%) in the alteplase arm and 128 (81.5%) in the aspirin arm achieved the primary outcome thereby concluding that the use of alteplase did not increase the chances of the same in this patient population.

COMMENT

The American Heart Association/American Stroke Association (AHA/ASA) recommend the administration of intravenous (IV) alteplase within 3 hours for patients with mild but disabling stroke symptoms but are indecisive about those with mild and nondisabling symptoms. This has posed a therapeutic dilemma: treat because they might worsen or do not treat because of risk of symptomatic intracerebral hemorrhage (sICH).

The PRISMS trial helped define the role of IV recombinant tissue plasminogen activator (rTPA) in this setting. The excellent outcome in the aspirin group and numerically similar outcomes between the two groups make it unlikely that IV rTPA would significantly improve functional outcome in patients with National Institutes of Health Stroke Scale (NIHSS) scores of 5 or lower with non-disabling deficits at presentation. However, the trial does not address the issue of what constitutes a "nondisabling" deficit in its entirety. Ambiguity and lack of consensus in this regard will continue to raise concerns regarding "missing" eligible patients for IV thrombolysis on the grounds of the deficits being "nondisabling".

ARTICLE 2

EXTEND: Thrombolysis Guided by Perfusion Imaging up to 9 Hours after Onset of Stroke

Ma H, Campbell BCV, Parsons MV, Churilov L, Levi CR, Hsu C, et al. EXTEND Investigators Collaborators. Thrombolysis guided by perfusion imaging up to 9 hours after onset of stroke.
N Engl J Med. 2019;380(19):1795-803.

Abstract

Randomized, placebo-controlled, multicenter trial involving patients with ischemic stroke who had hypoperfused but salvageable regions of brain detected on automated perfusion imaging. The patients were randomly assigned to receive intravenous alteplase or placebo between 4.5 and 9.0 hours after the onset of stroke or on awakening with stroke (if within 9 hours from the point of sleep). The primary outcome was a score of 0 or 1 on the modified Rankin scale.

225 patients were enrolled, 113 to the alteplase and 112 to the placebo group. The primary outcome occurred in 40 patients (35.4%) in the alteplase group and in 33 patients (29.5%) in the placebo group [adjusted risk ratio 1.44; 95% confidence interval (CI) 1.01–2.06; $p = 0.04$]. Symptomatic intracerebral hemorrhage occurred in seven patients (6.2%) in the alteplase group and in one patient (0.9%) in the placebo group (adjusted risk ratio 7.22; 95% CI 0.97–53.5; $p = 0.05$).

The use of alteplase between 4.5 and 9.0 hours after stroke onset resulted in a higher percentage of patients with minor or no neurologic deficits with more cases of symptomatic cerebral hemorrhage in the same group.

COMMENT

Thanks to this study, the era of time-based treatment of acute ischemic stroke with intravenous alteplase may finally be over. The use of alteplase is still limited to patients presenting within 4.5 hours of symptom onset. Although it was terminated after only two-thirds of the intended enrolment, the likelihood of a good outcome (modified Rankin Scale score of 0 or 1 at 90 days) was 44% higher in the alteplase group [adjusted risk ratio 1.44; 95% confidence interval (CI) 1.01–2.06; $p = 0.04$]. This is attributable to an image-guided approach to selecting patients (similar to mechanical thrombectomy trials performed many hours after stroke symptom onset). Patients were eligible if they had a mismatch between the core of infarction and potentially salvageable brain tissue in the penumbra. This trial presents a significant successful step in using an image-guided approach to extend the seemingly immutable time window for thrombolysis in acute ischemic stroke patients.

ARTICLE 3

Effect of Intravenous Tenecteplase Dose on Cerebral Reperfusion before Thrombectomy in Patients with Large Vessel Occlusion Ischemic Stroke: The EXTEND-IA TNK Part 2 Randomized Clinical Trial

Campbell BCV, Mitchell PJ, Churilov L, Yassi N, Kleinig TJ, Dowling RJ, et al. EXTEND-IA TNK Part 2 investigators. Effect of intravenous tenecteplase dose on cerebral reperfusion before thrombectomy in patients with large vessel occlusion ischemic stroke: The EXTEND-IA TNK Part 2 Randomized Clinical Trial.
JAMA. 2020;323(13):1257-65.

Abstract

Randomized clinical trial conducted in Australia and New Zealand with the objective of determining whether 0.40 mg/kg of tenecteplase safely improves reperfusion before endovascular thrombectomy over 0.25 mg/kg of tenecteplase in patients with large vessel occlusion (internal carotid, basilar or middle cerebral artery) ischemic stroke within 4.5 hours of symptom onset using standard intravenous thrombolysis eligibility criteria. The primary outcome was reperfusion of >50% of the involved ischemic territory prior to thrombectomy.

Adult patients ($n = 300$) with ischemic were enrolled with 150 patients in each arm with tenecteplase given as a bolus before endovascular thrombectomy. 29 patients (19.3%) in each arm achieved the primary outcome concluding that a dose of 0.40 mg/kg, compared with 0.25 mg/kg, of tenecteplase did not significantly improve cerebral reperfusion prior to endovascular thrombectomy.

COMMENT

The earlier study by the same group had established the superiority of bolus dose of tenecteplase at a dosage of 0.25 mg/kg body weight given intravenously in patients with acute ischemic stroke and large vessel occlusions. The percentage of patients requiring additional endovascular therapy (EVT) were lesser compared to the group who received standard alteplase.

The current study investigated the efficacy of 0.4 mg/kg dose of tenecteplase versus 0.25 mg/kg in similar trial design and found that a higher dose of tenecteplase did not result in an improved primary or secondary outcomes. Although not clinically significant, there was also a three-fold increase in rates of intracranial hemorrhage with the higher dose.

ENDOVASCULAR TREATMENT

ARTICLE 1

BASILAR: Assessment of Endovascular Treatment for Acute Basilar Artery Occlusion via Nation-wide Prospective Registry

Zi W, Qiu Z, Wu D, Li F, Liu H, Liu W, et al. Writing Group for the BASILAR Group. Assessment of endovascular treatment for acute basilar artery occlusion via a nationwide prospective registry.
JAMA Neurol. 2020;77(5):561-73.

Abstract

A nonrandomized cohort study was conducted across 47 centers in China to evaluate the association between endovascular treatment (EVT) and clinical outcome in patients with basilar artery occlusion. 829 patients were divided into EVT with standard medical treatment ($n = 647$) versus standard medical treatment alone ($n = 182$) with the primary endpoint being improvement in modified Rankin Scale (mRS) scores at 90 days.

The study found that mRS at 90 days was significantly better with EVT with standard medical treatment when done within 24 hours [adjusted odds ratio (OR) –3.08; $p < 0.001$].

COMMENT

The study assessed outcome of endovascular treatment (EVT) for Acute Basilar Artery Occlusion Study (BASILAR). Patients with radiologically proven basilar artery occlusion (BAO) within 24 hours were divided into those receiving standard medical treatment plus EVT and those only standard medical treatment. The results revealed significant improvement in functional outcomes with the EVT arm with BAO, indicating that the time window for intervention for posterior circulation extends up to 24 hours.

ARTICLE 2

Aspiration Thrombectomy versus Stent Retriever Thrombectomy as First-line Approach for Large Vessel Occlusion (COMAPSS): A Multicenter, Randomized, Open-label, Blinded Outcome, Non-inferiority Trial

Turk AS 3rd, Siddiqui A, Fifi JT, De Leacy RA, Fiorella DJ, Gu E, et al. Aspiration thrombectomy versus stent retriever thrombectomy as first-line approach for large vessel occlusion (COMPASS): A multicentre, randomised, open label, blinded outcome, non-inferiority trial.
Lancet. 2019;393(10175):998-1008.

Abstract

Randomized, multicenter, open-label, blinded outcome, noninferiority trial investigating whether patients with acute ischemic stroke and large vessel occlusion presenting within 6 hours of symptom onset and ASPECTS (Alberta Stroke Program Early CT Score) more than 6, treated with direct aspiration first pass have noninferior functional outcomes to those treated with a stent retriever as first line.

270 patients were enrolled; 134 in direct aspiration and 136 in the stent retriever group. The primary outcome, described as favorable functional outcome [modified Rankin Scale (mRS) of 0–2], was achieved in 69 patients (52%) in the aspiration arm and 67 patients (50%) in the stent retriever arm showing that the former was noninferior to the latter.

COMMENT

The null hypothesis for this study was that patients who are treated with aspiration as the first pass achieve inferior outcomes compared with those treated with a stent retriever first-line approach. It provided evidence that contact aspiration may be used as a noninferior alternative to thrombectomy with a stent retriever as first-line therapy in ischemic strokes with large vessel occlusions in the anterior circulation within 6 hours of symptom onset, provided that rescue therapy with stent retriever is performed where necessary.

ARTICLE 3

MR CLEAN-NO IV: A Randomized Trial of Intravenous Alteplase before Endovascular Treatment for Stroke

LeCouffe NE, Kappelhof M, Treurniet KM, Rinkel LA, Bruggeman AE, Berkhemer OA, et al. MR CLEAN–NO IV Investigators. A randomized trial of intravenous alteplase before endovascular treatment for stroke. *N Engl J Med. 2021;385(20):1833-44.*

Abstract

Randomized, open-label, multicenter trial in acute stroke patients within 4.5 hours of symptom onset [eligible both for thrombolysis and endovascular treatment (EVT)], with intracranial anterior circulation large vessel occlusion [internal carotid artery (ICA), M1-middle cerebral artery (MCA) or proximal M2-MCA], presenting directly to a hospital capable of providing EVT with National Institutes of Health Stroke Scale (NIHSS) score ≥2.

539 patients were enrolled (273 in EVT alone and 266 in alteplase plus EVT group) in the trial. The primary outcome was the modified Rankin Scale (mRS) score at the 3 months, which was 3 (2–5) in the EVT alone group and 2 (2–5) in the latter [odds ratio (OR) –0.84; 95% confidence interval (CI) 0.62–1.15; $p = 0.28$]. EVT alone neither showed superiority nor noninferiority. Mortality occurred in 20.5% patients when treated with EVT alone compared to 15.8% with EVT plus intravenous (IV) tissue plasminogen activator (TPA) [adjusted odds ratio (aOR) 1.39; 95% CI 0.84–2.30] symptomatic intracerebral hemorrhage occurred in 5.9% and 5.3% patients, respectively (aOR 1.30; 95% CI 0.60–2.81).

COMMENT

This trial evaluated the value of administration of intravenous alteplase prior to endovascular thrombectomy. The predominant hypothesis was that omitting thrombolysis with alteplase prior to endovascular treatment (EVT) would improve outcomes by decreasing the risk of intracerebral hemorrhage. However, this was not substantiated. Also, this trial only used alteplase as the thrombolytic agent. The results might have favored thrombolysis prior to EVT had tenecteplase been used considering higher recanalization rates with large vessel occlusion compared to alteplase (as documented by the EXTEND1A-TNK trial) precluding the need for EVT.

ARTICLE 4

Safety and Efficacy of Aspirin, Unfractionated Heparin, Both, or Neither during Endovascular Stroke Treatment (MR CLEAN-MED): An Open-label, Multicentre, Randomized Controlled Trial

van der Steen W, van de Graaf RA, Chalos V, Lingsma HF, van Doormaal PJ, Coutinho JM, et al. MR CLEAN-MED investigators. Safety and efficacy of aspirin, unfractionated heparin, both, or neither during endovascular stroke treatment (MR CLEAN-MED): An open-label, multicentre, randomised controlled trial. *Lancet. 2022;399(10329):1059-69.*

Abstract

Randomized, open-label, multicenter trial in acute stroke patients with endovascular treatment (EVT) done within 6 hours of symptom onset with intracranial anterior circulation large vessel occlusion [internal carotid artery (ICA), M1-middle cerebral artery (MCA) or proximal M2-MCA], with National Institutes of Health Stroke Scale (NIHSS) score ≥2, without intracerebral hemorrhage.

628 patients were enrolled and randomized to receive periprocedural intravenous 300 mg bolus of aspirin or no aspirin, unfractionated heparin (UFH) (either low dose: 5,000 IU bolus followed by 500 IU/h for 6 hours or moderate dose: 5,000 IU bolus followed by 1,250 IU/h for 6 hours) or no heparin. The trial was stopped prematurely due to safety concerns. The risk of symptomatic intracerebral hemorrhage (sICH) was higher in patients receiving than not receiving aspirin [14% vs. 7%; adjusted odds ratio (aOR) 1.95; 95% confidence interval (CI) 1.13–3.35, respectively] and patients receiving than not receiving UFH (13% vs. 7%; aOR 1.98; 95% CI 1.14–3.46). Both aspirin and UFH use led to a nonsignificant trend toward poorer modified Rankin Scale (mRS) scores (OR 0.91; 95% CI 0.69–1.21 and OR 0.81; 95% CI 0.61–1.08, respectively).

COMMENT

Anti-thrombotic agents are commonly used during endovascular procedures as they can theoretically decrease periprocedural thrombotic complications and prevent distal clot migration. However, this trial not only showed that this practice did not yield better functional results but also led to increased risk of symptomatic intracerebral hemorrhage. Therefore, this practice should be abolished till data proving its efficacy comes about.

ARTICLE 5

Safety and Efficacy of Intensive Blood Pressure Lowering after Successful Endovascular Therapy in Acute Ischaemic Stroke (BP-TARGET): A Multicentre, Open-label, Randomized Controlled Trial

Mazighi M, Richard S, Lapergue B, Sibon I, Gory B, Berge J, et al. BP-TARGET investigators. Safety and efficacy of intensive blood pressure lowering after successful endovascular therapy in acute ischaemic stroke (BP-TARGET): A multicentre, open-label, randomised controlled trial.
Lancet Neurol. 2021;20(4):265-74.

Abstract

Randomized, open-label, multicenter trial in acute stroke patients with intracranial anterior large vessel occlusion [internal carotid artery (ICA) or proximal M1-middle cerebral artery (MCA)], and successful endovascular treatment (EVT) [modified treatment in cerebral infarction (mTICI) 2b or 3] without hemorrhagic complications and systolic blood pressure (SBP) > 130 mm Hg post-EVT.

318 patients were enrolled and randomized to either intensive SBP target group (100–129 mm Hg) [intensive SBP target group (ISTG) 158 patients] or standard care SBP target group (130–185 mm Hg) [standard care SBP target group (SSTG) 160 patients]. These SBPs had to be attained within 1 hour postrandomization and maintained for at least 24 hours. The primary outcome was the rate of intraparenchymal hemorrhage radiologically and was observed in 42% of ISTG compared to 42% of SSTG [adjusted odds ratio (aOR) 0.96; 95% confidence interval (CI) 0.60–1.51; $p = 0.84$]. Hypotension and mortality occurred in 8% and 7% in the ISTG and 3% and 4% in the SSTG group, respectively.

COMMENT

Intensive systolic blood pressure (SBP) lowering postsuccessful endovascular treatment (EVT) did not result in reduced occurrence of intracerebral hemorrhages and was associated with a nonsignificant increase in hypotension episodes and mortality. This might be due to blood pressure variability poststroke and highlights the need to not treat SBP intensively, even after successful reperfusion post-EVT.

SECONDARY PREVENTION

ARTICLE 1

The Acute Stroke or Transient Ischemic Attack Treated with Ticagrelor and Aspirin for Prevention of Stroke and Death (THALES) Trial: Rationale and Design

Johnston SC, Amarenco P, Denison H, Evans SR, Himmelmann A, James S, et al. THALES Investigators. The acute stroke or transient ischemic attack treated with ticagrelor and aspirin for prevention of stroke and death (THALES) trial: Rationale and design.
Int J Stroke. 2019;14(7):745-51.

Abstract

Randomized, double-blinded, placebo-controlled, event driven study to evaluate whether ticagrelor combined with aspirin is superior to aspirin alone in preventing stroke or death in patients with nondisabling, noncardioembolic ischemic stroke or transient ischemic attack, with patients randomized within 24 hours of symptom onset. It is expected to enroll 13,000 patients in 45 centers worldwide with the primary efficacy outcome is the time to composite endpoint of stroke or death through 30-day follow-up.

COMMENT

The rationale and design was published in October, 2018. The trial investigated the combination of ticagrelor with aspirin in preventing recurrence of stroke or death in patients presenting with minor, noncardio-embolic ischemic stroke, or high risk (ABCD^2 of >5), transient ischemic attack. THALES randomized 13,000 patients at >450 sites world-wide with predominantly Asian population. Results are expected to be released soon.

ARTICLE 2

The ESUS Trials: NAVIGATE ESUS

Hart RG, Sharma M, Mundl H, Kasner SE, Bangdiwala SI, Berkowitz SD, et al. NAVIGATE ESUS Investigators. Rivaroxaban for stroke prevention after embolic stroke of undetermined source.
N Engl J Med. 2018;378(23):2191-201.

Abstract

Randomized controlled trial to evaluate the efficacy and safety of rivaroxaban (15 mg/day) with aspirin (100 mg/day) for prevention of stroke recurrence in patients with recent presumed embolic stroke without an identified cardioembolic source.

7,213 patients were enrolled: 3,609 in the rivaroxaban and 3,604 in the aspirin group. The primary efficacy outcome, evaluated as time-to-event analysis, was the first occurrence of ischemic or hemorrhagic stroke or systemic embolism. This occurred in 172 patients (5.2%) in the rivaroxaban group and 160 patients in the aspirin group (4.8%) proving the former not to be superior.

ARTICLE 3
RESPECT ESUS

Diener HC, Sacco RL, Easton JD, Granger CB, Bernstein RA, Uchiyama S, et al. RE-SPECT ESUS Steering Committee and Investigators. Dabigatran for prevention of stroke after embolic stroke of undetermined source.
N Engl J Med. 2019;380(20):1906-17.

Abstract

Randomized, multicenter, double-blinded trial comparing dabigatran (110 mg/150 mg BD) to aspirin (100 mg/day) is preventing stroke recurrence amongst patients who had an embolic stroke of undetermined source.

5,390 patients were enrolled: 2,695 in each arm and the primary outcome was recurrent stroke. Ischemic strokes occurred in 177 patients (6.6%) on dabigatran and 207 patients (7.7%) on aspirin, proving it to be nonsuperior.

COMMENT

In quick succession, usefulness of novel anticoagulants versus aspirin were published (RESPECT-ESUS, NAVIGATE-ESUS) in prevention of recurrence of stroke and death. Both trials did not document superiority of either rivaroxaban (15 mg/day) or dabigatran (110 mg BID) over aspirin. The saga of the true validity of the new clinical construct as ESUS and the optimal stroke prophylactic regimen for this entity continues.

ARTICLE 4

PRASTRO-II: Safety and Efficacy of Prasugrel in Elderly/Low Body Weight Japanese Patients with Ischemic Stroke: Randomized PRASTRO-II

Kitagawa K, Toyoda K, Kitazono T, Nishikawa M, Nanto S, Ikeda Y, et al. Safety and Efficacy of Prasugrel in Elderly/Low Body Weight Japanese Patients with Ischemic Stroke: Randomized PRASTRO-II.
Cerebrovasc Dis. 2020;49(2):152-9.

Abstract

Randomized, double-blinded, phase III study enrolling Japanese patients with noncardioembolic strokes with age ≥75 years and/or weight <50 kg. They were treated with either prasugrel 3.75 mg, prasugrel 2.5 mg or clopidogrel 50 mg and followed up for 48 weeks. The primary endpoint was a composite of occurrence of ischemic stroke, myocardial infarction, or death from vascular cause.

654 patients were enrolled: 216 in prasugrel 3.75 mg, 215 in prasugrel 2.5 mg, and 223 in the clopidogrel arm. No patients (0%) in the prasugrel 3.75 mg, 7 (3.3%) in the prasugrel 2.5 mg, and 8 (3.6%) in the clopidogrel arm met the primary endpoint. This study showed that prasugrel was safe and had lesser incidence of vascular endpoints when compared to clopidogrel in elderly/low body weight Japanese patients.

COMMENT

This study from Japan aimed to investigate the safety and efficacy of long-term prasugrel monotherapy for stroke prevention compared with clopidogrel in elderly and/or low body weight Japanese patients with noncardioembolic ischemic stroke and showed that it was both as safe and effective as clopidogrel. Though, trials in our population may be needed before it can become clinical practice in our country.

ARTICLE 5

Relationship of Spontaneous Microembolic Signals to Risk Stratifcation, Recurrence, Severity, and Mortality of Ischemic Stroke: A Prospective Study

Bazan R, Luvizutto GJ, Braga GP, Bazan SGZ, Hueb JC, de Freitas CCM, et al. Relationship of spontaneous microembolic signals to risk stratification, recurrence, severity, and mortality of ischemic stroke: A prospective study. *Ultrasound J. 2020;12(1):6.*

Abstract

Prospective cohort study to assess the prevalence of spontaneous microembolic signals (MES) in acute stroke and their relationship with risk stratification, stroke recurrence, morbidity, and mortality. MES presence was evaluated by transcranial Doppler (TCD) in patients with ischemic stroke within 48 hours and outcomes (risk stratification, morbidity, mortality, and recurrence of a stroke) were followed up for 6 months.

111 patients were studied and the MES frequency was found to be 7%. There was a significant relationship between MES and symptomatic carotid disease [odds ratio (OR) = 22.7; 95% confidence interval (CI) 4.1–125.7; $p = 0.009$]. It was observed that the stroke recurrence adjusted for prior stroke was higher and earlier among patients with MES detection.

COMMENT

Risk stratification with microembolic signals on transcranial Doppler has been demonstrated to be crucial for decision-making on intervention for even nonsignificant stenotic lesions in carotid artery. The presence of microembolic signals suggested an unstable plaque capable of early recurrence of stroke and therefore warranted more aggressive management.

ARTICLE 6

Early Prolonged Ambulatory Cardiac Monitoring in Stroke (EPACS): An Open-label Randomized Controlled Trial

Kaura A, Sztriha L, Chan FK, Aeron-Thomas J, Gall N, Piechowski-Jozwiak B, et al. Early prolonged ambulatory cardiac monitoring in stroke (EPACS): An open-label randomised controlled trial. *Eur J Med Res. 2019;24(1):25.*

Abstract

An open-label, randomized controlled trial comparing short duration Holter to a 14-day electrocardiogram (ECG) monitoring patch for the detection of paroxysmal atrial fibrillation (PAF).

90 patients were enrolled: 47 in the Holter group and 43 in the ECG patch group with the primary outcome being the detection of one or more episodes of ECG-documented PAF lasting at least 30 seconds within 90 days.

The rate of detection was 16.3% ($n = 7$) in the patch-based monitoring group compared to 2.1% ($n = 1$) in the short-duration Holter monitoring group, with an odds ratio of 8.9 [95% confidence interval (CI) 1.1–76.0; $p = 0.026$]. This translates into 10.8 more strokes avoided per year compared to current practice with Holter monitoring with an associated yearly saving in direct medical costs of £113,630, increasing to £162,491 over 5 years. The study concluded that early, prolonged, patch-based monitoring after a stroke/transient ischemic attack (TIA) is superior to short-duration Holter monitoring in the detection of PAF and likely cost-effective for preventing recurrent strokes.

COMMENT

There is level I evidence to use oral anticoagulation (OAC) for stroke prevention in patients with even short epochs (at least 30 seconds) of paroxysmal atrial fibrillation (AF). For optimal institution of OAC, demonstration of paroxysmal AF is imperative. Often, the single most important limiting factor is lack of adequate sensitivity of conventional 24 hours Holter monitoring for detection of AF. The current study demonstrates a cost-effective method of prolonged Holter monitoring to be able to diagnose significantly higher number of epochs of AF compared to conventional Holter monitoring.

NEUROPROTECTION

ARTICLE 1

ESCAPE-NA1: Efficacy and Safety of Nerinitide for the Treatment of Acute Ischemic Stroke

Hill MD, Goyal M, Menon BK, Nogueira RG, McTaggart RA, Demchuk AM, et al. ESCAPE-NA1 Investigators. Efficacy and safety of nerinetide for the treatment of acute ischaemic stroke (ESCAPE-NA1): A multicentre, double-blind, randomised controlled trial.
Lancet. 2020;395(10227):878-87.

Abstract

Randomized, double-blinded, multicentric, placebo-controlled trial done in 48 centers in eight countries. The trial enrolled acute ischemic stroke cases with ASPECTS (Alberta Stroke Program Early CT Score) more than four due to large vessel occlusion within 12 hours of symptom onset. Nerinitide was used in a dose of 2.6 mg/kg body weight (maximum 270 mg) and the primary endpoint was good functional outcome at 90 days defined by a modified Rankin Scale (mRS) of 0–2.

1,105 patients were enrolled; 549 in the nerinitide and 556 in the placebo arm. 61.4% (334) in the nerinitide and 59.2% (329) in the placebo arm achieved the primary outcome demonstrating that nerinitide did not improve the proportion of patients having a good functional outcome.

COMMENT

Yet another neuroprotective trial in patients undergoing endovascular thrombectomy using intravenous (IV) nerinetide, an eicosapeptide that interferes with postsynaptic density protein 95 within 12 hours treatment window was published in August, 2019. Compared to placebo, IV nerinetide did not offer additional benefit [adjusted risk ratio 1.04; 95% confidence interval (CI) 0.96–1.14; $p = 0.35$].

ARTICLE 2

Randomized, Controlled, Dose Escalation Trial of a Protease-activated Receptor-1 Agonist in Acute Ischemic Stroke: Final Results of the RHAPSODY Trial

Lyden P, Pryor KE, Coffey CS, Cudkowicz M, Conwit R, Jadhav A, et al. NeuroNEXT Clinical Trials Network NN104 Investigators. Final results of the RHAPSODY trial: A multi-center, phase 2 trial using a continual reassessment method to determine the safety and tolerability of 3K3A-APC, a recombinant variant of human activated protein C, in combination with tissue plasminogen activator, mechanical thrombectomy or both in moderate to severe acute ischemic stroke. *Ann Neurol. 2019;85(1):125-36.*

Abstract

Randomized, controlled, blinded trial to determine the maximally tolerated dose (MTD) of 3K3A-activated protein C (APC) in ischemic stroke patients using tiers of 120, 240, 360, and 540 µg/kg and their vasculoprotective effect following revascularization by either intravenous tissue plasminogen activator (tPA) or intra-arterial mechanical thrombectomy, or both. Vasculoprotection was assessed as microbleed and intracranial hemorrhage (ICH) rates.

110 patients were enrolled and there was no difference in prespecified ICH rates. Exploratory analyses revealed that 3K3A-APC reduced ICH rates from 86.5% in placebo arm to 67.4% in the combined treatment arm ($p = 0.046$), and total hemorrhage volume from an average of 2.1 ± 5.8 mL in placebo to 0.8 ± 2.1 mL in the combined treatment arms ($p = 0.066$). This trial showed a trend toward lower hemorrhage rate in an exploratory analysis.

COMMENT

RHAPSODY was a dose finding study using protease-activated receptor 1 agonist by activated protein C (3k3A-APC) evaluating their vasculoprotection, as assessed by the occurrence of microbleed and intracranial hemorrhage rates. Though not powered for any definitive conclusion, the study showed a trend toward lower hemorrhagic rate.

ARTICLE 3

A Multicentre, Randomized, Sham-controlled Trial on Remote Ischemic Conditioning in Patients with Acute Stroke (RESIST): Rationale and Study Design

Blauenfeldt RA, Hjort N, Gude MF, Behrndtz AB, Fisher M, Valentin JB, et al. A multicentre, randomised, sham-controlled trial on remote ischemic conditioning in patients with acute stroke (RESIST) - rationale and study design. *Eur Stroke J. 2020;5(1):94-101.*

Abstract

Randomized, prospective, patient-assessor blinded, multicenter, sham-controlled study enrolling adult patients with a putative stroke identified prehospital with stroke duration <4 hours, who are independent in activities of daily living.

Patients in the treatment arm will receive five cycles of 5 minutes each of cuff inflation to 200–285 mm Hg followed by deflation for 5 minutes on the presumption that this remote ischemic preconditioning might improve functional outcome in stroke patients (both ischemic and hemorrhagic). The sample size is 1,000 patients and the outcome will be assessed on the modified Rankin Scale (mRS).

COMMENT

This trial is designed to evaluate whether a prehospital intervention in acute stroke patients (ischemic and hemorrhagic) as a "neuroprotectant" would increase the odds of bettering stroke outcomes. This trial has a study sample of 1,500 patients who are <4 hours of stroke onset. The trial is currently ongoing.

STROKE RECOVERY

ARTICLE 1

The SHINE Randomized Clinical Trial: Intensive versus Standard Treatment of Hyperglycemia and Functional Outcome in Patients with Acute Ischemic Stroke

Johnston KC, Bruno A, Pauls Q, Hall CE, Barrett KM, Barsan W, et al. Intensive vs standard treatment of hyperglycemia and functional outcome in patients with acute ischemic stroke. The SHINE Randomized Clinical Trial. *JAMA. 2019;322(4):326-35.*

Abstract

Randomized clinical trial enrolling acute stroke patients within 12 hours of symptom onset and hyperglycemia (blood sugar levels ≥ 110 mg/dL if diabetic and ≥150 mg/dL if not), in 63 USA centers enrolling 1,151 patients between 2012 and 2018. Intensive control group ($n = 581$) received continuous intravenous insulin infusion with target blood sugar levels between 80 and 130 mg/dL and standard treatment group ($n = 570$) received subcutaneous insulin according to sliding scale to maintain blood sugar levels between 80 and 179 mg/dL for up to 72 hours poststroke.

Primary outcome was the number of patients with a favorable clinical outcome at 90 days [modified Rankin Scale (mRS) 0–2]. This was achieved by 20.5% ($n = 119$) in the intensive control group and 21.6% ($n = 123$) in the standard treatment group. Occurrence of hypoglycemia was 11.2% ($n = 65$) and 3.2% ($n = 18$) in the intensive and standard treatment groups, respectively.

Intensive glucose control found no evidence of favorable clinical outcome.

COMMENT

Hyperglycemia is an established independent adverse stroke outcome modifier both in terms of increased infarct growth and enhanced propensity to hemorrhagic transformation of the infarct. Approximately 40% of patients with acute ischemic stroke have hyperglycemia and this study was conducted to assess whether aggressive treatment of the same improved outcomes following an ischemic stroke. This trial found no benefit of the same.

ARTICLE 2

PROSCIS-B: Serum Anti-N-methyl-D-aspartate-receptor Antibodies and Long-term Clinical Outcome after Stroke

Sperber PS, Siegerink B, Huo S, Rohmann JL, Piper SK, Prüss H, et al. Serum anti-NMDA (N-methyl-D-aspartate)-receptor antibodies and long-term clinical outcome after stroke (PROSCIS-B).
Stroke. 2019;50(11):3213-9.

Abstract

Data from the prospective cohort with incident stroke-Berlin was used and anti-N-methyl-D-aspartate receptor 1 (NMDAR1) antibodies were measured within 1 week of stroke. The outcomes assessed with modified Rankin Scale (mRS) at 1 year and combined endpoint of stroke, myocardial infarction, and all-cause mortality within 3 years.

583 patients were enrolled and 13% ($n = 76$) were found to be antibody positive.

Antibody status was not found to be associated with functional outcome [confidence interval (CI) 0.77–2.09]. Seropositivity, however, was associated with increased incidence of secondary vascular event or death [hazard ratio (HR) 1.83; CI 1.10–3.05] with worse outcomes in patients with high titres.

COMMENT

Anti-N-methyl-D-aspartate (NMDA) receptor drugs were studied with great enthusiasm two decades ago on the premise that NMDA excitotoxicity contributed to poor poststroke recovery. However, none of those trials was positive. In confirmation with above hypothesis the presence of anti-NMDA receptor GluN1 (NR1) antibodies was presumed to be neuroprotective and facilitate functional recovery poststroke. It was concluded that NMDA receptor-1 (NMDAR-1) antibody seropositivity was not associated with improved functional outcome at 1 year poststroke and a high titre (>1:320) antibody level was associated with poor functional outcome and with increased cardiovascular risk factors.

ARTICLE 3

RESTORE BRAIN Study

Chabriat H, Bassetti CL, Marx U, Picarel-Blanchot F, Sors A, Gruget C, et al. Randomized efficacy and safety trial with oral S 44819 after recent ischemic cerebral event (RESTORE BRAIN study): A placebo-controlled phase II study. *Trials. 2020;21(1):136.*

Abstract

Randomized, double-blinded, parallel group, placebo-controlled, phase II multicenter study which enrolled ischemic stroke patients with onset 3–8 days prior, with a National Institutes of Health Stroke Scale (NIHSS) between 7 and 20 and aged between 18 and 85 years.

The sample size is 580 and the primary objective is to prove the efficacy by means of functional recovery measured on modified Rankin Scale (mRS) at 90 days, of either of the doses of S44819 (150 mg or 300 mg BD) over placebo along with standard medical care.

COMMENT

In an ongoing effort to enhance neural plasticity and optimize poststroke recovery, a unique approach was undertaken in the above study. Based on the premise that sustained hypoexcitability seen in the peri-infarct cortex on account of increased activity of GABAergic neurons can be reversed by suing a selective antagonist of $GABA_A$ receptor-mediated activity. S44819 is a potent and selective antagonist of $GABA_A$-$\alpha 5$ receptor. The trial has completed recruitment and awaiting results.

ARTICLE 4

Effects of Fluoxetine on Outcomes at 12 Months after Acute Stroke: Results from EFFECTS, a Randomized Controlled Trial

Lundström E, Isaksson E, Norin NG, Näsman P, Wester P, Mårtensson B, et al. Effects of fluoxetine on outcomes at 12 months after acute stroke: Results from EFFECTS, a randomized controlled trial. *Stroke. 2021;52(10):3082-7.*

Abstract

Randomized, placebo-controlled, double-blinded, investigator-led trial which enrolled patients with acute stroke (ischemic or hemorrhagic) in the prior 2–15 days to receive either 20 mg fluoxetine or placebo for 6 months and were evaluated at 12 months postrandomization.

1,500 patients were recruited (750 in each arm) but the distribution of modified Rankin Scale (mRS) was found to be similar in both groups [adjusted odds ratio (aOR) 0.92; 95% confidence interval (CI) 0.76–1.10]. Patients on fluoxetine scored statistically worse on memory and communication when compared to placebo.

COMMENT

The FLAME trial and a subsequent Cochrane meta-analysis had concluded that selective serotonin reuptake inhibitors could reduce poststroke motor disability, generating much interest in this class of drugs. However, EFFECTS trial concluded that fluoxetine once daily for 6 months not only had no effect on the functional outcome of the patients at both 6 and 12 months but also was associated with worse performance on memory and communication scales.

MOBILE STROKE UNITS

ARTICLE 1

Prospective, Multicentre, Controlled Trial of Mobile Stroke Units

Grotta JC, Yamal JM, Parker SA, Rajan SS, Gonzales NR, Jones WJ, et al. Prospective, multicenter, controlled trial of mobile stroke units.
N Engl J Med. 2021;385(11):971-81.

Abstract

Observational, multicenter, prospective, alternating-week trial comparing outcomes of acute ischemic strokes within 4.5 hours of onset, managed by mobile stroke units (MSUs) versus emergency medical services (EMSs). Their primary objective was the score on utility-weighted modified Rankin Scale (mRS) (range 0–1; higher scores indicate a better outcome).

1,515 patients were enrolled, of which 1,047 were eligible for thrombolysis. The median time to thrombolysis was 72 minutes and 108 minutes in the MSU and EMS groups, respectively. 97.1% in the MSU group were thrombolysed compared to 79.5% in the EMS group. The mean utility-weighted mRS scores were 0.72 in the MSU compared to 0.66 in the EMS group [adjusted odds ratio (aOR) for score ≥0.91–2.43; 95% confidence interval (CI) 1.75–3.36; $p < 0.001$]. Nearly all secondary outcomes also favored MSUs, including mortality at 90 days.

COMMENT

Time is brain and therefore quicker thrombolysis is likely to lead to better clinical outcomes. This was proven further in context of mobile stroke units (MSUs) where in-ambulance computed tomography helped in earlier diagnosis of ischemic stroke/ruling out hemorrhagic stroke, and lesser symptom onset to needle time. MSUs might therefore become the future of improved and enhanced stroke care.

Section 4: Epilepsy

Section Editor: Viswanathan LG, Sinha S

ARTICLE 1

Epilepsy Outcome at Four Years in a Randomized Clinical Trial Comparing Oral Prednisolone and Intramuscular ACTH in West Syndrome

Wanigasinghe J, Arambepola C, Ranganathan SS, Jayasundara K, Weerasinghe A, Wickramarachchi P. Epilepsy outcome at four years in a randomized clinical trial comparing oral prednisolone and intramuscular ACTH in West syndrome.
Pediatr Neurol. 2021;119:22-6.

Abstract

Objective: This study aimed to examine the role of oral steroids versus adrenocorticotropic hormone (ACTH) in controlling spasms in West syndrome.

Methods: The Sri Lanka Infantile Spasm Study is a prospective clinical trial aimed to evaluate the response to intramuscular ACTH compared with oral prednisolone. A previous study reported response through the age of 12 months. However, this study provides 4-year follow-up data.

Results: Of a total sample of 97 children, 13 had died, 19 could not be traced or contacted, and only 65 were available for follow-up at 4 years. Of the 65 children, 37 (57%) children continued to have seizures and 28 children were free of seizures. In the children with ongoing epilepsy, 32% continued to experience spasms, either alone or in combination with other types of seizures. Types of epilepsies observed in these children were focal epilepsy (59.4%), mixed focal and generalized epilepsy (24%), generalized epilepsy only (10.8%), and unknown (5%). Most of the children who were still having epilepsy (66.7%) were controlled with seizure medication. No significant difference was observed in the rate of epilepsy or spasms or control by medication between those treated with ACTH or oral prednisolone. Control of spasms at day 14 did not affect the 4-year spasm or epilepsy outcome.

Conclusion: Most of the children diagnosed with West syndrome continued to have seizures at the age of 4 years, though most were controlled with antiseizure medication. In addition, the long-term risk of developing epilepsy or its control was the same regardless of whether ACTH or prednisolone was used as initial treatment.

COMMENT

The ideal first-line treatment for infantile spasms is still up for debate. Hormonal treatments were found to have considerably better control of spasms on day 14 than vigabatrin in the United Kingdom Infantile Spasms Study (UKISS).[1] The authors have discussed the 4-year follow-up data of the Sri Lanka Infantile Spasm Study which was a prospective clinical trial that pitted intramuscular adrenocorticotropic hormone (ACTH) against oral prednisolone. They had observed there was no difference between the two with respect to control of seizures over 4 years. The spasm control at day 14 did not influence the epilepsy outcomes over the long term. Though there is reasonable evidence for administering steroids to reduce the frequency of seizures, long-term effects of steroid therapy on epileptic encephalopathy is largely unknown.[2] The International Collaborative Infantile Spasm Study involving 377 children, evaluated the effect of vigabatrin plus steroid treatment as a combination therapy for infantile spasms. Due to the possibility of vigabatrin-induced visual problems, the initial benefit of combination therapy becomes unclear in the absence of a clear long-term benefit.[3] Intuitively, one may hypothesize that its role in this regard is minimal as steroids do not modify the underlying disease process. It is rather more plausible that the cause of the epileptic encephalopathy may influence the long-term prognosis both epilepsy and development wise rather than steroid therapy.

ARTICLE 2

Safety and Tolerability of Transdermal Cannabidiol Gel in Children with Developmental and Epileptic Encephalopathies: A Nonrandomized Controlled Trial

Scheffer IE, Hulihan J, Messenheimer J, Ali S, Keenan N, Griesser J, et al. Safety and tolerability of transdermal cannabidiol gel in children with developmental and epileptic encephalopathies: A nonrandomized controlled trial. *JAMA Netw Open. 2021;4(9):e2123930.*

Abstract

Objective: This study aimed to examine the tolerability and safety of cannabidiol (CBD) transdermal gel in children with developmental and epileptic encephalopathies (DEEs) and to evaluate its impact on seizure frequency, sleep, and quality of life.

Methods: This nonrandomized controlled trial was conducted at two centers in Australia and New Zealand from April, 2018 to July, 2019. Inclusion criteria involved children and adolescents aged 3–18 years with DEEs and were receiving a stable regimen of one to four antiseizure medications. Patients entered a flexible dosing maintenance period of 5.5 months, after 1-month baseline and titration periods, for a total 6.5 month treatment period. Data were analyzed throughout the 6.5 months of the treatment. CBD transdermal gel was applied twice daily at doses of 125–500 mg for 6.5 months.

Results: Safety and tolerability of the transdermal gel were assessed by reported adverse events (AEs) and skin examination. Median percent change from baseline to monthly (28-day) frequency of focal impaired awareness seizures (FIAS) and tonic-clonic seizures (TCS) over a period of 6.5 months was the primary outcome of this study.

Of 48 patients [mean age 10.5, standard deviation (SD) 3.8 years; number of boys: 26, 54%], 29 (60%) patients had at least one treatment-related AE over 6.5 months. Furthermore, 96% (44/46) of the treatment-related AEs were mild or moderate. Application-site dryness, application-site pain, and somnolence [each reported by 4 (8%) patients] were the reported treatment-related AEs in at least 5% of the patients. Diarrhea was reported as the only treatment-related gastrointestinal AE, which was reported in a single patient. Treatment with CBD gel was associated with reduction in the frequency of FIAS and TCS. Analysis of 33 patients with FIAS and TCS showed a median monthly reduction in seizures of 58% [interquartile range (IQR) −5.3% to 81.8%] at 5 months and 43.5% (IQR −23.8% to 57.5%) over the entire 6.5-month period. Improvements in social or interpersonal engagement and irritability (33/43, 77% participants); alertness, energy, and sleep (23/43, 53%); and cognition or concentration (20/43, 47%) were observed by the parents and caregivers.

Conclusion: In conclusion, CBD transdermal gel is a safe, well-tolerated treatment for children with DEEs, and is associated with reduction in frequency of FIAS and TCS and disease burden.

COMMENT

Cannabidiol (CBD) in epilepsy has generated a lot of research interest, especially in individuals with refractory and difficult to treat epilepsy.[4] This study aims to assess the safety and tolerability of transdermal CBD in children with developmental and epileptic encephalopathy (DEE). Children with DEE may have trouble taking medication orally and this can adversely impact drug adherence. Transdermal drug administration avoids first pass metabolism and effectively results in uniform drug levels in blood. This improves drug efficacy, reduces the dosage required, and avoids peak concentration-related side effects. Though this study was unblinded and did not have a control group, the authors observed transdermal application was safe. Not only did the seizure frequency reduce but caregivers also noticed some improvement in cognition and alertness. The absence of a control group makes it difficult to establish the effect size. Add-on CBD was proven to be effective in controlling seizures associated with Lennox–Gastaut syndrome (LGS) and Dravet syndrome (DS) in phase-3 clinical trials in recent times.[3,5,6] CBD as an adjuvant therapy to antiseizure medications (ASMs) and nonpharmacological treatments in children with drug-resistant epilepsy appears to be efficacious in reducing seizure duration and frequency, and may have a favorable impact on quality of life as reported by families.

ARTICLE 3

Cost-effectiveness of Adrenocorticotropic Hormone versus Oral Steroids for Infantile Spasms

Sánchez Fernández I, Amengual-Gual M, Gaínza-Lein M, Barcia Aguilar C, Bergin AM, Yuskaitis CJ, et al. Cost-effectiveness of adrenocorticotropic hormone versus oral steroids for infantile spasms.
Epilepsia. 2021;62(2):347-57.

Abstract

Objective: In this study, the efficacy and cost-effectiveness of adrenocorticotropic hormone (ACTH) and oral steroids as first-line treatment for resolution of infantile spasms was explored.

Methods: A decision analysis model was populated with effectiveness data from a systematic review and meta-analysis of preexisting literature and cost data from publicly available prices. Effectiveness was defined as the probability of resolution of clinical spasms 14 days after initiation of treatment.

Results: In total, 21 studies with a total of 968 patients were included in the study. There was no statistically significant difference in the effectiveness of ACTH as compared with oral steroids [0.70, 95% confidence interval (CI) 0.60–0.79 vs. 0.63, 95% CI 0.56–0.70; $p = 0.28$]. Considering only three available randomized trials consisting of 185 patients, the odds ratio of resolution of spasms at 14 days with ACTH compared with high-dose prednisolone (4–8 mg/kg/day) was 0.92 (95% CI 0.34–2.52; $p = 0.87$). When adjusted for potential publication bias, the estimates became more favorable to high-dose prednisolone. In United States currency, high-dose prednisolone was a more cost-effective treatment, at an incremental cost-effectiveness ratio (ICER) of US $333 per case of spasms resolved, followed by ACTH, with an ICER of US $1,432,200 per case of spasms resolved. The results obtained were robust to multiple sensitivity analyses and different assumptions. Prednisolone at 4–8 mg/kg/day was found more cost-effective than ACTH under a wide range of assumptions.

Conclusion: Existing evidence does not support the superiority of ACTH in terms of efficacy and, especially, cost-effectiveness for resolution of infantile spasms 2 weeks after initiation of treatment.

COMMENT

Adrenocorticotropic hormone (ACTH) has been the mainstay of treatment for infantile spasms/West syndrome (WS). Available evidence has demonstrated that ACTH as well as steroids reduces infantile spasm frequency and also results in resolution of hypsarrhythmia when treatment is successful.[7] The purported advantage that ACTH has over steroids is its ability to also interact with ACTH receptors and interaction with these receptors may also alter epileptogenesis. However, clear evidence to support these claims is lacking. The high cost and lack of availability of ACTH are its inherent disadvantages.

Varying doses of steroid therapy administered orally or parenterally (low to high) have also been shown to improve seizure outcomes in WS. In this study, oral steroids have had comparable efficacy as compared to ACTH. High-dose prednisolone had the lowest incremental cost-effectiveness ratio (ICER) at per case of spasms resolved. These findings held up to multiple sensitivity analyses and assumptions and prednisolone was definitely cost effect. Studies from India have supported the use of steroids in WS and other epileptic encephalopathies (EEs) and various steroid regimens have been used. Chatterjee et al. reported a large retrospective study documenting the successful use of intravenous pulse methylprednisolone (IVMP) in EE.[2] A randomized trial from Northern India comparing IVMP versus oral steroids observed the oral steroids arm did not observe any significant difference between these two modalities.[8] Due to the heterogeneity in the etiology and variable clinical course, prognostication using group statistics from such trials is difficult. It is possibly safe to say that steroids in some form are indicated in this patient age group; however, the dose, duration, and type of steroid to be used are still in contention and provide grounds for future trials.

ARTICLE 4

The SANTÉ Study at 10 Years of Follow-up: Effectiveness, Safety, and Sudden Unexpected Death in Epilepsy

Salanova V, Sperling MR, Gross RE, Irwin CP, Vollhaber JA, Giftakis JE, et al.; SANTÉ Study Group. The SANTÉ study at 10 years of follow-up: Effectiveness, safety, and sudden unexpected death in epilepsy. *Epilepsia. 2021;62(6):1306-17.*

Abstract

Objective: This study aimed to evaluate the safety and efficacy of deep brain stimulation (DBS) of anterior nucleus of the thalamus after 7 and 10 years, and to report the incidence of sudden unexpected death in epilepsy (SUDEP) and overall mortality in adults in the Stimulation of the Anterior Nucleus of the Thalamus for Epilepsy (SANTÉ) study.

Methods: After the blinded and unblinded phases of 3 months and 9 months, respectively, participants continued to be assessed during long-term follow-up (LTFU) and later a continued therapy access phase (CAP) to characterize adverse events and the incidence of SUDEP. Stimulus parameter and medication changes were allowed.

Results: A total of 110 implanted participants accumulated a total of 938 device-years of experience (69 subjects during the LTFU phase and 61 subjects in the CAP phase). Before study closure, 57 active participants continued therapy at 14 study centers, with follow-up of at least 10 (maximum 14) years. At 7 years, median percent reduction in seizure frequency from baseline was 75% ($p < 0.001$), with no outcome differences related to prior vagus nerve stimulation (VNS) or resective surgery. Focal to bilateral tonic-clonic, the most severe seizure type, was reported to be reduced by 71%. Adding new antiseizure medications did not affect the pattern of seizure reduction over time. Overall, there were no unanticipated serious adverse events in the study. The definite-plus-probable SUDEP rate, based on SANTÉ study experience (2 deaths in 938 years) and previous pilot studies (0 deaths in 76 years), indicated a rate of 2.0 deaths for 1,000 person-years. The overall mortality was 6.9 deaths per 1,000 person-years.

Conclusion: Overall, the findings report that the long-term efficacy and safety profiles of the DBS system for epilepsy are favorable and show stable outcomes. Improvement in frequency of the most severe seizure type may reduce risk of SUDEP. The rate of SUDEP with DBS (2.0) is comparable with other neuromodulation treatments (i.e., VNS and responsive neurostimulation) for drug-resistant focal epilepsy.

COMMENT

Refractory epilepsy that is not amenable for resective epilepsy surgeries can be truly challenging to treat. Neuromodulation has offered an alternative treatment option for such patients. The main contention for deep brain stimulation (DBS) as a successful antiepileptic therapy is the same as it is for movement disorders: within the target structure, possible cellular inhibition or excitement (neuromodulation).[9,10] As with any neuromodulatory technique [i.e., vagus nerve stimulation (VNS)/DBS, etc.], it is now known that with time, outcomes improve. This 10-year follow-up of the Stimulation of the Anterior Nucleus of the Thalamus for Epilepsy (SANTÉ) trial has reposed faith in that notion with 75% reduction in seizure frequency noted after 7 years of implantation. 7-year retention was 66%, with discontinuations due to lack of benefit (24%), death (6%), and implant site infection. (5%). The mean response rate was 74%, with 8% of patients were seizure free for 2 years or more. Last observation carried forward and other sensitivity methods were used to analyze the impact of missing data. Controlling for patient attrition, new autism spectrum disorders (ASDs), past VNS therapy, or epileptogenic zone location had no impact on the results. Notably, patients with uni- or bitemporal lobe seizures had higher effectiveness. Concerningly, mental disorders, which are prevalent comorbidities in drug-resistant epilepsy, may limit utilization of this therapy. Depression was noted in 37.3% of participants, 67% of whom had a history of depression and suicidality in 10%. Memory impairment was noted in 30% of subjects, 50% of whom already had memory issues, although no comprehensive neuropsychological test was conducted. These adverse events (AEs) were highly prevalent yet resulted in few discontinuations. The long-term follow-up (LTFU) data from the SANTÉ trial[11] is encouraging; however, there are many more questions—the optimal stimulation parameters, choosing the appropriate site, and if there is a difference in outcome between DBS versus other neuromodulatory techniques.

ARTICLE 5

Identifying Seizure Risk Factors: A Comparison of Sleep, Weather, and Temporal Features using a Bayesian Forecast

Payne DE, Dell KL, Karoly PJ, Kremen V, Gerla V, Kuhlmann L, et al. Identifying seizure risk factors: A comparison of sleep, weather, and temporal features using a Bayesian forecast.
Epilepsia. 2021;62(2):371-82.

Abstract

Objective: Most of the algorithms that forecast seizures rely on features that are specific to recordings of an electroencephalogram (EEG). Various environmental and physiological factors, such as weather and sleep, have been claimed to influence brain activity and occurrence of seizures but have not been fully investigated as prior information for forecasting seizures in a patient-specific analysis. This study aimed to quantify whether sleep, weather, and temporal factors (time of day, day of week, and lunar phase) can provide predictive prior probabilities that may be used to advance the forecasting of seizures.

Methods: This study performed a post-hoc analysis on data from eight patients with a total of 12.2 years of continuous intracranial electroencephalographic recordings (average = 1.5 years, range = 1.0–2.1 years) that were collected in a prospective trial. In addition, patients had sleep scoring and location-specific weather data. Histograms of future seizure likelihood were generated for each feature. A Bayesian approach was used to combine different factors into an overall forecast of seizure likelihood for measuring the predictive utility of individual factors. Area under the receiver operating curve was used to compare the performance of different feature combinations. However, performance evaluation was pseudoprospective.

Results: For the eight patients who were included in the study, seizures could be predicted above chance accuracy using sleep (five patients), weather (two patients), and temporal features (six patients). Forecasts using combined features performed significantly better than chance in six patients. For four of these patients, combined forecasts outperformed any individual feature.

Conclusion: To conclude, data with regard to environmental and physiological factors, including sleep, weather, and temporal features, provide significant predictive information on seizures forecasts. Although both the forecasts and the algorithms that use invasive intracranial electroencephalography did not perform, the results were significantly above chance. Furthermore, complementary signal features derived from an individual's previous seizure records may provide useful information to boost the detection of traditional seizures or augment the forecasting algorithms. Most importantly, many predictive features used in this study can be measured noninvasively.

COMMENT

Meteorological events have long been assumed to affect health, but reliable scientific proof is lacking. Accurate prediction models that can reliably forecast seizure recurrence is also inadequate. Most algorithms deal with data obtained from patient-centric data. There is a growing body of evidence that indicts environmental factors in the occurrence of seizures.[12-14] This study is a post-hoc analysis that attempts to describe a seizure model with intracranial electroencephalogram (EEG), sleep, and environmental data. The authors investigated sleep, temporal variables (clock and calendar time), and weather as seizure predictors. In order to examine seizure forecasting for different feature categories, continuous long-term EEG recordings were used. Though intracranial EEG data improved performance of the algorithms, forecasting was possible to a certain extent using noninvasive data and historical seizure records from seizure diaries. Of all the studied variables, time of the day was most significant in forecasting seizures and weather indicators did not perform well. The results from this study provide complementary features that can be used in conjunction with or in lieu of invasively measured features. Better understanding patient-specific risk variables may lead to clinical seizure forecasting for epilepsy patients in the future using deep-learning/artificial intelligence (AI)-enabled applications.

ARTICLE 6

The SANAD II Study of the Effectiveness and Cost-effectiveness of Valproate versus Levetiracetam for Newly Diagnosed Generalized and Unclassifiable Epilepsy: An Open-label, Non-inferiority, Multicenter, Phase 4, Randomized Controlled Trial

Marson A, Burnside G, Appleton R, Smith D, Leach JP, Sills G, et al.; SANAD II collaborators. The SANAD II study of the effectiveness and cost-effectiveness of valproate versus levetiracetam for newly diagnosed generalised and unclassifiable epilepsy: An open-label, non-inferiority, multicentre, phase 4, randomised controlled trial. *Lancet. 2021;397(10282):1375-86.*

Abstract

Objective: This study aimed to compare the long-term efficacy and cost-effectiveness of levetiracetam (LEV) compared with valproate in patients with a newly diagnosed generalized epilepsy or unclassified epilepsy. Valproate is a first-line treatment for patients with newly diagnosed idiopathic generalized or unclassified epilepsy. However, it is not advisable for women of childbearing potential because of its teratogenicity. LEV is increasingly prescribed for these patient populations despite paucity of evidence about its clinical efficacy or cost-effectiveness.

Methods: This study is an open-label, randomized controlled trial (RCT) to compare LEV with valproate as a first-line treatment for patients with generalized or unclassified epilepsy. Adult and pediatric neurology services (69 centers overall) across the United Kingdom recruited participants who were aged ≥5 years (with no upper age limit) and reported ≥2 unprovoked generalized or unclassifiable seizures. Participants were randomly allocated in a 1:1 ratio to receive either LEV or valproate, using a minimization program with a random element utilizing factor. The treatment allocation was known to the participants and investigators. Initial advisable maintenance doses were 500 mg twice a day for LEV and valproate for participants who were aged ≥12 years and 25 mg/kg for valproate and 40 mg/kg for LEV for participants aged 5–12 years. Both drugs were administered orally. SANAD-II was designed to compare the noninferiority of LEV with valproate for the primary outcome time to 12-month remission. The noninferiority limit was a hazard ratio (HR) of 1.314, which equates to an absolute difference of 10%. A HR >1 indicated that an event was more likely on valproate. All participants were included in the intention-to-treat (ITT) analysis. Per-protocol (PP) analyses excluded participants with major protocol deviations and those who were subsequently diagnosed as not having epilepsy. All participants who received one dose of any of the drug under study were included in the safety analyses.

Results: A total of 520 participants were recruited for the study between April 30, 2013, and August 2, 2016, and were followed up for a period of 2 years. Of these, 260 (50%) participants were randomly allocated to receive LEV and 260 (50%) participants were allocated to receive valproate. The ITT analysis included all participants and the PP analysis included 255 participants randomly allocated to valproate and 254 randomly allocated to LEV. Median age of participants was 13.9 years (range 5.0–94.4). Overall, 65% of the participants were male and 35% of the participants were female. Of 520 participants, 397 reported to have generalized epilepsy, whereas 123 had unclassified epilepsy. LEV did not meet the criteria for noninferiority in the ITT analysis of time to 12-month remission [HR 1.19 (95% CI 0.96–1.47); noninferiority margin 1.314]. The PP analysis showed that the 12-month remission was superior with valproate than with LEV. There were two deaths, one in each group, which were unrelated to trial treatments. Adverse reactions were reported by 96 (37%) participants randomly assigned to valproate and 107 (42%) participants randomly assigned to LEV. LEV was dominated by valproate in the cost-utility analysis, with a negative incremental net health benefit of −0.040 (95% central range −0.175 to 0.037) and a probability of 0.17 of being cost-effective at a threshold of £20 000 per quality-adjusted life year. Cost-effectiveness was based on differences between treatment groups in costs and quality-adjusted life year.

Conclusion: It was found that LEV was neither clinically effective nor cost-effective as compared with valproate. Furthermore, these results inform the discussions pertaining to benefit and harm of avoiding valproate in girls and women of childbearing potential.

COMMENT

With the advent of newer antiseizure medications, the burgeoning question has been are they better than the older drugs? Surprisingly, the results of SANAD-II did not lend much support to the use of levetiracetam (LEV) in generalized and unclassifiable epilepsy. In light of its favorable adverse effect profile, few drug interactions and reasonable efficacy in many seizure types; LEV has gained popularity since its introduction in 1999. Morso, it was proven to be safe for women in childbearing, pregnancy, and lactation.[15] On the other hand, LEV is associated with an increased risk of reversible neuropsychiatric adverse effects that may occur in up to 10–13% of adults. In this randomized controlled trial (RCT), LEV was shown to be inferior to valproic acid (VPA) in the time to achieve long-term (1 and 2 year) seizure remission (12-month seizure freedom: LEV: 24%; VPA: 33%). Surprisingly, there was no difference in treatment failure due to side effects. These findings lead the authors to recommend VPA as the first-line medication in generalized epilepsy. However, women in the childbearing age group will remain an exception to this recommendation. A prior randomized trial[16] and a meta-analysis[17] had reported that LEV was inferior to sodium channel blockers (carbamazepine and lamotrigine) in focal epilepsy and to VPA in generalized epilepsy. The "user-friendliness" of LEV has probably precluded the thorough consideration of its efficacy when starting first-line management for many including non-neurologists. If we are to go by the SANAD-II results, LEV may not be the obvious effective choice in the long term.

ARTICLE 7

Prevention of Epilepsy in Infants with Tuberous Sclerosis Complex in the EPISTOP Trial

Kotulska K, Kwiatkowski DJ, Curatolo P, Weschke B, Riney K, Jansen F, et al. EPISTOP Investigators. Prevention of epilepsy in infants with tuberous sclerosis complex in the EPISTOP trial.
Ann Neurol. 2021;89(2):304-14.

Abstract

Objective: Epilepsy develops in 70–90% of children with tuberous sclerosis complex (TSC) and is often resistant to treatment medications. However, recently, the concept of preventive antiepileptic treatment to alter the natural history of epilepsy has been proposed. EPISTOP was a clinical trial designed to compare preventive with conventional antiepileptic treatment in infants with TSC.

Methods: In this multicenter study, 94 infants with TSC without any history of seizures were followed with monthly video electroencephalography (EEG). The infants received vigabatrin either as a conventional antiepileptic treatment, started after the first electrographic or clinical seizure, or preventively when an epileptiform EEG activity was detected before seizures. At 6 sites, participants were randomly allocated to treatment in a 1:1 ratio in a randomized controlled trial (RCT). At 4 sites, treatment allocation was fixed; this was denoted an open-label trial (OLT). Participants were followed up to 2 years of age. Time to first clinical seizure was defined as the primary endpoint.

Results: Epileptiform EEG abnormalities were identified before seizures in 54 participants. Of these, 27 participants were included in the RCT and 27 participants were included in the OLT. The time to the first clinical seizure was significantly longer with preventive than conventional treatment [RCT 364 days (95% confidence interval (CI) 223–535] vs. 124 days (95% CI 33–149); OLT 426 days (95% CI 258–628) vs. 106 days (95% CI 11–149)]. At 24 months, our pooled analysis showed that the preventive treatment reduced the risk of clinical seizures [odds ratio (OR) 0.21; $p = 0.032$), drug-resistant epilepsy (OR 0.23; $p = 0.022$), and infantile spasms (OR 0; $p < 0.001$). No adverse events related to preventive treatment were observed.

Conclusion: This study concluded that the preventive treatment with vigabatrin was safe, modified the natural history of seizures in TSC, thereby reducing the risk and severity of epilepsy.

COMMENT

The "holy grail" of epilepsy treatment is to stop the process of epileptogenesis. A majority of patients with tuberous sclerosis complex (TSC) suffer from epilepsy and is usually refractory to conventional treatment. A growing body of evidence has supported the notion that the natural history of epilepsy could be modified with medical treatment. Vigabatrin is the first line medication for TSC-associated spasms or seizures in the first year of life. Also, vigabatrin appears to block mammalian target of rapamycin (mTOR) activation in animal experiments, suggesting a dual involvement in epileptogenesis.[18] Vigabatrin may be used presymptomatically or in the presence of epileptiform abnormalities on electroencephalography (EEG). In this case, epileptiform discharges on EEG were 100% predictive of epilepsy onset in a group of 40 TSC patients.[19] In the EPISTOP trial, vigabatrin was given to subset of children with TSC who also had EEG abnormalities before the first episode of seizure. This group was compared with patients who received treatment after the first episode. After 24 months, it was observed that preventive treatment significantly reduced the odds of developing clinical seizures, drug resistant epilepsy, and spasms. In fact, none of the children who received preventive therapy suffered from infantile spasms. Secondary outcomes for neurodevelopmental measures were not met. There were no adverse events related to preventive treatment. In TSC, early onset of epilepsy is a predictor of poor neurodevelopmental outcomes.[20] EPISTOP study has remarkably demonstrated that a simple intervention may alter the natural history of epilepsy in TSC, however, number of patients were small and real-world experience of preventive therapy in TSC may throw more light on its efficacy.

ARTICLE 8

When Should a Brain MRI be Performed in Children with New-onset Seizures? Results of a Large Prospective Trial

Hourani R, Nasreddine W, Dirani M, Hmaimess G, Sabbagh S, El Tourjuman O, et al. When should a brain MRI be performed in children with new-onset seizures? Results of a large prospective trial.
AJNR Am J Neuroradiol. 2021;42(9):1695-701.

Abstract

Objective: There is a scarcity of data with regard to the incidence of structural brain lesions in children with new onset unprovoked seizures. This study aimed to determine the frequencies and types of epileptogenic lesions detected on a dedicated epilepsy protocol magnetic resonance (MR) imaging according to age group, presence of developmental delay, and number and types of seizures.

Methods: This study included children between the age group of 6 months and 18 years and with new-onset unprovoked seizures. The frequencies and types of epileptogenic lesions were determined and then stratified according to sex, age groups, presence of developmental delay, and number and types of seizures at presentation. Multivariate analysis was used to identify variables significantly associated with the presence of epileptogenic lesions.

Results: A total of 1,000 children were included in the study. An epileptogenic lesion was identified in 26% of the children. Malformations of cortical development were the most common lesion (32%), followed by hypoxic-ischemic injury (20%), and vascular etiologies (16%). Univariate analysis showed a significant increase in the frequency of epileptogenic lesions with a decrease in age, presence of developmental delay, and number and types of seizures at presentation. Presence of developmental delay and type of seizures at presentation remained significant in a multivariate analysis.

Conclusion: This study reported a relatively high rate of epileptogenic lesions in children with new-onset seizures. Furthermore, presence of developmental delay and specific seizure types were associated with a higher likelihood of detecting an epileptogenic lesion on neuroimaging. This study meets the requirements of the study design as per the recommendations of the Practice Committee of the American Academy of Neurology. The authors hope that these results will help the relevant societies and committees in drafting guidelines for neuroimaging for children with new-onset seizures.

COMMENT

In resource-limited settings, imaging modalities may not be easily accessible or affordable. According to the International League Against Epilepsy (ILAE) Subcommittee for Pediatric Neuroimaging, over half of children with new-onset focal seizures have abnormal neuroimaging, which offers information on etiology and localization.[21] This study by

Hourani et al., aimed to identify the subset of children with new-onset seizures who would benefit most from immediate neuroimaging. The authors prospectively enrolled a thousand children aged between 6 and 18 months into the study. About a quarter of children (26%) were observed to have epileptogenic lesions upon imaging (most common being malformations of cortical development followed by hypoxic ischemic sequelae). Delayed development and seizure types (focal) were significant predictors for imaging abnormalities when multivariate analysis was used. Other studies have also recommended imaging when the first seizure is prolonged or status epilepticus.[22] Structural neuroimaging is useful in the diagnosis, management, and therapy of epilepsy in children. Detecting underlying brain lesions that may be linked to a child's seizure disease or neurodevelopmental deficit early in the course of illness may lead to improved outcomes. This study adds evidence to recommend imaging after the first episode of seizure when children have comorbid developmental delay or the first episode was a focal seizure.

ARTICLE 9

Improved Everyday Executive Functioning Following Profound Reduction in Seizure Frequency with Fenfluramine: Analysis from a Phase 3 Long-term Extension Study in Children/Young Adults with Dravet Syndrome

Bishop KI, Isquith PK, Gioia GA, Gammaitoni AR, Farfel G, Galer BS, et al. Improved everyday executive functioning following profound reduction in seizure frequency with fenfluramine: Analysis from a phase 3 long-term extension study in children/young adults with Dravet syndrome.
Epilepsy Behav. 2021;121(Pt A):108024.

Abstract

Objective: Individuals with Dravet syndrome (DS) experience frequent pharmacoresistant seizures that begin in infancy. Most of these individuals exhibit poor neurodevelopmental outcomes including motor function difficulties, behavioral problems, and cognitive impairment. Cognitive deficits in children with DS have been associated with frequency of seizures and use of antiseizure medication (ASM).

Recent research in children and young adults with DS has begun to explore the role of executive functions (EFs), as these include higher order cognitive functions and may mediate the relationship between risk factors and cognitive impairment. Current conceptualizations, however, of EFs involve broader self-regulation of cognitive, behavioral, and emotional domains. This study aimed to explore relationships between reduction in convulsive seizure frequency and everyday EFs in a group of children and young adults with DS who were treated with adjunctive fenfluramine for 1 year.

Methods: This is a post-hoc analysis of data from children and young adults with DS who were aged 5–18 years and participated in a phase 3 randomized, placebo-controlled clinical trial (core study) followed by completion of at least 1 year of fenfluramine treatment in an open-label extension (OLE) study. Eligible children and young adults started the OLE study at 0.2 mg/kg/day fenfluramine and were titrated to optimal seizure control and tolerability (maximum daily dose: 26 mg/day). Parents/Caregivers documented the convulsive seizure frequency per 28 days data [i.e., monthly convulsive seizure frequency (MCSF)] in an electronic diary. In addition, a parent or a caregiver for all the participants filled the Behavior Rating Inventory of Executive Function (BRIEF®) parent form, a questionnaire recording the perceptions of parents or caregivers with regard to the everyday EFs. This was included as a safety measure to determine treatment-related adverse effects on EFs during the trial. Ratings on BRIEF® were mapped to the new edition, the BRIEF®2 parent form, and were used to calculate T-scores for the emotion regulation index (ERI), cognitive regulation index (CRI), behavior regulation index (BRI), and global executive composite (GEC). Furthermore, changes in BRIEF®2 T-scores from baseline in the core study to year 1 of the OLE study were calculated. Spearman's Rho correlation coefficient was used to assess the associations between change in BRIEF®2 indexes or composite T-scores and percent change in MCSF. Children and young adults were divided into two groups (<50% and ≥50% MCSF reduction) based on percent MCSF reduction achieved from prerandomization baseline in the core study to year 1 of the OLE study. Mann–Whitney U test was used to compare the changes in the distribution of BRIEF®2 indexes or composite T-scores between MCSF reduction groups. The proportions of children and young adults in these groups who showed clinically significant improvement in everyday EFs, defined as reliable change index (RCI) values ≥95% certainty relative to a reference population of neurotypically developing healthy volunteers, were then evaluated by cross-tabulations and Somers' D tests ($p \leq 0.05$). In cases where a significant improvement in an index score was found, post-hoc analyses using the same statistical methods were performed to assess the individual BRIEF®2 scales composing that index. Supplemental analyses examined the proportions of patients in MCSF reduction groups <25% and ≥75% who achieved clinically significant improvement or worsening in everyday EFs using RCI values ≥95% certainty and ≥80% certainty, respectively, in relation to the reference population.

Results: At the time of analysis, a total of 58 children and young adults (mean age 11, SD 4 years) had reached OLE year 1 of fenfluramine treatment with a 75% median percent reduction in seizure frequency from the baseline. Overall, a significant correlation between change in MCSF and change in BRIEF®2 T-scores was found for ERI ($p = 0.008$), but no significant correlation was observed for BRI, CRI, or GEC ($p > 0.05$). At OLE year 1, 78% ($n = 45$) of the participants had ≥50% MCSF reduction ($n = 29$; 50% achieved ≥75% MCSF reduction) and 22% ($n = 13$) of the total participants had <50% MCSF reduction ($n = 7$; 12% showed <25% MCSF reduction). The ≥50% MCSF reduction group was more likely to achieve clinically significant improvement (RCI ≥ 95% certainty) in ERI ($p = 0.002$) and in CRI ($p = 0.001$) as compared to the <50% MCSF reduction group. There were no significant differences in the proportions of participants in these two groups showing clinically meaningful worsening (RCI ≥ 80% certainty) on the BRIEF®2 indexes/composite.

Conclusion: The magnitude of reduction in MCSF after long-term treatment with adjunctive fenfluramine was associated with clinically meaningful levels of improvement in everyday EFs in children and young adults with DS. Overall, 78% of the children and young adults treated with adjunctive fenfluramine for 1 year in the OLE study achieved ≥50% reduction in MCSF, for a magnitude of efficacy associated with a significantly greater likelihood of experiencing clinically meaningful improvement in emotion regulation and cognitive regulation.

COMMENT

Dravet syndrome (DS) is a devastating epilepsy syndrome of childhood. Therapeutic options are limited to avoidance of sodium channel blockers and stiripentol and recently, cannabidiol derivatives have been added to this list. Randomized controlled trials (RCTs) have explored the possibility of using fenfluramine in DS with good results.[23,24] Fenfluramine is a serotonergic drug which has been used since the 1960s as an anorexigenic drug for combating obesity. In 2020, it was approved by the Food and Drug Administration (FDA) for DS after a RCT showed promising results in 2019. The modulatory action on the sigma-1 receptor is hypothesized to contribute to its antiseizure activity. This paper summarized the results of the open-label section of the earlier RCT and was a post-hoc analysis. The authors have observed significant reduction of ≥50% in mean convulsive seizure frequency in 78% of patients. In addition, there was a greater likelihood of achieving better cognitive and emotional regulation. The greatest impediment for widespread adoption of fenfluramine is its potential risk to cause cardiac valvulopathy and pulmonary hypertension. Data from long-term follow up studies from Belgium have suggested that fenfluramine was safe as none of the patients developed such side effects.[25,26] Though disease modifying therapies in DS are wanting, adjunctive treatment with fenfluramine has provided meaningful clinical benefit for these patients.

ARTICLE 10

Virtual Epilepsy Clinics: A Canadian Comprehensive Epilepsy Center Experience pre-COVID and during the COVID-19 Pandemic Period

Aleboyeh S, Appireddy R, Winston GP, Lomax LB, Shukla G. Virtual epilepsy clinics—A Canadian comprehensive epilepsy center experience pre-COVID and during the COVID-19 pandemic period.
Epilepsy Res. 2021;176:106689.

Abstract

Objective: This study aimed to assess the role of prior experience with virtual care (through e-visits) in maintaining continuity in ambulatory epilepsy care during an unprecedented coronavirus disease 2019 (COVID-19) pandemic situation and thus comparing in-person versus e-visit clinic uptake.

Methods: This is an observational study on virtual epilepsy care (through e-visits) over 2 years, during a pre-COVID period (14 months) continuing into the COVID-19 pandemic period (10 months). A physician survey and a patient satisfaction survey were completed for a small sample of patients observed during the study period ($n = 53$). Descriptive statistics were used to analyze the outcomes of e-visits.

Results: The findings revealed that the median numbers of epilepsy clinic visits conducted during the COVID-19 pandemic period (27.5 new and 113 follow-up) were similar to the median uptake during the pre-COVID period (28 new and 116 follow-up). Prior experience with e-visits for epilepsy resulted in smooth transition to the pandemic period with many other advantages. Despite technical difficulties and major components of history and management being still easily implemented, most of the e-visits were successful. The results from surveys conducted in patients supported that virtual epilepsy clinics saved a significant amount of time and money, which was in line with our health-economic analysis.

Conclusion: This is one of the first few reports of fully integrated virtual care in a comprehensive epilepsy clinic starting much before the beginning of the COVID-19 pandemic. The results of this study support the feasibility of using virtual care to deliver specialized outpatient care in a comprehensive epilepsy center.

COMMENT

The coronavirus disease 2019 (COVID-19) has disrupted every sphere of life and healthcare delivery was crippled across the globe. This study observed that compared to "in-person" clinics, using e-visits for ambulatory epilepsy care is clinically viable, convenient, and cost-efficient. When the COVID-19 pandemic struck, the experience acquired aided resource efficiency and the subsequent quick adoption of virtually totally virtual care. As the center was already practicing telemedicine, there was a seamless transition and ensured that this susceptible patient population received uninterrupted care. However, almost half of the e-visits (49%) faced some form of technical problem, albeit minor. The authors felt that patients and caregivers who consult at their center find "in-person" visits emotionally and physically difficult, especially if they travel great distances to see the hospital. This is especially important in patients with epilepsy when a substantial percentage of people are restricted from driving. A similar paradigm of virtual care implementation can be replicated at other centers. The author's team recommends first asking patients about their willingness to participate in a virtual visit during in-person visits. Before the COVID-19 pandemic, teleconsultation was an uncommon practice in India. Almost all major hospitals and neurologists began offering teleconsultation within 2 months of the outbreak. Approximately half of the neurologists surveyed in an Indian study said they used teleconsultation regularly.[27] In the same survey that was conducted in multiple centers across the country, three-quarters of patients were ready for teleconsultation. Because India has one of the largest mobile phone populations in the world, this can be leveraged to improve primary and secondary treatment gaps in India and other low- and middle-income countries (LAMIC). Finally, clinicians can benefit from the use of standardized checklists, as well as questionnaires for patients to provide feedback.[28]

REFERENCES (Epilepsy)

1. Lux AL, Edwards SW, Hancock E, Johnson AL, Kennedy CR, Newton RW, et al. The United Kingdom Infantile Spasms Study comparing vigabatrin with prednisolone or tetracosactide at 14 days: a multicentre, randomised controlled trial. Lancet. 2004;364(9447):1773-8.
2. Chatterjee A, Mundlamuri RC, Kenchaiah R, Asranna A, Nagappa M, Bindu PS, et al. Role of pulse methylprednisolone in epileptic encephalopathy: A retrospective observational analysis. Epilepsy Res. 2021;173:106611.
3. O'Callaghan FJK, Edwards SW, Alber FD, Hancock E, Johnson AL, Kennedy CR, et al. Safety and effectiveness of hormonal treatment versus hormonal treatment with vigabatrin for infantile spasms (ICISS): a randomised, multicentre, open-label trial. Lancet Neurol. 2017;16(1):33-42.
4. Caraballo R, Demirdjian G, Reyes G, Huaman M, Gutierrez R. Effectiveness of cannabidiol in a prospective cohort of children with drug-resistant epileptic encephalopathy in Argentina. Seizure. 2020;80:75-80.
5. Devinsky O, Patel AD, Cross JH, Villanueva V, Wirrell EC, Privitera M, et al. Effect of Cannabidiol on Drop Seizures in the Lennox-Gastaut Syndrome. N Engl J Med. 2018;378(20):1888-97.
6. Caraballo R, Reyes G, Demirdjian G, Huaman M, Gutierrez R. Long-term use of cannabidiol-enriched medical cannabis in a prospective cohort of children with drug-resistant developmental and epileptic encephalopathy. Seizure. 2022;95:56-63.
7. Guang S, Mao L, Zhong L, Liu F, Pan Z, Yin F, et al. Hormonal Therapy for Infantile Spasms: A Systematic Review and Meta-Analysis. Front Neurol. 2022;13:772333.
8. Kapoor D, Sharma S, Garg D, Samaddar S, Panda I, Patra B, et al. Intravenous Methylprednisolone Versus Oral Prednisolone for West Syndrome: A Randomized Open-Label Trial. Indian J Pediatr. 2021;88(8):778-84.
9. Zangiabadi N, Ladino LD, Sina F, Orozco-Hernández JP, Carter A, Téllez-Zenteno JF. Deep Brain Stimulation and Drug-Resistant Epilepsy: A Review of the Literature. Front Neurol. 2019;10:601.
10. Hamani C, Hodaie M, Lozano AM. Present and future of deep brain stimulation for refractory epilepsy. Acta Neurochir (Wien). 2005;147(3):227-9.
11. Fisher R, Salanova V, Witt T, Worth R, Henry T, Gross R, et al. Electrical stimulation of the anterior nucleus of thalamus for treatment of refractory epilepsy. Epilepsia. 2010;51(5):899-908.
12. Karoly PJ, Ung H, Grayden DB, Kuhlmann L, Leyde K, Cook MJ, et al. The circadian profile of epilepsy improves seizure forecasting. Brain. 2017;140(8):2169-82.
13. Rakers F, Walther M, Schiffner R, Rupprecht S, Rasche M, Kockler M, et al. Weather as a risk factor for epileptic seizures: A case-crossover study. Epilepsia. 2017;58(7):1287-95.
14. Baud MO, Kleen JK, Mirro EA, Andrechak JC, King-Stephens D, Chang EF, et al. Multi-day rhythms modulate seizure risk in epilepsy. Nat Commun. 2018;9(1):88.
15. Meador KJ, Baker GA, Browning N, Cohen MJ, Bromley RL, Clayton-Smith J, et al. Fetal antiepileptic drug exposure and cognitive outcomes at age 6 years (NEAD study): a prospective observational study. Lancet Neurol. 2013;12(3):244-52.
16. Trinka E, Marson AG, Van Paesschen W, Kälviäinen R, Marovac J, Duncan B, et al. KOMET: an unblinded, randomised, two parallel-group, stratified trial comparing the effectiveness of levetiracetam with controlled-release carbamazepine and extended-release sodium valproate as monotherapy in patients with newly diagnosed epilepsy. J Neurol Neurosurg Psychiatry. 2013;84(10):1138-47.
17. Nevitt SJ, Sudell M, Weston J, Tudur Smith C, Marson AG. Antiepileptic drug monotherapy for epilepsy: a network

meta-analysis of individual participant data. Cochrane Database Syst Rev. 2017;6:CD011412.
18. Zhang B, McDaniel SS, Rensing NR, Wong M. Vigabatrin inhibits seizures and mTOR pathway activation in a mouse model of tuberous sclerosis complex. PLoS One. 2013;8(2):e57445.
19. Wu JY, Peters JM, Goyal M, Krueger D, Sahin M, Northrup H, et al. Clinical Electroencephalographic Biomarker for Impending Epilepsy in Asymptomatic Tuberous Sclerosis Complex Infants. Pediatr Neurol. 2016;54:29-34.
20. Capal JK, Bernardino-Cuesta B, Horn PS, Murray D, Byars AW, Bing NM, et al. TACERN Study Group. Influence of Seizures on Early Development in Tuberous Sclerosis Complex. Epilepsy Behav. 2017;70(Pt A):245-52.
21. Gaillard WD, Chiron C, Cross JH, Harvey AS, Kuzniecky R, Hertz-Pannier L, et al. ILAE. Guidelines for imaging infants and children with recent-onset epilepsy. Epilepsia. 2009;50(9):2147-53.
22. Al-shami R, Khair AM, Elseid M, Ibrahim K, Al-Ahmad A, Elsetouhy A, et al. Neuro-imaging evaluation after the first afebrile seizure in children: A retrospective observational study. Seizure. 2016;43:26-31.
23. Lagae L, Sullivan J, Knupp K, Laux L, Polster T, Nikanorova M, et al. FAiRE DS Study Group. Fenfluramine hydrochloride for the treatment of seizures in Dravet syndrome: a randomised, double-blind, placebo-controlled trial. Lancet. 2019;394(10216):2243-54.
24. Nabbout R, Mistry A, Zuberi S, Villeneuve N, Gil-Nagel A, Sanchez-Carpintero R, et al. Fenfluramine for Treatment-Resistant Seizures in Patients With Dravet Syndrome Receiving Stiripentol-Inclusive Regimens: A Randomized Clinical Trial. JAMA Neurol. 2020;77(3):300-8.
25 Ceulemans B, Boel M, Leyssens K, Rossem CV, Neels P, Jorens PG, et al. Successful use of fenfluramine as an add-on treatment for Dravet syndrome. Epilepsia. 2012;53(7):1131-9.
26. Ceulemans B, Schoonjans AS, Marchau F, Paelinck BP, Lagae L. Five-year extended follow-up status of 10 patients with Dravet syndrome treated with fenfluramine. Epilepsia. 2016;57(7):e129-34.
27. Rathore C, Baheti N, Bansal AR, Jabeen SA, Gopinath S, Jagtap S, et al. Impact of COVID-19 pandemic on epilepsy practice in India: A tripartite survey. Seizure. 2021;86: 60-7.
28. Hatcher-Martin JM, Adams JL, Anderson ER, Bove R, Burrus TM, Chehrenama M, et al. Telemedicine in neurology: Telemedicine Work Group of the American Academy of Neurology update. Neurology. 2020;94(1):30-8.

Section 5: Movement Disorders

Section Editors: Hrishikesh Kumar, Prashanth LK

Associate Editors: Adreesh Mukherjee, Ajith Cherian, Divya KP, Elavarasi A, Heli Shah, Jacky Ganguly, Jaslovleen Kaur, Mitesh Chandarana, Srinivas Raju, Suvorit Subhas Bhowmick

ARTICLE 1

Effects of Statins on Dopamine Loss and Prognosis in Parkinson's Disease

Jeong SH, Lee HS, Chung SJ, Yoo HS, Jung JH, Baik K, et al. Effects of statins on dopamine loss and prognosis in Parkinson's disease.
Brain. 2021;144(10):3191-200.

Abstract

The study investigated whether the previous statin use influence baseline nigrostriatal dopamine loss during diagnosis and longitudinal motor and cognitive outcomes in patients with Parkinson's disease (PD).

Five hundred untreated PD patients underwent dopamine transporter (DAT) imaging and were classified into two groups as per the prior use of statins: patients with [PD-statin (+)] and without [PD-statin (−)] statin use. Multivariate linear regression was used to compare DAT availability between these two groups. Linear mixed model and survival analysis were performed to assess longitudinal changes in levodopa equivalent dose (LED) and Parkinson's disease dementia (PDD) conversion between the groups. Additionally, mediation analysis was performed to examine the effect of total cholesterol. The PD-statin (+) group showed: (1) lower baseline DAT availability in the anterior, posterior, and ventral putamen; (2) faster longitudinal increase in LED, (3) higher risk of conversion to PDD compared to the PD-statin (−) group, and (4) the effect was independent of total cholesterol levels.

Limitations: (1) Total cholesterol level was measured instead of biomarkers specific for brain cholesterol level, (2) selection bias, as statin is prescribed to those who already have vascular risk factors, (3) increase in LED may not directly reflect progression of PD, (4) duration and dose of statin was unknown prior to diagnosis of PD, and (5) the study was done in a single center in Korea encompassing single ethnic background.

Comment: The effect of statins on PD is controversial. Cholesterol lowering effect is the main confounding factor. This is the first study showing that statin use itself can have direct detrimental effects on baseline nigral density and longitudinal outcome in PD, not related to total cholesterol level.

COMMENT

Statins are key in lipid lowering and have anti-inflammatory effects.[1] The effects and role of statin in Parkinson's disease (PD), which is also prorogated to be a result of oxidative stress, remains unanswered. The meta-analysis of statins for PD,[2] had left with many questions unanswered. This current study by Seong Ho[3] gives one of the critical answers about whether statins can have direct detrimental effects on nigral density and final outcome on PD. Albeit the authors have been able to indicate the changes further studies addressing dose, duration, and other confounding factors would be required in near future. This study does open windows on assessment of direct effect of statins on PD.

ARTICLE 2

Onset of Skin, Gut, and Genitourinary Prodromal Parkinson's Disease: A Study of 1.5 Million Veterans

Scott GD, Lim MM, Drake MG, Woltjer R, Quinn JF. Onset of Skin, Gut, and Genitourinary Prodromal Parkinson's Disease: A Study of 1.5 Million Veterans.
Mov Disord. 2021;36(9):2094-103.

Abstract

This study emphasizes the long duration between the first manifestations of peripheral dysfunction and diagnosis of Parkinson's disease (PD) highlighting a window of opportunity for future potential disease-modifying therapies. Identification of these systems holds potential as early targets for further investigation in PD, including mechanisms, early diagnostic screening, and potential new sites for pathological sampling. These results offer a long window of opportunity to assay accessible organs for early PD research.

The authors of this study report on the onset of prodromal PD features using the medical records database from the largest integrated healthcare system in the United States, the Veterans Affairs Corporate Data Warehouse. Patients with PD ($n = 303,693$) were identified using diagnostic codes in the medical records database of the United States Veterans Affairs healthcare system and were compared 4:1 with matched controls. Disorder prevalence and estimated onset times were assessed for 20 years preceding diagnosis.

They found that the earliest measured differences and estimated onset times of dysfunction occurred 15–20 years before PD diagnosis. Smell and taste dysfunction occurred 20.9 years before diagnosis, followed closely by gastroesophageal reflux, sexual dysfunction, and gastroparesis.

In this study, the earliest significantly increased prodromal disorders were gastroesophageal reflux, sexual dysfunction, and esophageal dyskinesia at 17, 16, and 15 years before diagnosis. Estimated onset times for each disorder occurred 5.5 ± 3.4 years before the first measured increase. Onset times for constipation and urinary dysfunction were notably longer by 7 and

9 years compared to prior studies in sleep disorder patients. Dermatophytosis and prostatic hypertrophy were identified as new high prevalence prodromal disorders.

Limitations: Underestimation of disorder prevalence because of coding insensitivity, weaker detection of groupwise differences because of contamination by false-positive PD cases described previously in the VA population.

COMMENT

Nonmotor symptoms (NMS) such as gastrointestinal, genitourinary, and skin disorders manifest decades before diagnosis of Parkinson's disease (PD), emphasizing their potential as sites for developing early diagnostic testing and understanding pathogenesis.[4,5] Onset of disorders in peripheral organs often precedes the clinical diagnosis of PD by at least two decades. Involved organ systems are easily accessible for sampling and may provide new insights into pathogenesis and early diagnosis of prodromal PD. These data add to the alluring prospect of identifying and treating PD before significant brain damage has occurred. In future studies, more emphasize on the NMS is required for proper early interventions.

ARTICLE 3

Safety and Efficacy of Mevidalen in Lewy Body Dementia: A Phase 2, Randomized, Placebo-controlled Trial

Biglan K, Munsie L, Svensson KA, Ardayfio P, Pugh M, Sims J, et al. Safety and Efficacy of Mevidalen in Lewy Body Dementia: A Phase 2, Randomized, Placebo-controlled Trial.
Mov Disord. 2022;37(3):513-24.

Abstract

The safety and efficacy of Mevidalen, a selective positive allosteric modulator of the dopamine D1 receptor, as treatment for cognition in Lewy body dementia was assessed in PRESENCE, a 12-week study. Participants ($n = 344$) were randomly assigned (1:1:1:1) to daily doses (10, 30, or 75 mg) or placebo. Primary outcome measure was change from baseline on Cognitive Drug Research Continuity of Attention composite score. Secondary outcomes included Alzheimer's Disease Assessment Scale-cognitive subscale 13, the Movement Disorder Society-Sponsored Revision of the Unified Parkinson's Disease Rating Scale (MDS-UPDRS), and Alzheimer's Disease Cooperative Study-Clinical Global Impression of Change (ADCS-CGIC). However, Mevidalen failed to meet primary or secondary cognition endpoints but resulted in significant, dose-dependent improvement of MDS-UPDRS, and ADCS-CGIC scores. Increases in blood pressure and cardiovascular adverse events were pronounced at 75 mg dose.

COMMENT

Lewy body dementia present with wide variety of symptoms from cognition, parkinsonism, behavioral issues, and autonomic disorders. Due to varied domains involvement and pathophysiological process, decent treatment modules are limited.[6] Mevidalen, a selective positive allosteric modulator of D1 receptor was assumed to help the cognitive aspects of Lewy body dementia. However, in this phase-2 randomized controlled trial (RCT), it failed to meet the primary/secondary endpoints, indicating the complexity of pathophysiology. This does open up for restrateging the therapy options and newer targets for consideration. It might also indicate that we should try to look for more upstream targets for possible interventions.

ARTICLE 4

Clinical Study of 668 Indian Subjects with Juvenile, Young, and Early Onset Parkinson's Disease

Kukkle PL, Goyal V, Geetha TS, Mridula KR, Kumar H, Borgohain R, et al. Parkinson Research Alliance of India (PRAI). Clinical Study of 668 Indian Subjects with Juvenile, Young, and Early Onset Parkinson's Disease.
Can J Neurol Sci. 2022;49(1):93-101.

Abstract

Kukkle et al. have described a series of 668 patients with Parkinson's disease (PD) with onset <50 years of age. They compared the clinical features, motor and nonmotor symptoms at onset, treatment trends, and temporal profile of development of motor complications including dyskinesias and motor fluctuations between juvenile onset (<20 years), young onset (20–39 years), and early onset (40–49 years) PD. They found differences in presenting symptoms as compared to the west, with tremor being the most common symptom in >75% of patients. The limitations are lack of genetic data and the cross-sectional nature of the study.

COMMENT

Young onset Parkinson's disease (YOPD) is a varied cohort with variable cutoff over the last few decades. The current early onset Parkinson's disease (EOPD) task force recommends to consider all under the 50 as EOPD and hence amalgamating YOPD into a bigger umbrella.[7] Is there a clinical or genetic differences between these cohorts, remains unanswered. This pan India study of YOPD, gives insights into clinical profile of YOPD from Indian cohort and in addition, the authors have shown that the clinical differences do exit between <40 years and >40 years onset.[8] Probably, this needs to be further supported by genetic analysis. A decadewise analysis/big data analysis is required to see if any age groups can be differentiated for YOPD/EOPD or this would continue as a gray zone area.

ARTICLE 5

Non-invasive Vagus Nerve Stimulation Improves Clinical and Molecular Biomarkers of Parkinson's Disease in Patients with Freezing of Gait

Mondal B, Choudhury S, Banerjee R, Roy A, Chatterjee K, Basu P, et al. Non-invasive vagus nerve stimulation improves clinical and molecular biomarkers of Parkinson's disease in patients with freezing of gait.
NPJ Parkinsons Dis. 2021;7(1):46.

Abstract

It is a randomized, double blind, sham-controlled crossover trial to examine the efficacy of cervical noninvasive vagus nerve stimulation (nVNS) as an adjunct to standard treatment in Parkinson's disease (PD) patients with gait freezing. Thirty-three such patients were enrolled in the study, and randomized into active nVNS and sham stimulation groups in 1:1 ratio. The treatment consisted of two, 2-minute stimulation intervals delivered 5–10 minutes apart to the left vagus nerve, delivered at 3 prespecified times every day for 1 month followed by a 1 month washout period followed by crossover to alternative treatment. Each patient was assessed four times over a 12-week study period. They also measured serum markers of inflammation [interleukin-6 (IL-6), IL-10, and tumor necrosis factor-alpha (TNF-α)], oxidative stress, and brain-derived neurotrophic factor (BDNF). nVNS therapy showed statistically significant increases in gait velocity and step length, and reduction in stance time along with significant improvement in mean Unified Parkinson's Disease Rating Scale-part III (UPDRS-III) score, fall efficacy scale, and freezing of gait questionnaire. nVNS significantly reduced TNF-α levels and increased the concentrations of reduced glutathione and BDNF from baseline.

This study has provided first preliminary evidence for the efficacy and safety of nVNS as an adjunct in treating gait and motor symptoms in PD patients and reducing serum inflammatory markers. Moreover, it also provided the first evidence that nVNS downregulates major proinflammatory cytokines, upregulates BDNF and antioxidant markers and it may have disease-modifying effects in PD.

Limitations: (1) A relatively high number of dropouts from the initial study arm due to multiple study visits over a short time period. (2) Long-term effects of intervention could not be established due to short study duration. (3) Molecular biomarkers could not be tested in all trial participants. (4) Practical issues related to nVNS delivery in older populations.

COMMENT

Gait remains one of the major hurdle in management of Parkinson's disease (PD) and Parkinsonian disorders. Noninvasive vagal nerve stimulation has caught the eye with possible answers to the gait issues.[9,10] This study from India provides preliminary evidence for efficacy and safety of vagus nerve stimulation (VNS) and as an adjunct therapy for PD. The study has also looked into the possible biomarkers of inflammation changes with VNS, giving a better insight on VNS effects. The study will pave way for long-term analysis studies. Further studies with larger cohort and multicentric randomized controlled trial (RCT) studies would help to give an answer for possible use of VNS in gait issues.

ARTICLE 6

Divergent Pallidal Pathways Underlying Distinct Parkinsonian Behavioral Deficits

Lilascharoen V, Wang EH, Do N, Pate SC, Tran AN, Yoon CD, et al. Divergent pallidal pathways underlying distinct Parkinsonian behavioral deficits.
Nat Neurosci. 2021;24(4):504-15.

Abstract

The pathophysiology of Parkinson's disease (PD) has always been revolving around the basal ganglia thalamocortical circuit. This study focused on the distinct role of parvalbumin neurons in globus pallidus externa (GPe-PV) and its innervations to substantia nigra pars reticulata (SNr) and parafascicular (PF) thalamus. They used dopamine depleted mice, and viral vectors to label the targeted GPe-PV neurons and studied the afferent and efferent pathways, electrophysiological properties, locomotion, and behavioral functions using various task-related activities. They demonstrated that while GPe-SNr neurons control motor functions, GPe-PF has a major role in the reversal learning which affects cognition. These findings provide a novel framework for understanding the circuit basis of varying PD-related motor and nonmotor symptoms, and therefore, better strategies for the treatment.

COMMENT

Neurology as a field is slowly changing from localization based pathology to circuit-based disorders, as any aberration in the circuit pathway can cause similar phenotypes. Parkinson's disease, albeit put as an basal ganglionic disorder, the clinical phenotypes can be due to various connections associated corticobasal ganglia and corticocerebellar circuits.[11,12] Various nuclei, in these path would be playing critical roles in various symptoms.[11] Many of these are still unexplored. Currently, Lilascharoen et al. have looked into the district role of parvalbumin neurons in globus pallidus externa (GPe-PV) and its effect on clinical symptoms. The findings that these GPe-PV neurons have effects on cognition, could give an insights into the variable phenotypes and possible genetic insights/therapeutic interventions.

ARTICLE 7

Detection of α-synuclein in CSF by RT-QuIC in Patients with Isolated Rapid-eye-movement Sleep Behavior Disorder: A Longitudinal Observational Study

Iranzo A, Fairfoul G, Ayudhaya ACN, Serradell M, Gelpi E, Vilaseca I, et al. Detection of α-synuclein in CSF by RT-QuIC in patients with isolated rapid-eye-movement sleep behaviour disorder: A longitudinal observational study. *Lancet Neurol. 2021;20(3):203-12.*

Abstract

A major challenge in developing targeted disease-modifying therapy (precision medicine) for Parkinson's disease (PD) and dementia with Lewy bodies (DLBs) is identifying individuals at risk. Iranzo et al. reported longitudinal follow-up (for 7.3 ± 2.9 years) of 52 patients with isolated rapid eye movement sleep behavior disorder (IRBD) and 40 healthy controls, who underwent real-time quaking-induced conversion (RT-QuIC) analysis of cerebrospinal fluid (CSF) for the detection of misfolded α-synuclein. They found that 32 (62%) participants, of whom 31 (97%) were α-synuclein positive, developed PD or DLB. In IRBD, detection of misfolded α-synuclein in the CSF by RT-QuIC analysis has sensitivity and specificity of 90%. If findings are replicated, this biomarker could be used to enrich IRBD cohorts in neuroprotective trials targeting α-synuclein.

COMMENT

Reliable diagnostic marker for Parkinson's disease (PD) is a dire requirement for early disease modification therapies.[13,14] There quest for an ideal biomarker, which can predict clinical syndrome and prognosticate PD is ongoing. In the current study, Iranzo et al. have looked into the isolated rapid eye movement sleep behavior disorder (IRBD) patients for misfolded α-synuclein using RT-QuIC. The patients with positive results had an high sensitivity and specificity. This could pave way for early predictor of IRBD cohort who might develop PD/DLB. However, given the requirement for significant invasive intervention [cerebrospinal fluid (CSF)], whether any less invasive biomarkers can give the same or better answers, needs to be awaited.

ARTICLE 8

Predictors of Short-term Impulsive and Compulsive Behavior after Subthalamic Stimulation in Parkinson Disease

Sauerbier A, Loehrer P, Jost ST, Heil S, Petry-Schmelzer JN, Herberg J, et al. EUROPAR and the International Parkinson and Movement Disorders Society Non-Motor Parkinson's Disease Study Group. Predictors of short-term impulsive and compulsive behaviour after subthalamic stimulation in Parkinson disease.
J Neurol Neurosurg Psychiatry. 2021;92(12):1313-8.

Abstract

A prospective, open-label, multicenter study was done on Parkinson's disease (PD) patients undergoing bilateral subthalamic nucleus-deep brain stimulation (STN-DBS) on clinical predictors of impulsive and compulsive behaviors (ICBs). 55 patients aged 61.7 years with 9.8 years PD duration were assessed preoperatively and at 6-month postoperatively. Clinical scales included the Questionnaire for Impulsive-Compulsive Disorders in PD-Rating Scale (QUIP-RS), nonmotor symptoms scale (NMSS), levodopa-equivalent daily dose total (LEDD-total), and dopamine agonists (LEDD-DA). QUIP-RS cut-offs and psychiatric assessments identified patients with preoperative ICB. Higher baseline QUIP-RS and lower baseline LEDD-DA were associated with greater QUIP-RS improvements. The "QUIP-RS worsening" group had severe baseline impairment in the NMSS attention/memory domain emphasizing the need for nonmotor assessments in patients undergoing STN-DBS.

COMMENT

Impulse control disorders (ICDs) are well recognized in Parkinson's disease (PD) and highlighted as secondary to medications and surgical interventions.[15,16] Given the importance of interventions contributing to ICD, proper patient's selection and red flagging who might develop ICD with interventions becomes very important. This prospective study looked in the ICD features in deep brain stimulation (DBS) cohort. The highlighting of worsening of ICD features in people with other impaired nonmotor symptoms (NMS) domains (cognitive domain—attention/memory), does help to fine tune the patient selections and close follow up in postoperative care. This concept will help in bringing personalized medicine.

ARTICLE 9

Gene Therapy in Movement Disorders: A Systematic Review of Ongoing and Completed Clinical Trials

Merola A, Kobayashi N, Romagnolo A, Wright BA, Artusi CA, Imbalzano G, et al. Gene Therapy in Movement Disorders: A Systematic Review of Ongoing and Completed Clinical Trials.
Front Neurol. 2021;12:648532.

Abstract

In this systematic review, the methodology and selection is of recommended standard with bias elimination. The article mainly contains Parkinson's disease (PD), Huntington disease (HD), and amino acid decarboxylase (AADC) deficiency human trials with several other ongoing trials. The relative delivery and safety of the gene therapy have been established. Results in PD are promising with relative motor Unified Parkinson's Disease Rating Scale-part III (UPDRS III) improvement and metabolic pet imaging changes. HD trials showed no improvement but post hoc analysis showed reduction in cerebrospinal fluid mutant huntingtin (CSF mHTT) and improvement in Unified Huntington's Disease Rating Scale (UHDRS). AADC deficiency trials showed improvement in motor scores especially in younger subjects and improvement were seen in swallowing/respiration/dystonia/oculogyric crisis and improvement in cognition in all. Limitation of the study is small sample size with no control group and no long-term safety and clinical data. Overall this article summarizes all the human gene therapy trials in the movement disorders up to 2021. It gives us insights into the future directions for therapeutic benefits and further trials and advancement for better outcomes.

COMMENT

Efforts to change the course of management of Parkinson's disease (PD) from symptomatic therapies to disease-modifying therapies have been going on for last few decades.[17] Among the various disease-modifying therapies being tried, the gene therapy is of the prominent therapies, which can have implications of various degenerative disorders. This article gives an update on current status of various human gene therapies, especially for movement disorders and the future directions of studies.

ARTICLE 10

Assessment of Botulinum Neurotoxin Injection for Dystonic Hand Tremor: A Randomized Clinical Trial

Rajan R, Srivastava AK, Anandapadmanabhan R, Saini A, Upadhyay A, Gupta A, et al. Assessment of Botulinum Neurotoxin Injection for Dystonic Hand Tremor: A Randomized Clinical Trial.
JAMA Neurol. 2021;78(3):302-11.

Abstract

Placebo-controlled, parallel-group randomized clinical trial of botulinum neurotoxin (BoNT) injection in patients with upper-extremity dystonic tremor (DT) with individualized dosing. Primary outcome was the total score on the Fahn–Tolosa–Marin Tremor Rating Scale (FTM-TRS) at 6 weeks after intervention. In the intention-to-treat group, FTM-TRS total score was significantly lower in the BoNT group at 6 and 12 weeks. Dynamometer-assessed grip strength was similar in both groups. BoNT injections were superior to placebo in upper-extremity DT. An individualized dosing approach was beneficial without unacceptable adverse effects.

Placebo effects might be significant for interventions such as BoNT.

This well-designed study provides level 1 evidence to support the use of BoNT injections in upper-extremity DT.

COMMENT

Botulinum toxins are well-accepted therapies for various dystonic syndromes. Among the various disorders, there was paucity for high quality clinical evidence studies on botulinum toxin for upper limb dystonic tremors (DTs), given the significant disability associated with it.[18,19] This placebo controlled parallel group randomized clinical trial by Rajan et al. fills that gap with unequivocal evidence to support botulinum toxin for dystonic upper limb tremors.

REFERENCES (Movement Disorders)

1. Sandwith L, Forget P. Statins in Healthy Adults: A Meta-Analysis. Medicina (Kaunas). 2021;57(6):585.
2. Yan J, Qiao L, Tian J, Liu A, Wu J, Huang J, et al. Effect of statins on Parkinson's disease: A systematic review and meta-analysis. Medicine. 2019;98(12):e14852.
3. Jeong SH, Lee HS, Chung SJ, Yoo HS, Jung JH, Baik K, et al. Effects of statins on dopamine loss and prognosis in Parkinson's disease. Brain. 2021;144(10):3191-200.
4. Konno T, Al-Shaikh RH, Deutschländer AB, Uitti RJ. Biomarkers of Nonmotor Symptoms in Parkinson's Disease. Int Rev Neurobiol. 2017;133:259-89.
5. Pont-Sunyer C, Hotter A, Gaig C, Seppi K, Compta Y, Katzenschlager R, et al. The onset of nonmotor symptoms in Parkinson's disease (the ONSET PD study). Mov Disord. 2015;30(2):229-37.

6. Taylor JP, McKeith IG, Burn DJ, Boeve BF, Weintraub D, Bamford C, et al. New evidence on the management of Lewy body dementia. Lancet Neurol. 2020;19(2):157-69.
7. Mehanna R, Smilowska K, Fleisher J, Post B, Hatano T, Pimentel Piemonte ME, et al. Age Cutoff for Early-Onset Parkinson's Disease: Recommendations from the International Parkinson and Movement Disorder Society Task Force on Early Onset Parkinson's Disease. Mov Disord Clin Pract. 2022;9(7):869-78.
8. Kukkle PL, Goyal V, Geetha TS, Mridula KR, Kumar H, Borgohain R, et al. Parkinson Research Alliance of India (PRAI). Clinical Study of 668 Indian Subjects with Juvenile, Young, and Early Onset Parkinson's Disease. Can J Neurol Sci. 2022;49(1):93-101.
9. Mondal B, Choudhury S, Simon B, Baker MR, Kumar H. Noninvasive vagus nerve stimulation improves gait and reduces freezing of gait in Parkinson's disease. Mov Disord. 2019;34(6):917-8.
10. Marano M, Anzini G, Musumeci G, Magliozzi A, Pozzilli V, Capone F, et al. Transcutaneous Auricular Vagus Stimulation Improves Gait and Reaction Time in Parkinson's Disease. Mov Disord. 2022.
11. Martinu K, Monchi O. Cortico-basal ganglia and cortico-cerebellar circuits in Parkinson's disease: pathophysiology or compensation? Behav Neurosci. 2013;127(2):222-36.
12. Rosin B, Nevet A, Elias S, Rivlin-Etzion M, Israel Z, Bergman H. Physiology and pathophysiology of the basal ganglia-thalamo-cortical networks. Parkinsonism Relat Disord. 2007;13(Suppl 3):S437-9.
13. Marek K, Chowdhury S, Siderowf A, Lasch S, Coffey CS, Caspell-Garcia C, et al. Parkinson's Progression Markers Initiative. The Parkinson's progression markers initiative (PPMI)—establishing a PD biomarker cohort. Ann Clin Transl Neurol. 2018;5(12):1460-77.
14. Parnetti L, Gaetani L, Eusebi P, Paciotti S, Hansson O, El-Agnaf O, et al. CSF and blood biomarkers for Parkinson's disease. Lancet Neurol. 2019;18(6):573-86.
15. Zhang JF, Wang XX, Feng Y, Fekete R, Jankovic J, Wu YC. Impulse Control Disorders in Parkinson's Disease: Epidemiology, Pathogenesis and Therapeutic Strategies. Front Psychiatry. 2021;12:635494.
16. Razmkon A, Abdollahifard S, Rezaei H, Bahadori AR, Roshanshad A, Jaafari N. Effect of deep brain stimulation on impulse control behaviors of Parkinson's disease patients: A systematic review and meta-analysis. InterdiscNeurosurg. 2021;26:101361.
17. Axelsen TM, Woldbye DPD. Gene Therapy for Parkinson's Disease, An Update. J Parkinsons Dis. 2018;8(2):195-215.
18. Chen S. Clinical uses of botulinum neurotoxins: current indications, limitations and future developments. Toxins (Basel). 2012;4(10):913-39.
19. Niemann N, Jankovic J. Botulinum Toxin for the Treatment of Hand Tremor. Toxins (Basel). 2018;10(7):299.

Section 6: Ataxia

Section Editors: Pramod Kumar Pal, Achal Kumar Srivastava

Associate Editor: Divya M Radhakrishnan

ARTICLE 1

SCA2 in the Indian Population: Unified Haplotype and Variable Phenotypic Patterns in a Large Case Series

Sonakar AK, Shamim U, Srivastava MP, Faruq M, Srivastava AK. SCA2 in the Indian population: Unified haplotype and variable phenotypic patterns in a large case series.
Parkinsonism Relat Disord. 2021;89:139-45.

Abstract

Background: Spinocerebellar ataxia type 2 (SCA2) is one of the most common autosomal dominant ataxia in India and displays great clinical and genetic diversity.[1] Studying a larger ethnically heterogeneous population of SCA2 can help to understand the pathogenesis of the disease. Whereas studying a homogenous population of SCA2 with a common genetic and environmental backdrop can give insight into its phenotypic variability.

Aim: The aim of this study was to describe the clinical and genetic characteristics of SCA2 patients from India.

Methods: Patients with genetically proven SCA2 ($n = 436$) enrolled in the ataxia clinic of a tertiary care neurology center were recruited for this study. The cohort comprised 347 cases from 347 unrelated families from India, one large endogamous Banjara community from Saharanpur, Northern India, and one south Indian family from Belgaum, Karnataka. The DNA samples of controls were taken from Indian Genome Variation Consortium, CSIR-IGIB (Council of Scientific and Industrial Research-Institute of Genomics and Integrative Biology) ($n = 306$) and unaffected individuals of Banjara population ($n = 9$). All participants had a detailed clinical evaluation, and genetic analysis included analysis of two novel single nucleotide polymorphism (SNP) markers (rs695871 and rs695872 located 177 bp and 106 bp upstream of CAG sequence in Exon 1 of ATXN2) and CAG repeat length estimation.

Results: The most frequent clinical features observed in SCA2 cohort were gait ataxia (61.6%), dysarthria (55%), upper limb ataxia (48.8%), and slow saccades (36.7%). Extrapyramidal features (14.4%) and hyporeflexia (10.1%) were less common features. Age of onset and age at examination showed a significant association with slow saccades and upper limb incoordination. Similarly, disease duration and CAG repeat length had a significant association with slow saccades and upper limb ataxia. An inverse correlation was observed between age of onset and CAG repeat length. The data of the two marker haplotypes revealed a complete association of C-C haplotype with CAG repeats expansion in ATXN2.

Conclusion: This study revealed the clinical and genetic aspects of a large ethnically heterogeneous Indian SCA2 cohort. Slow saccades and hyporeflexia were less frequent in the present cohort compared with other populations. The presence of CC haplotype in all the participants represents a common origin within all subpopulations and the role of this haplotype in the pathogenesis of SCA2.

COMMENT

Strengths
- The study had a larger sample size with ethnical and geographical diversity, and described the characteristics of a large endogamous community with a high frequency of spinocerebellar ataxia type 2 (SCA2).
- The study also confirmed the existence of a common CC haplotype across all the subpopulations of SCA2.

Limitation
The study was limited by the unavailability of clinical information from a substantial number of participants.

ARTICLE 2

Cognitive Impairment in Spinocerebellar Ataxia Type 12

Agarwal A, Kaur H, Agarwal A, Nehra A, Pandey S, Garg A, et al. Cognitive impairment in spinocerebellar ataxia type 12. *Parkinsonism Relat Disord. 2021;85:52-6.*

Abstract

Background: Cognitive impairment is a well-known feature in many spinocerebellar ataxias (SCAs).[2-4] However, cognitive dysfunction in SCA12 has not been evaluated in larger studies.

Aim: This study aimed to evaluate the cognitive impairment in patients with genetically proven SCA12.

Methods: This cross-sectional study was conducted in a tertiary care center of Northern India. Patients ($n = 30$, 20 males) with genetically confirmed SCA12 from unrelated families and 30 healthy controls with matched age, gender, and education were recruited. All study participants had cognitive assessment using a battery of validated tests assessing various neurocognitive domains.

Results: The mean age of the patients and disease duration were 51.6 ± 8.0 and 5.3 ± 3.0 years, and mean International Cooperative Ataxia Rating Scale (ICARS) score was 29.8 ± 12. Compared to the controls, patients with SCA12 significantly lower scores in tests for executive function and new learning ability. Patients with SCA12 had performed poorly in tests assessing other neurocognitive domain compared to the matched controls; but the difference was not statistically significant. No correlation was observed between cognitive dysfunction and age, age at onset, disease duration, CAG repeat length, or ataxia severity.

Conclusion: The clinical spectrum of SCA12 comprises cognitive impairment. Significant executive dysfunction and impairment of new learning ability may be seen in the early part of the disease.

COMMENT

Strength
First and largest study assessing the cognitive dysfunction in spinocerebellar ataxia type 12 (SCA12).

Limitations
- Cognitive dysfunction was not corroborated with structural or functional imaging.
- The study tested only limited cognitive domains; social cognition and language assessment were not part of the study.

ARTICLE 3

Cognitive Impairment and its Neuroimaging Correlates in Spinocerebellar Ataxia 2

Stezin A, Bhardwaj S, Hegde S, Jain S, Bharath RD, Saini J, et al. Cognitive impairment and its neuroimaging correlates in spinocerebellar ataxia 2.
Parkinsonism Relat Disord. 2021;85:78-83.

Abstract

Background: Cognitive impairment is a well-recognized feature of spinocerebellar ataxia type 2 (SCA2).[2,5] Marked cognitive impairment due to the involvement of frontal-subcortical circuits is reported in various studies of SCA2.[6] However, the severity, progression, interindividual variability, and the neural substrates responsible for the cognitive impairment are not explored well.

Aim: This study aimed to assess and classify the cognitive impairment, and to identify the neuroimaging (grey matter) correlates in patients with SCA2.

Methods: The study was conducted at the National Institute of Mental Health and Neurosciences (NIMHANS), India. 35 patients with SCA2 and 30 healthy controls matched for age, gender, and education were recruited. All the participants had a comprehensive cognitive assessment using validated neuropsychological tests. The various domains evaluated include attention, learning and memory, language and fluency, executive functions, and visuomotor constructive ability. Patients were then categorized into SCA2 with and without cognitive impairment. Those with cognitive deficits are further classified as multidomain if ≥3 domains were affected, and limited domain if cognitive impairment affected ≤2 domains. Voxel-based morphometry was used to identify the grey matter changes in patients with cognitive impairment.

Results: The mean age at onset, disease duration, the Scale for the Assessment and Rating of Ataxia (SARA) score were 28.7 ± 8.51 (years), 66.7 ± 44.1 (months), and 16.1 ± 4.9 (points), respectively. Cognitive impairment was seen 71.4% of patients despite the short duration of disease; multi- and limited domain cognitive impairment were seen in 42.7% and 28.5%, respectively. Visuomotor construction and focused attention were the most frequent domain affected in the multidomain cognitive impairment group, whereas language and fluency domain were the most common domain affected in the limited domain cognitive impairment group. SCA2 patients with cognitive impairment showed significant grey matter atrophy of posterior cerebellum, bilateral sensorimotor cortex, and left superior frontal cortex compared to those with no cognitive impairment [family-wise error (FWE) $p < 0.05$]. Compared to the limited domain cognitive impairment group, patients with multidomain cognitive impairment group had more atrophy of left angular gyrus (FWE corrected $p < 0.05$).

Conclusion: Cognitive impairment may be detected on neuropsychological evaluation even in the initial phases of SCA2. Patients with cognitive dysfunction show grey matter atrophy cerebellum and frontal lobes, suggesting pathological involvement of cerebello-fronto-cortical pathways.

COMMENT

Strengths

- This study classified the participants based on the domains affected, and identified different severity levels of cognitive dysfunction associated with spinocerebellar ataxia type 2 (SCA2).
- The study had a relatively larger sample size.

Limitation

The study had a cross-sectional design and the worsening of cognitive function across time was not studied.

ARTICLE 4

Motor and Cognitive Outcomes of Cerebello-spinal Stimulation in Neurodegenerative Ataxia

Benussi A, Cantoni V, Manes M, Libri I, Dell'Era V, Datta A, et al. Motor and cognitive outcomes of cerebello-spinal stimulation in neurodegenerative ataxia.
Brain. 2021;144(8):2310-21.

Abstract

Background: The treatment of neurodegenerative cerebellar ataxia remains symptomatic. Cerebellar transcranial direct current stimulation (tDCS) has shown to improve motor functions in neurodegenerative ataxias by enhancing neuroplasticity.[7] The results of a previous pilot study from the authors' group showed beneficial effects of cerebello-spinal tDCS on motor symptoms in these patients.[8]

Aim: The aim of the study was to investigate the efficacy of cerebello-spinal tDCS in improving the motor and cognitive functions in patients with neurodegenerative ataxia.

Methods: The study had a randomized double-blind sham-controlled design with an open-label phase. At baseline (T0), patients were randomized to receive either the placebo (sham tDCS) stimulation or an anodal cerebellar and a cathodal spinal (real tDCS) stimulation for 5 days a week for 2 weeks (T1). This randomized sham-controlled phase had a 12-week follow-up and at the 12th week follow-up, all the patients received a real tDCS for 5 days a week for 2 weeks; the open-label phase had a follow-up at 14th week (T3), 24th week (T4), 36th week (T5), and 52nd week. Patients underwent a clinical, cognitive, neurophysiological, and quality of life (QoL) assessment at each time point (T0–T6). Transcranial magnetic stimulation (TMS) was used to assess the connectivity between motor and cerebellar cortex. The coprimary outcome measures were a change in the Scale for the Assessment and Rating of Ataxia (SARA), International Cooperative Ataxia Rating Scale (ICARS), and Cerebellar Cognitive Affective Syndrome Scale (CCASS) scores from baseline. The secondary outcome measures were a change in cerebellar inhibition (CBI) and SF-36 QoL scale from baseline.

Results: Sixty-one patients were randomized to receive real ($n = 33$) or sham ($n = 28$) stimulation. There was significant improvement in motor scores [SARA, mean difference (MD) 3.1 (2.3–3.9), $p < 0.001$; ICARS, MD: 8.7 (6.5–10.8), $p < 0.001$], in cognition [CCASS, MD −5.9 (−9.3 to −2.5), $p < 0.001$], in SF-36 [MD −88.8 (−121.5 to −56.2), $p < 0.001$], and CBI [MD 0.11 (0.08–0.14), $p < 0.001$] after real tDCS both at short and long term. Compared to single real tDCS, double real tDCS treatment showed better efficacy. The cognitive and motor improvement showed a correlation with the restoration of CBI. The improvement in motor scores and cognitive scores was independent of the disease subtype. Motor score improvement inversely correlated with the disease duration.

Conclusion: Repeated sessions of cerebello-spinal tDCS were effective in improving the motor and cognitive functions in neurodegenerative cerebellar ataxia. Cerebello-spinal tDCS can be a potential treatment with long-term efficacy in patients with these disorders.

COMMENT

Strength

This trial has overcome the shortcomings of the previous studies. It had a larger sample size with a double-blind, randomized, placebo-controlled phase followed by an open-label phase. This allowed determining the effects of repeated sessions of tDCS over time.

Limitation

The study included different diseases and had relatively small heterogeneous groups. Thus, one needs to interpret the results with caution.

Future Perspective

Future studies should focus on examining the efficacy of tDCS in at-home settings.

ARTICLE 5

Quantitative Evaluation of Cerebellar Function in Multiple System Atrophy with Transcranial Magnetic Stimulation

Shirota Y, Hanajima R, Shimizu T, Terao Y, Tsuji S, Ugawa Y. Quantitative evaluation of cerebellar function in multiple system atrophy with transcranial magnetic stimulation.
Cerebellum. 2022;21(2):219-24.

Abstract

Background: The objective assessment of cerebellar dysfunction in multiple system atrophy (MSA) is challenging because of the overlapping features like parkinsonism. Cerebellar inhibition (CBI) can be a quantitative measure of cerebellar function, and the degree of CBI can reflect the severity of ataxia.[9] Less CBI was observed in cases of moderate neurodegenerative as compared to mild cases.[9] The CBI is examined by transcranial magnetic stimulation (TMS). The inhibition of the primary motor cortex (M1) by the cerebellar TMS is reflected as a reduced amplitude of motor-evoked potential (MEP).[10]

Aim: This study aimed to quantify the cerebellar dysfunction in patients with cerebellar type of MSA (MSA-C) and to evaluate the correlation between disease severity and the degree of CBI.

Methods: 10 right-handed healthy subjects and 25 patients with MSA-C were recruited for the study. MEP was recorded from the first dorsal interosseous muscle on the more affected side by stimulating the hand area of M1. The cerebellar TMS (conditioning stimulus) was delivered over the midpoint between inion and mastoid process, ipsilateral to the recording site. CBI was quantified as the degree of reduction in the amplitude in the presence of conditioning stimulus as compared to isolated M1 stimulation. Correlation of CBI with the International Cooperative Ataxia Rating Scale (ICARS) was also assessed.

Results: Patients with MSA-C had higher MEP ratio than the healthy volunteers, implying a lower CBI in the patients. Correlation between the degree of CBI and ICARS subtotal score of the tested hand was significant ($r = 0.60$, $p = 0.002$). ICARS total score ($r = 0.672$, $p < 0.001$) and sub scores ($r = 0.641$, $p = 0.001$) had a significant correlation with disease duration.

Conclusion: Cerebellar inhibition is a good index of cerebellar dysfunction and has the potential to assess disease severity in MSA-C. The utility of CBI as a promising biomarker of disease progression needs to be explored in larger clinical trials.

COMMENT

Limitations
- Diagnosis of multiple system atrophy (MSA) in this study was not neuropathological.
- The study had a small sample size, and the results were not correlated with advanced neuroimaging.

Future Perspective
Application of CBI should be tested in larger clinical trials, including both parkinsonian type of MSA (MSA-P) and cerebellar type of MSA (MSA-C) patients, and the results should be correlated with advanced neuroimaging findings.

ARTICLE 6

Nicotinamide Riboside Improves Ataxia Scores and Immunoglobulin Levels in Ataxia Telangiectasia

Veenhuis SJ, van Os NJ, Janssen AJ, van Gerven MH, Coene KL, Engelke UF, et al. Nicotinamide riboside improves ataxia scores and immunoglobulin levels in ataxia telangiectasia.
Mov Disord. 2021;36(12):2951-7.

Abstract

Background: The treatment of ataxia telangiectasia (A-T) remains symptomatic to date.[11] Nicotinamide riboside (NR) is a precursor of nicotinamide adenine dinucleotide (NAD+), a substrate that plays a crucial role in DNA a repair.[12] NR has shown to improve the neurological outcome and survival in animal models of A-T.[13]

Aim: This study aimed to evaluate the efficacy of NR in patients with A-T.

Methods: This proof of concept, open-label, single center study was conducted in the Netherlands. 24 patients with A-T received NR (25 mg/kg/day) for 4 consecutive months followed by 2-months washout period. The effects of NR on ataxia rating scales [Scale for the Assessment and Rating of Ataxia (SARA) and International Cooperative Ataxia Rating Scale (ICARS)], dysarthria, the Nine-Hole Peg Test (9HPT), quality of life, and laboratory parameters including the untargeted metabolomics were assessed.

Results: The mean age of the participants was 17.5 ± 15 years and 17 were of <18 years. Amongst the 24, 18 had the classical A-T phenotype, and the rest had variant A-T. During the intervention, the mean ataxia scores, SARA (−2.4) and ICARS (−10.1) improved. The ataxia scores worsened after withdrawal of NR. The serum immunoglobulin G (IgG) concentration in the classic A-T patients increased throughout the study period, whereas IgA and IgM increased during the treatment period only. Compared to baseline, NR metabolites showed increased plasma levels at the end of the intervention period. There were no significant adverse effects on the participants.

Conclusion: In patients with A-T, treatment with NR was safe and resulted in symptomatic improvement in ataxia and serum Ig levels.

COMMENT

Strength

This study reported the effect of nicotinamide riboside (NR) on purine metabolism for the first time.

Limitations

- This study had a small sample size and was not powered to find the dose, resulting in a probable overestimation of clinical effects.

- The study had no control group and thus the possibility of the placebo effect on the outcome parameters cannot be excluded.

Future Perspective

Large longitudinal, multicenter, placebo-controlled trials are required to investigate the effect of NR treatment on the disease course of ataxia telangiectasia (A-T).

ARTICLE 7

Safety and Efficacy of Acetyl-DL-leucine in Certain Types of Cerebellar Ataxia: The ALCAT Randomized Clinical Crossover Trial

Feil K, Adrion C, Boesch S, Doss S, Giordano I, Hengel H, et al. Safety and efficacy of acetyl-DL-leucine in certain types of cerebellar ataxia: The ALCAT randomized clinical crossover trial.
JAMA Netw Open. 2021;4(12):e2135841.

Abstract

Background: No convincing disease modifying or symptomatic therapy is available to treat degenerative cerebellar ataxia.[14] Treatment with Acetyl-DL-leucine has shown an improvement of ataxia scores and gait in a series of patients with cerebellar ataxia.[15,16]

Aim: The acetyl-DL-leucine on cerebellar ataxia (ALCAT) trial aimed to examine whether treatment with acetyl-DL-leucine is efficacious and safe in patients with cerebellar ataxia of various causes.

Methods: The ALCAT trial was a multicentric double-blind placebo-controlled crossover trial. The eligible patients were ≥18 years of age, diagnosed with cerebellar ataxia of different etiologies (hereditary/nonhereditary/unknown) and had the Scale for the Assessment and Rating of Ataxia (SARA) total score of at least 3. Patients with Friedreich ataxia, clinically likely multiple system atrophy and rapidly progressive ataxia were excluded. Eligible patients were randomized to either of the two sequences; active (acetyl-DL-leucine, 5 g/day, after 14 days up-titration) followed by matching placebo (A-P), each for 42 days divided by 28 days washout period or vice versa (P-A). The primary outcome was the period-dependent absolute change in the total score of SARA from baseline to sixth week. The secondary outcome measures included EuroQol–5 dimensions-5 level (EQ-5D-5L), the Z score of the Spinocerebellar Ataxia Functional Index (SCAFI), beck depression inventory (BDI-II) and Fatigue Severity Scale (FSS).

Results: One hundred and eight patients were randomly assigned to one of the two sequences. The mean age of participants and total score of SARA was 54.8 ± 14.4 years 13.33 ± 5.57 points, respectively. The absolute change in the SARA score from the baseline to sixth week was not significant between the two treatment groups [mean difference: 0.23; 95% confidence interval (CI) –0.40 to –0.85 points; $p = 0.48$]. Secondary outcome analysis showed no benefit of acetyl-DL-leucine over the placebo.

Conclusion: In patients with cerebellar ataxia, 6 weeks of treatment of acetyl-DL-leucine was not superior to placebo. Acetyl-DL-leucine was well tolerated. The study provided valuable information about the treatment duration and placebo effects in patients with progressive ataxia.

COMMENT

Strength

Largest multicentric randomized control trial with good treatment adherence and low lost to follow-up.

Limitations

- This trial was not powered to detect heterogeneity and the treatment benefit in various ataxia subgroups.
- Trial had a short treatment period.
- Patient-centered outcome measures were not considered while evaluating the treatment benefit.
- The investigators involved in the study performed ataxia rating, increasing the risk of bias.

Future Perspective

The findings from ALCAT trial call for further trials investigating the long-term efficacy of acetyl-DL-leucine for symptomatic therapy in clearly defined ataxia population.

ARTICLE 8

Developments and Validation of a Patient-reported Outcome Measure of Ataxia

Schmahmann JD, Pierce S, MacMore J, L'Italien GJ. Development and validation of a patient-reported outcome measure of ataxia.
Mov Disord. 2021;36(10):2367-77.

Abstract

Background: Assessment of cerebellar ataxia largely depends on tools like clinical rating scales, wearable sensors, gait laboratory, biomarkers, and neuroimaging. However, the existing assessment methods are oblivious to patients' inputs about his/her disease. Patient-reported symptoms and activities could provide better insight into the disease and its progression.[17] Patient-reported outcome measures (PROMs) are also essential for evaluating the treatment response.[18] There are no existing PROMs specific to ataxia developed with the involvement of patients.

Aim: The aim of this study was to develop and validate a PROM for cerebellar ataxia (PROM-ataxia).

Methods: The PROM-ataxia was developed in five phases:

1. Development of conceptual framework, item pool development, and domain selection: An extensive online survey was conducted to collect patient's symptoms, activities, and experience related to ataxia; 147 ataxia patients completed the survey. A 70-item PROM-ataxia was developed from the responses, with 0–4 scoring on a Likert scale.
2. The cognitive debrief with in-person patient focus groups: For assessment of readability, comprehension, content validity, and relevance of each item. 17 patients grouped by ataxia severity participated in cognitive debrief.
3. Psychometric scale validation: 78 anonymized ataxia patients completed the psychometric scale validations, including the internal consistency, test–retest reliability, item versus total score correlations, and responsiveness to disease severity.
4. (A) Validation against external measures and (B) supplementary assessment of responsiveness: External validation of PROM-ataxia against the existing ataxia clinical rating scales and quality of life (QoL) scales were done in 20 patients. The phase 4 also determined the total PROM-ataxia scores for each level of ataxia severity.
5. Development of PROM-ataxia short form (10-item scale)

Results: During the conceptual framework development, 3,855 symptoms were identified and after eliminating the redundancy, a three-domain (physical, mental health, activities of daily living) 70-item PROM-ataxia was generated. PROM-ataxia was comprehensible, relevant to the disease, and had a high internal consistency, item versus total score correlation, and test–retest reliability. Responsiveness to ataxia severity stages was significant for all three domains.

The total PROM-ataxia score showed a significant correlation with three levels of ataxia severity ($r = 0.58$, $p < 0.0001$). Validation of the PROM-ataxia was performed against the established measures of emotional well-being, QoL, and motor ataxia. The correlation between PROM-ataxia short form (10-item) and the rest of the items of PROM-ataxia (60-items) was strong ($R^2 = 0.82$) ($p < 0.0001$).

Conclusion: The PROM-ataxia is a 70-item questionnaire generated in collaboration with ataxia patient groups. The scale is valid, reliable, and shows good correlation with ataxia severity.

COMMENT

Strengths

- The patient-reported outcome measure (PROM-ataxia) is the first cerebellar ataxia specific rating scale incorporating patients' inputs.
- The PROM-ataxia has the potential of improving care and wellbeing of ataxia patients. It can serve as a promising tool in natural history studies and clinical trials.

Limitations

- The proportion of cerebellar type of multiple system atrophy (MSA-C) and Friedreich's ataxia were marginal in this study, affecting the external validity.
- The PROM-ataxia is an adult scale and further studies involving the pediatric focus group might be required.

ARTICLE 9

Serum Neurofilament Light Chain as a Severity Marker for Spinocerebellar Ataxia

Shin HR, Moon J, Lee WJ, Lee HS, Kim EY, Shin S, et al. Serum neurofilament light chain as a severity marker for spinocerebellar ataxia.
Sci Rep. 2021;11(1):1-7.

Abstract

Background: Spinocerebellar ataxia (SCA) comprises a heterogeneous group of autosomal dominant (AD) ataxia with variable disease severity and prognosis.[19] There is no widely accepted biomarker to assess the progression of SCA. Serum neurofilament light chain (NfL) has been identified as a potential biomarker in various neurodegenerative diseases.[20]

Aim: The aim of this study was to assess whether serum NfL could represent the neuronal damage in AD-SCA.

Methods: This study was conducted in the Neurology Outpatient Clinic of Seoul National University Hospital. Patients diagnosed with AD-SCA, enrolled in another clinical trial (NCT03932669) were reviewed to collect the clinical and demographic details, Scale for the Assessment and Rating of Ataxia (SARA) score, and magnetic resonance imaging (MRI) brain characteristics. Serum NfL was determined using electrochemiluminescence (ECL) immunoassay. Controls were included from one orthostatic tolerance cohort. Serum NfL level of AD-SCA patients was compared with healthy control from two prior NfL.

Results: Serum NfL was measured in 49 patients with AD-SCA and was higher than controls (109.5 vs. 41.1 pg/mL) ($p < 0.001$). A significant positive correlation was observed between serum NfL level and the disease duration, trinucleotide repeat number, disease duration/age X trinucleotide repeat number, and SARA score.

Conclusion: Serum NfL was higher in patients with AD-SCA compared to controls and correlated with disease severity. Serum NfL can be a promising biomarker for monitoring the disease progression and severity in AD-SCA.

COMMENT

Limitations
- Sample size was too small to perform validation and subgroup analysis. Also, the sample size limited the analysis of correlation between serum neurofilament light chain (NfL) and cerebellar atrophy.
- Limited analysis of the correlation between trinucleotide repeats number and serum NfL because of the variability in the repeat size across the subtypes of spinocerebellar ataxia (SCA).
- Patients in the preclinical phase were not included in the study.
- The control group was not completely healthy.

Future Perspective
Further research with large longitudinal multicenter cohorts of SCA patients, including those in the preclinical stage with validation, is required to establish serum NfL as a biomarker for autosomal dominant (AD)-SCA.

ARTICLE 10

Fampridine and Acetazolamide in EA2 and Related Familial EA: A Prospective Randomized Placebo-controlled Trial

Muth C, Teufel J, Schöls L, Synofzik M, Franke C, Timmann D, et al. Fampridine and acetazolamide in EA2 and related familial EA: A prospective randomized placebo-controlled trial.
Neurol Clin Pract. 2021;11(4):e438-e446.

Abstract

Background: Episodic ataxia type 2 (EA2) is an inherited disorder caused by mutations in *CACNA1A* gene and the only recommended medications for EA2 are acetazolamide and 4-aminopyridine (4-AP).[21] The American Academy of Neurology recommends 4-AP for treatment of EA2 based on the results from a double-blind placebo-controlled crossover trial.[22] Acetazolamide treatment can avoid or reduce the attacks of EA2.[23] The efficacy of acetazolamide and fampridine (prolonged-release form of 4-AP) has not been proven in randomized controlled trials.

Aim: The aim of this study was to investigate the safety and efficacy of treatment with acetazolamide and fampridine in patients with EA2.

Methods: Episodic Ataxia Type 2 TREAtment Trial (EAT2TREAT) was a phase 3, randomized, double-blind, placebo-controlled crossover trial. All eligible patients (≥ 18 years) with genetically proven EA2 or familial EAs were recruited to receive each of the treatment options for 12 weeks each in a three-period crossover design. Patients received acetazolamide 250 mg three times daily, fampridine 10 mg twice daily, and a placebo in one of the six possible treatment sequences. Between the first and second treatment, there was a washout of 4 weeks. The primary outcome was the number of attacks during the last 30 days within the treatment period. The secondary outcome measures were the median duration and severity of the attacks in the last 30 days within the treatment period. Other secondary measures included the changes in the coefficient of variability of maximal walking speed, Scale for the Assessment and Rating of Ataxia (SARA) score, Vestibular Disorders Activities of Daily Living Scale (VDADL), and EuroQol in five dimensions with five-level scale (EQ-5D-5L) at the end of treatment period and at 4 weeks of follow-up after the treatment period compared to baseline. Adverse events were documented throughout the study period.

Results: 30 patients were randomized to receive one of the six treatment sequences; 18/30 had CACNA1A mutation, 7 were negative for mutation, and 5 were not tested. Compared to placebo, fampridine and acetazolamide decreased the number of attacks to 63% [95% confidence interval (CI) 54–74%] and 52% (95% CI 46–60%), respectively. The secondary outcome analysis showed no significant effect of fampridine and acetazolamide compared to placebo. The adverse events were reported with fampridine, acetazolamide, and placebo treatment were 26.5% (sensory symptoms and paresthesia most frequently), 44.9% (taste disturbances and gastrointestinal symptoms most frequently), and 28.6%, respectively.

Conclusion: In patients with EA2 and related EA, fampridine and acetazolamide had comparable efficacy in reducing the number of attacks. Compared to acetazolamide 750 mg/day, fampridine 20 mg/day had a lesser number of adverse effects. The EAT2TREAT trial provides class II evidence.

COMMENT

Limitation
Only 18 patients in this study had a genetically defined diagnosis of episodic ataxia type 2 (EA2).

Future Perspective
- Further studies that directly compare fampridine and acetazolamide or test the efficacy of a combination of these agents should be planned, as the mechanism of action is different.
- As EA has the onset in infancy and childhood, efficacy and safety of these drugs should be tested in the pediatric population as well.

REFERENCES (Ataxia)

1. Saleem Q, Choudhry S, Mukerji M, Bashyam L, Padma M, Chakravarthy A, et al. Molecular analysis of autosomal dominant hereditary ataxias in the Indian population: high frequency of SCA2 and evidence for a common founder mutation. Hum Genet. 2000;106(2):179-87.
2. Bürk K, Globas C, Bösch S, Klockgether T, Zühlke C, Daum I, et al. Cognitive deficits in spinocerebellar ataxia type 1, 2, and 3. J Neurol. 2003;250(2):207-11.
3. Suenaga M, Kawai Y, Watanabe H, Atsuta N, Ito M, Tanaka F, et al. Cognitive impairment in spinocerebellar ataxia type 6. J Neurol Neurosurg Psychiatry. 2008;79(5):496-9.
4. Choudhury S, Chatterjee S, Chatterjee K, Banerjee R, Humby J, Mondal B, et al. Clinical characterization of genetically diagnosed cases of spinocerebellar ataxia type 12 from India. Mov Disord Clin Pract. 2017;5(1):39-46.
5. Lindsay E, Storey E. Cognitive changes in the spinocerebellar ataxias due to expanded polyglutamine tracts: a survey of the literature. Brain Sci. 2017;7(7):83.
6. Storey E, Forrest SM, Shaw JH, Mitchell P, Gardner RM. Spinocerebellar ataxia type 2: clinical features of a pedigree displaying prominent frontal-executive dysfunction. Arch Neurol. 1999;56(1):43-50.
7. Chen TX, Yang CY, Willson G, Lin CC, Kuo SH. The efficacy and safety of transcranial direct current stimulation for cerebellar ataxia: a systematic review and meta-analysis. Cerebellum. 2021;20(1):124-33.
8. Benussi A, Borroni B. Author response: Cerebello-spinal tDCS in ataxia: A randomized, double-blind, sham-controlled, crossover trial. Neurology. 2019;92(23):1122.
9. Ugawa Y, Terao Y, Hanajima R, Sakai K, Furubayashi T, Machii K, et al. Magnetic stimulation over the cerebellum in patients with ataxia. Electroencephalogr Clin Neurophysiol. 1997;104(5):453-8.
10. Ugawa Y, Terao Y, Hanajima R, Sakai K, Furubayashi T, Machii K, et al. Magnetic stimulation over the cerebellum in patients with ataxia. Electroencephalogr Clin Neurophysiol. 1997;104(5):453-8.
11. van Os NJ, Haaxma CA, van der Flier M, Merkus PJ, van Deuren M, de Groot IJ, et al.; A-T Study Group. Ataxia-telangiectasia: recommendations for multidisciplinary treatment. Dev Med Child Neurol. 2017;59(7):680-9.
12. Weidele K, Beneke S, Bürkle A. The NAD+ precursor nicotinic acid improves genomic integrity in human peripheral blood mononuclear cells after X-irradiation. DNA Repair (Amst). 2017;52:12-23.
13. Fang EF, Kassahun H, Croteau DL, Scheibye-Knudsen M, Marosi K, Lu H, et al. NAD+ replenishment improves lifespan and healthspan in ataxia telangiectasia models via mitophagy and DNA repair. Cell Metab. 2016;24(4):566-81.
14. Gandini J, Manto M, Brémovà-Ertl T, Feil K, Strupp M. The neurological update: therapies for cerebellar ataxias in 2020. J Neurol. 2020;267(4):1211-20.
15. Strupp M, Teufel J, Habs M, Feuerecker R, Muth C, van de Warrenburg BP, et al. Effects of acetyl-DL-leucine in patients with cerebellar ataxia: a case series. J Neurol. 2013;260(10):2556-61.
16. Schniepp R, Strupp M, Wuehr M, Jahn K, Dieterich M, Brandt T, et al. Acetyl-DL-leucine improves gait variability in patients with cerebellar ataxia-a case series. Cerebellum Ataxias. 2016;3:8.
17. Black N, Jenkinson C. Measuring patients' experiences and outcomes. BMJ. 2009;339:b2495.
18. Wiering B, de Boer D, Delnoij D. Patient involvement in the development of patient-reported outcome measures:

The developers' perspective. BMC Health Serv Res. 2017;17(1):635.
19. Klockgether T, Mariotti C, Paulson HL. Spinocerebellar ataxia. Nat Rev Dis Primers. 2019;5(1):25.
20. Zetterberg H. Neurofilament light: a dynamic cross-disease fluid biomarker for neurodegeneration. Neuron. 2016;91(1):1-3.
21. Denier C, Ducros A, Vahedi KA, Joutel A, Thierry P, Ritz A, et al. High prevalence of CACNA1A truncations and broader clinical spectrum in episodic ataxia type 2. Neurology. 1999;52(9):1816-21.
22. Strupp M, Kalla R, Claassen J, Adrion C, Mansmann U, Klopstock T, et al. A randomized trial of 4-aminopyridine in EA2 and related familial episodic ataxias. Neurology. 2011;77(3):269-75.
23. Strupp M, Zwergal A, Brandt T. Episodic ataxia type 2. Neurotherapeutics. 2007;4(2):267-73.

Section 7: Dementia and Cognition

Section Editors: Suvarna Alladi, Atanu Biswas, Faheem Arshad

Associate Editor: S Sandeep Kumar

ARTICLE 1

Estimation of the Global Prevalence of Dementia in 2019 and Forecasted Prevalence in 2050: An Analysis for the Global Burden of Disease Study 2019

GBD 2019 Dementia Forecasting Collaborators. Estimation of the global prevalence of dementia in 2019 and forecasted prevalence in 2050: An analysis for the Global Burden of Disease Study 2019. *Lancet Public Health. 2022;7(2):e105-e125.*

Abstract

Background: It is anticipated that there will be more dementia patients as a result of projected trends in population growth and ageing. The significance of possibly modifiable risk factors for dementia has also been strongly supported by studies. Planning for public health and allocating scarce resources require a thorough understanding of the distribution and size of predicted increase. By generating estimates at the country level and include data on a few key risk factors, the present study aimed to improve on earlier predictions of dementia prevalence.

Methods: Using relative risks and projected risk factor prevalence, we predicted the prevalence of dementia attributable to the three dementia risk factors included in the Global Burden of Diseases (GBD), Injuries, and Risk Factors Study 2019 (high body mass index, high fasting plasma glucose, and smoking) from 2019 to 2050. We did this both globally and by world region and country. We next predicted the prevalence of dementia not caused by GBD hazards using linear regression models with schooling as an additional predictor. We performed a decomposition analysis to determine the relative contributions of future developments in GBD risk factors, education, population growth, and population ageing.

Findings: According to our projection, there will be 152.8 (130.8–175.9) million cases of dementia worldwide by 2050, up from 57.4 (95% confidence interval 50.4–65.1) million cases in 2019. Age-standardized both-sex prevalence remained steady between 2019 and 2050 [global percentage change of 0.1% (-7.5 to 10.8)], despite expected increases in the number of dementia sufferers. According to our estimates, there were 1.69 (1.64–1.73) times as many women as males worldwide who had dementia in 2019. We anticipate this trend to last until 2050, when it will increase to 1.67 (1.52–1.85). There was geographic heterogeneity in the projected increases across the various nations and regions, with the highest percentage increases in North Africa and the Middle East [367% (329–403)] and eastern sub-Saharan Africa [357% (323–395)] and the lowest percentage changes in high-income Asia Pacific [53% (41–67)] and Western Europe. Although their relative importance varied by world region, projected increases in cases could largely be attributed to population growth and population ageing, with population growth being most responsible for increases in sub-Saharan Africa and population ageing being most responsible for increases in East Asia.

Interpretation: Dementia is becoming more prevalent, which emphasizes the need for public health planning initiatives and policies to address this group's requirements. Estimates at the national level can help guide planning and decision-making processes. In order to address the anticipated rise in the number of people afflicted by dementia, multifaceted strategies will be essential. These strategies should include scaling up treatments to address modifiable risk factors and investing in research on biological causes.

COMMENT

This study estimated prevalence of dementia in all countries in different geographical areas in 2019. Although several other studies have attempted to estimate prevalence,[1] the Global Burden of Diseases (GBD) estimate appears plausible due to its robust methodology and universal coverage. The article gives projected numbers of dementia sufferers in different countries in 2050 and percentage of rise from that in the year 2019. Dementia rates are growing at alarming proportion in all regions of the world and are related to population aging. In some geographic areas this increment is due to population growth as in sub-Saharan Africa. This estimate is a wakeup call for all of us. Policy-makers need to take public health measures for risk reduction and creating public awareness urgently. There is also a growing need to invest in creating infrastructure to provide management to these huge numbers of dementia sufferers in near future.

ARTICLE 2

Validation of ICMR Neurocognitive Toolbox for Dementia in the Linguistically Diverse Context of India

Verma M, Tripathi M, Nehra A, Paplikar A, Varghese F, Alladi S, et al. Validation of ICMR neurocognitive toolbox for dementia in the linguistically diverse context of India.
Front Neurol. 2021;12:661269.

Abstract

Objective: The growing prevalence of dementia, especially in low- and middle-income countries (LMICs), has raised the need for a unified cognitive screening tool that can aid its early detection. The linguistically and educationally diverse population in India contributes to challenges in diagnosis. The present study aimed to assess the validity and diagnostic accuracy of the Indian Council of Medical Research-Neurocognitive Toolbox (ICMR-NCTB), a comprehensive neuropsychological test battery adapted in five languages, for the diagnosis of dementia.

Methods: A multidisciplinary group of experts developed the ICMR-NCTB based on reviewing the existing tools and incorporation of culturally appropriate modifications. The finalized tests of the major cognitive domains of attention, executive functions, memory, language, and visuospatial skills were then adapted and translated into five Indian languages: Hindi, Bengali, Telugu, Kannada, and Malayalam. 354 participants were recruited, including 222 controls and 132 dementia patients. The sensitivity and specificity of the adapted tests were established for the diagnosis of dementia.

Result: A significant difference in the mean (median) performance scores between healthy controls and patients with dementia was observed on all tests of ICMR-NCTB. The area under the curve for majority of the tests included in the ICMR-NCTB ranged from 0.73 to 1.00, and the sensitivity and specificity of the ICMR-NCTB tests ranged from 70 to 100% and 70.7 to 100%, respectively, to identify dementia across all five languages.

Conclusion: The ICMR-NCTB is a valid instrument to diagnose dementia across five Indian languages, with good diagnostic accuracy. The toolbox was effective in overcoming the challenge of linguistic diversity. The study has wide implications to address the problem of a high disease burden and low diagnostic rate of dementia in LMICs like India.

COMMENT

Challenges to diagnosis to dementia are cultural, linguistic, and educationally heterogeneity across the world, and especially so in India. In India, there are at least 5.29 million people living with dementia currently. The linguistically and educationally diverse population in India contributes to challenges in diagnosis. Harmonizing diagnosis across diversity is crucial for developing effective intervention strategies. The cognitive test battery known as Indian Council of Medical Research-Neurocognitive Toolbox (ICMR-NCTB)[2] was adapted and validated in five Indian languages (Hindi, Bengali, Telugu, Kannada, and Malayalam) to diagnose dementia and other cognitive disorders. The tests of ICMR-NCTB showed high sensitivity and the specificity at optimal cutoff scores, suggesting the ability of the tests to diagnose dementia in Indian languages. The test battery has wide implications to address the problem of a high disease burden and low diagnostic rate of dementia in low- and middle-income countries (LMICs) like India.

ARTICLE 3

Progression of Subjective Cognitive Decline to MCI or Dementia in Relation to Biomarkers for Alzheimer's Disease: A Meta-analysis

Rostamzadeh A, Bohr L, Wagner M, Baethge C, Jessen F. Progression of subjective cognitive decline to MCI or dementia in relation to biomarkers for Alzheimer disease: A meta-analysis.
Neurology. 2022;10.1212/WNL.0000000000201072.

Abstract

Background and Objective: The risk of mild cognitive impairment (MCI) or dementia in individuals with subjective cognitive decline (SCD) and biomarkers indicating Alzheimer's disease (AD) pathology in comparison to individuals with SCD without biomarker evidence for AD is critical to delineate the potential role of biomarkers assessment in this group. We performed a meta-analysis of studies on this topic.

Methods: Three databases (PUBMED, PsycINFO, and Cochrane) were searched from inception to May 7, 2021. Search strings included the terms: SCD, biomarker, amyloid, tau, risk, Alzheimer, MCI, and dementia. Following PRISMA and Cochrane guidelines, two researchers independently performed literature search, data collection, and data extraction. We summarized odds ratios (ORs) in random-effects meta-analyses and calculated sensitivity, specificity, positive and negative predictive values (PPVs, NPVs), and likelihood ratios. The primary outcome was the OR of progressing from SCD to MCI or dementia in cases with biomarkers indicative of AD pathology relative to the chance of progression in cases with biomarkers indicating no AD pathology.

Result: Out of 4,147 studies screened, 8 studies were selected. The risk of bias analysis revealed low risk of bias in all studies. The prevalence of abnormal biomarkers ranged between 15.6 and 35.4% for amyloid, 11.1–33.7% for p-tau, 12.4–46.3% for t-tau, and 7.8–24.4% for full AD pathology (amyloid pathology with either increased p-tau or t-tau). The chance of clinical progression was increased in cases of amyloid pathology only [OR 5.89; 95% confidence interval (CI) 2.33–14.90], elevated p-tau (OR 3.99; 95% CI 2.34–6.85), elevated t-tau (OR 2.26; 95% CI 1.14–4.48), and full AD pathology (OR 11.36; 95% CI 1.97–65.41). The latter showed a PPV of 59.7% (95% CI 48.8–69.3%) and a NPV of 89.4% (95% CI 86.7–91.7%), whereas amyloid pathology only showed a PPV of 28.2% (95% CI 23.7–32.2%), and a NPV of 94.9% (95% CI 93.4–96.2%).

Discussion: Individuals with SCD and full AD pathology have a substantially increased risk of developing MCI or dementia in comparison with individuals with SCD without AD pathology.

COMMENT

Subjective cognitive decline (SCD) is a risk factor for dementia. There is emerging evidence that a biological characterization of cognitive decline and dementia is important for developing preventive and treatment strategies. This meta-analysis summarizes the current literature on Alzheimer's disease (AD) biomarker-associated progression to mild cognitive impairment (MCI) or dementia in SCD. It suggests that compared to SCD without AD biomarker abnormalities, the chance of cognitive decline to MCI or dementia in SCD is highest when combined with amyloid pathology with elevated p-tau or t-tau, indicating full AD pathology is present. This underscores the need for fluid biomarkers for the diagnosis of dementia years in advance of the onset of clinical symptoms.[3]

ARTICLE 4

Longitudinal Cognitive Changes in Genetic Frontotemporal Dementia within the GENFI Cohort

Poos JM, MacDougall A, van den Berg E, Jiskoot LC, Papma JM, van der Ende EL, et al.; Genetic FTD Initiative (GENFI). Longitudinal cognitive changes in genetic frontotemporal dementia within the GENFI cohort. *Neurology. 2022;99(3):e281-e295.*

Abstract

Background and Objective: There are currently ongoing disease-modifying trials for genetic frontotemporal dementia (FTD), however, sensitive cognitive outcome assessments are missing. By examining cognitive deterioration in a sizable cohort of genetic carriers of the FTD pathogenic mutation and by examining whether gene-specific differences are influenced by illness stage, the goal of this study was to discover such cognitive assessments in early stage FTD (asymptomatic, prodromal, and symptomatic).

Methods: As part of the genetic FTD initiative, a prospective multicenter cohort study, carriers of *C9orf72*, *GRN*, and *MAPT* pathogenic variants as well as controls had an annual neuropsychological evaluation spanning eight cognitive domains. Using the global clinical dementia rating (CDR) and National Alzheimer's Coordinating Center (NACC) frontotemporal lobar degeneration (FTLD) score (0, 0.5, or 1), pathogenic variant carriers were sorted by illness stage. The differences between genetic groups and illness stages as well as the three-way interaction between time, genetic group, and disease stage were examined using linear mixed-effects models.

Result: There were a total of 207 carriers of the pathogenic *C9orf72*, *GRN*, and *MAPT* variants, along with 206 controls. From CDR + NACC FTLD 0 onward, *C9orf72* pathogenic variant carriers showed worse performance on verbal fluency, executive function, and attention, with only a little reduction over time (i.e., disease progression). Lower memory function at CDR plus NACC FTLD 0.5, a gradual loss in language from the CDR plus NACC FTLD 0.5 stage onward, and executive dysfunction that emerged quickly at CDR plus NACC FTLD 1 were all characteristics of the cognitive profile in *MAPT* pathogenic variant carriers. Verbal fluency and visuoconstruction in *GRN* pathogenic variant carriers decreased at the CDR plus NACC FTLD 0.5 stage, and other cognitive domains began to degrade gradually at the CDR plus NACC FTLD 1 stage.

Discussion: In the asymptomatic and prodromal stages of hereditary FTD, we verified cognitive deterioration. At baseline, assessments for attention, executive function, language, and memory clearly distinguished genetic groups from controls, but the rate of change over time varied by genetic group and disease stage. This demonstrates the relevance of neuropsychological testing in monitoring the development and progression of clinical symptoms and may help clinical trials choose sensitive endpoints for assessing the effectiveness of treatment as well as define the ideal window for treatment initiation.

COMMENT

Frontotemporal dementia (FTD) is a complex group of disorders with heterogeneity in clinical, imaging, and genetic profiles. Recent advances suggest that understanding genetic mechanisms will contribute to understanding prognosis and developing specific treatments. This longitudinal study investigated a large cohort of all three major causes of genetic FTD (*MAPT, GRN,* and *C9orf72*) over a 5-year period. They observed significant differences in the tests of attention, executive function, language, and memory between genetic and healthy controls at baseline. This demonstrates the relevance of detailed cognitive assessment in monitoring and progression of clinical symptoms and may help clinical trials in selecting sensitive endpoints for measuring treatment effectiveness. The gene-specific cognitive composite scores have also been used, which have resulted in lower estimated sample sizes to detect a treatment effect.[4]

ARTICLE 5

Longitudinal Changes in Hearing and Visual Impairments and Risk of Dementia in Older Adults in the United States

Hwang PH, Longstreth WT Jr, Thielke SM, Francis CE, Carone M, Kuller LH, et al. Longitudinal changes in hearing and visual impairments and risk of dementia in older adults in the United States.
JAMA Netw Open. 2022;5(5):e2210734.

Abstract

Importance: Hearing and vision problems are individually associated with increased dementia risk, but the impact of having concurrent hearing and vision deficits, i.e., dual sensory impairment (DSI), on risk of dementia, including its major subtypes Alzheimer's disease (AD) and vascular dementia (VaD), is not well known.

Objective: To evaluate whether DSI is associated with incident dementia in older adults.

Design, Setting, and Participants: This prospective cohort study from the Cardiovascular Health Study (CHS) was conducted between 1992 and 1999, with as many as 8 years of follow-up. The multicenter, population-based sample was recruited from Medicare eligibility files in four US communities with academic medical centers. Of 5,888 participants aged 65 years and older in CHS, 3,602 underwent cranial magnetic resonance imaging and completed the modified Mini-Mental State Examination in 1992–1994 as part of the CHS Cognition Study. A total of 227 participants were excluded due to prevalent dementia, leaving a total of 3,375 participants without dementia at study baseline. The study hypothesis was that DSI would be associated with increased risk of dementia compared with no sensory impairment. The association between the duration of DSI with risk of dementia was also evaluated. Data analysis was conducted from November, 2019 to February, 2020.

Exposures: Hearing and vision impairments were collected via self-report at baseline and as many as 5 follow-up visits.

Main Outcomes and Measures: All-cause dementia, AD, and VaD, classified by a multidisciplinary committee using standardized criteria.

Result: A total of 2,927 participants with information on hearing and vision at all available study visits were included in the analysis {mean [standard deviation (SD)] age, 74.6 (4.8) years; 1,704 (58.2%) women; 455 (15.5%) African American or Black; 2,472 (85.5%) White}. Compared with no sensory impairment, DSI was associated with increased risk of all-cause dementia [hazard ratio (HR) 2.60; 95% confidence interval (CI) 1.66–2.06; $p < 0.001$], AD (HR 3.67; 95% CI 2.04–6.60; $p < 0.001$) but not VaD (HR 2.03; 95% CI 1.00–4.09; $p = 0.05$).

Conclusion and Relevance: In this cohort study, DSI was associated with increased risk of dementia, particularly AD. Evaluation of hearing and vision in older adults may help to identify those at high risk of developing dementia.

COMMENT

Dual sensory impairment (vision and hearing impairment) has been identified as a potential risk factor for cognitive decline and dementia that can, in many cases, be corrected and thereby sustain cognitive function. The present study contributes to an increasing body of recent literature indicating an association between dual sensory impairment and dementia in older adults. The study elaborates the existing hypotheses that associates sensory impairments and dementia such as sensory deprivation theory[5] and common causative pathways. This cohort study emphasizes that sensory impairment is associated with dementia and may help diagnose dementia in early stages. There is a need to further understand underlying mechanisms that associates sensory impairments, cognitive impairments, and dementia[6] and investigate the bidirectional relationship that will have implications for preventive and therapeutic measures for sensory impairments.

ARTICLE 6

Sex Differences in the Genetic Architecture of Cognitive Resilience to Alzheimer's Disease

Eissman JM, Dumitrescu L, Mahoney ER, Smith AN, Mukherjee S, Lee ML, et al.; Alzheimer's Disease Neuroimaging Initiative (ADNI), Alzheimer's Disease Genetics Consortium (ADGC), A4 Study Team. Sex differences in the genetic architecture of cognitive resilience to Alzheimer's disease.
Brain. 2022;145(7):2541-54.

Abstract

Approximately 30% of elderly adults are cognitively unimpaired at time of death despite the presence of Alzheimer's disease neuropathology at autopsy. Studying individuals who are resilient to the cognitive consequences of Alzheimer's disease neuropathology may uncover novel therapeutic targets to treat Alzheimer's disease. It is well established that there are sex differences in response to Alzheimer's disease pathology, and growing evidence suggests that genetic factors may contribute to these differences. Taken together, we sought to elucidate sex-specific genetic drivers of resilience. We extended our recent large scale genomic analysis of resilience in which we harmonized cognitive data across four cohorts of cognitive ageing, in vivo amyloid positron emission tomography (PET) across two cohorts, and autopsy measures of amyloid neuritic plaque burden across two cohorts. These data were leveraged to build robust, continuous resilience phenotypes. With these phenotypes, we performed sex-stratified [n (males) = 2,093, n (females) = 2,931] and sex-interaction [n (both sexes) = 5,024] genome-wide association studies (GWAS), gene and pathway-based tests, and genetic correlation analyses to clarify the variants, genes, and molecular pathways that relate to resilience in a sex-specific manner. Estimated among cognitively normal individuals of both sexes, resilience was 20–25% heritable, and when estimated in either sex among cognitively normal individuals, resilience was 15–44% heritable. In our GWAS, we identified a female-specific locus on chromosome 10 [rs827389, β (females) = 0.08, p (females) = 5.76×10^{-09}; β (males) = -0.01, p (males) = 0.70; β (interaction) = 0.09, p (interaction) = 1.01×10^{-04}] in which the minor allele was associated with higher resilience scores among females. This locus is located within chromatin loops that interact with promoters of genes involved in RNA processing, including GATA3. Finally, our genetic correlation analyses revealed shared genetic architecture between resilience phenotypes and other complex traits, including a female-specific association with frontotemporal dementia and male-specific associations with heart rate variability traits. We also observed opposing associations between sexes for multiple sclerosis, such that more resilient females had a lower genetic susceptibility to multiple sclerosis, and more resilient males had a higher genetic susceptibility to multiple sclerosis. Overall, we identified sex differences in the genetic architecture of resilience, identified a female-specific resilience locus and highlighted numerous sex-specific molecular pathways that may underly resilience to Alzheimer's disease pathology. This study illustrates the need to conduct sex-aware genomic analyses to identify novel targets that are unidentified in sex-agnostic models. Our findings support the theory that the most successful treatment for an individual with Alzheimer's disease may be personalized based on their biological sex and genetic context.

COMMENT

Emerging evidence in the understanding of Alzheimer's disease (AD) indicate that biological significance of sex tends to impact the neuropathological and clinical pathway of AD.[1] The current study indicates that sex differences in cognitive resilience to amyloid pathology may be influenced by genetic factors. The study also indicates that improvement of cognitive resilience to AD pathology may be dependent on both biological sex and the genetic conditions.[7]

A female-specific resilience locus was identified that may underly resilience to AD pathology through sex-specific molecular pathways. It is increasingly important to investigate sex-specific genetic influencers on dementia risk and protection,[8] and future dementia studies need to include an increased emphasis on sex stratification and sex interactions to validate and contribute to understanding of this complex relationship.

ARTICLE 7

Longitudinal Study of the Effect of a 5-year Exercise Intervention on Structural Brain Complexity in Older Adults. A Generation 100 Substudy

Pani J, Marzi C, Stensvold D, Wisløff U, Håberg AK, Diciotti S. Longitudinal study of the effect of a 5-year exercise intervention on structural brain complexity in older adults. A Generation 100 substudy.
Neuroimage. 2022;256:119226.

Abstract

Dementia risk factors have been linked closely to physical inactivity. The risk of dementia has been demonstrated to decrease with high levels of cardiorespiratory fitness (CRF). The exact way that exercise affects the health of the brain, meanwhile, is still up for debate. An index called fractal dimension (FD) measures how complex the brain's structure is. This study looked at 105 healthy older individuals who were a subset of the Generation 100 Study's randomized controlled trial to see how a 5-year exercise regimen affected the structural complexity of the brain as evaluated by the FD. Randomly assigned groups of controls, moderate intensity continuous training, and high-intensity interval training were created for the participants. At the baseline and at the 1, 3, and 5-year follow-up, brain magnetic resonance imaging (MRI) and CRF were both obtained. FreeSurfer was used to extract the cortical thickness and volume data, and the grey and white matter of the brain, cerebellum, and cerebral cortex were computed using FD. Ergospirometry was used to evaluate CRF as peak oxygen uptake (VO_2 peak) during graded maximal exertion testing. We looked into exercise group differences and potential CRF effects on the complexity of the brain's structural organization using linear mixed models. If there was a significant correlation between CRF and FD, associations between changes over time in CRF and FD were conducted. Group membership had no impact on the structural complexity. However, we discovered a significant correlation between CRF and the FDs of the cerebral and temporal lobe grey matter ($p < 0.001$). Cortical thickness did not experience this effect, indicating that FD is a more sensitive indicator of structural alterations. From baseline to the 5-year follow-up, the change in temporal lobe grey matter FD was correlated with the change in CRF ($p < 0.05$). There was no correlation between CRF and FD in the cerebral grey matter. These findings showed that structural complexity loss in regions vulnerable to ageing and age-related disease was prevented by entering old life with high and preserved CRF levels.

COMMENT

Physical exercise is an established neuroprotective factor against dementia.[1] This longitudinal study provided exercise intervention for older adults over 5 years and found that fractal dimension as a measure of brain structural complexity increases with better cardiorespiratory fitness (CRF) especially in the temporal lobe. This indicates that maintaining a good CRF through physical exercise can protect the brain from structural decline due to neurodegenerative diseases.[9]

ARTICLE 8

Yoga Prevents Gray Matter Atrophy in Women at Risk for Alzheimer's Disease: A Randomized Controlled Trial

Krause-Sorio B, Siddarth P, Kilpatrick L, Milillo MM, Aguilar-Faustino Y, Ercoli L, et al. Yoga prevents gray matter atrophy in women at risk for Alzheimer's disease: A randomized controlled trial.
J Alzheimers Dis. 2022;87(2):569-81.

Abstract

Background: Subjective cognitive decline (SCD), female sex, and cardiovascular risk factors (CVRFs) are recognized risk factors for Alzheimer's disease (AD) development. In older persons with mild cognitive impairment, yoga has been shown to improve depression, resilience, memory, and executive functioning. It has also been shown to raise hippocampus choline concentrations and modify brain connectivity.

Objective: In this trial (NCT03503669), we examined the effects of memory training and yoga on changes in brain grey matter volume (GMV) in older women with SCD and CVRFs after 3 months of yoga [memory enhancement training (MET)].

Methods: 12 weeks of *Kundalini Yoga* and *Kirtan Kriya* (KY + KK) were completed by 11 women [mean age = 61.45, standard deviation (SD) = 6.58] with CVRF and SCD, while 11 women (mean age = 64.55, SD = 6.41) received MET. T1-weighted magnetic resonance imaging (MRI) scans and baseline and 12-week assessments of anxiety, resilience, stress, and depression were also performed (Siemens 3T Prisma scanner). We examined group differences in GMV change using FreeSurfer 6.0 and Monte-Carlo simulations with alpha = 0.05. A region-of-interest study of the hippocampus and amygdala was conducted.

Result: The GMV in the left prefrontal, pre- and postcentral, supramarginal, superior temporal, and pericalcarine cortices, as well as the banks of the superior temporal sulcus, the pars opercularis, and the right paracentral, postcentral, superior, and inferior parietal cortices, decreased in the presence of MET compared to KY + KK. Yoga resulted with a rise in the right hippocampus volume, however, this gain did not last corrections.

Conclusion: Even over brief periods of time, yoga training may have neuroprotective advantages relative to MET in avoiding neurodegenerative alterations and cognitive deterioration. Future studies will focus on modifications in functional connections between the two groups.

COMMENT

Subjective cognitive decline (SCD), cardiovascular health, and female sex are considered as risk factors for developing Alzheimer's disease.[10-12] This randomized controlled trial demonstrated that yoga training for 3 months among older female adults with SCD and cardiovascular risk factors improves grey matter volume in the left hemispheric regions as well as right hippocampus. This emphasize the need for adopting lifestyle changes that are neuroprotective against neurodegeneration and cognitive decline.

ARTICLE 9

Clinical Characteristics with Inflammation Profiling of Long COVID and Association with 1-year Recovery Following Hospitalization in the UK: A Prospective Observational Study

PHOSP-COVID Collaborative Group. Clinical characteristics with inflammation profiling of long COVID and association with 1-year recovery following hospitalisation in the UK: A prospective observational study.
Lancet Respir Med. 2022;10(8):761-75.

Abstract

Background: For patients with protracted COVID, there are no efficient pharmaceutical or nonpharmacological therapies available. By describing the underlying inflammatory profiles of the previously described recovery clusters at 5 months after hospital discharge, we aimed to describe recovery for COVID-19 1 year after hospital discharge, identify factors associated with patient-perceived recovery, and identify potential therapeutic targets.

Methods: The posthospitalization COVID-19 study (PHOSP-COVID) is a prospective, longitudinal cohort study that enrolls persons (aged 18 years) who have COVID-19 and have been released from the hospital throughout the UK. At 5 months and 1 year after hospital discharge, recovery was assessed using patient-reported outcome measures, physical performance, and organ function, and stratified by both patient-perceived recovery and recovery cluster. At 1 year, patient-perceived recovery was modeled using hierarchical logistic regression. The clustering large applications k-medoids approach was used to analyze clinical outcomes at 5 months. At the 5-month visit, inflammatory protein profiling was performed on plasma. The ISRCTN registry number for this study is ISRCTN10980107, and recruitment is ongoing.

Finding: A total of 2,320 patients who were released from the hospital between March 7, 2020 and April 18, 2021, were evaluated 5 months after discharge, and 807 (32%) of those patients returned for both the 5-month and 1-year assessments. The mean age of these 807 patients was 58.7 years (SD 12.5), and 279 (35.6%) of the female patients and 505 (64%) of the male patients underwent invasive mechanical breathing (WHO class 7–9). Between 5 months [501 (25%) of 1965] and 1 year [232 (28%) of 804], the percentage of patients claiming full recovery remained constant. Female sex [odds ratio 0.68 (95% CI 0.46–0.99)], obesity [0.50 (0.34–0.74)], and invasive mechanical breathing [0.42 (0.23–0.76)] were linked with a lower likelihood of reporting full recovery at one year. The four previously reported clusters—very severe, severe, moderate with cognitive impairment, and mild—relating to the severity of physical health, mental health, and cognitive impairment at five months—were confirmed by a cluster analysis ($n = 1,636$). In both the extremely severe and the moderate with cognitive impairment clusters compared to the mild cluster, we discovered elevated levels of inflammatory mediators of tissue damage and repair, including interleukin-6 (IL-6) concentration, which was elevated in both groups ($n = 626$ people). We discovered a significant deficit in the median EQ-5D-5L utility index before COVID-19 [retrospective assessment; 0.88 (IQR 0.74–1.00)], at 5 months [0.74 (0.64–0.88)], and at 1 year [0.75 (0.62–0.88)] with only minor improvements across all outcome measures at 1 year after discharge in the entire cohort and within each of the four clusters.

Interpretation: 1 year after discharge, the COVID-19 hospitalization still had significant effects on a number of health categories, and only a small portion of our group reported feeling entirely recovered. At 1 year compared to before hospital admission, the patient's reported quality of life in terms of their health was lower. Obesity and systemic inflammation are potentially curable conditions that demand additional study in clinical trials.

COMMENT

The recent COVID-19 has had a devastating impact on health of societies globally. In addition to effects related to acute infection, the long-term consequences are being recognized. This prospective study tried to assess the recovery, characterized the sequelae, and identify potential targets for intervention by describing associated risk factors and inflammatory profiles of patients, 1 year after their hospital discharge for COVID-19 infection. The most common symptoms as per this study are fatigue, muscle pain, poor sleep, physically slowing down, and breathlessness. They also clustered the symptomatic patients with very severe, severe, moderate with cognitive impairment, and mild. This study also demonstrated significant difference between systematic inflammatory markers between various clusters with higher levels of interleukin-6 (IL 6) in patients with very severe and moderate with cognitive impairment clusters than in mild cluster. Female gender, obesity, and reduced exercise were associated with severity of cluster.[13] The study contributes to growing literature confirming chronic consequences of COVID-19 infection and yields insights into underlying mechanisms.

ARTICLE 10

Cognition, Behavior, and Caregiver Stress in Dementia during the COVID-19 Pandemic: An Indian Perspective

Rajagopalan J, Arshad F, Thomas PT, Varghese F, Hurzuk S, Hoskeri RM, et al. Cognition, behavior, and caregiver stress in dementia during the COVID-19 pandemic: An Indian Perspective.
Dement Geriatr Cogn Disord. 2022;51(1):90-100.

Abstract

Objective: Little is known regarding the cognitive and behavioral status of patients with dementia and their caregivers in lower middle-income countries during the COVID-19 pandemic. This study aimed to understand the impact of the pandemic on persons with dementia and their caregivers in India.

Methods: This was an observational study. A cohort of 66 persons with dementia and their caregivers were evaluated during the COVID-19 pandemic in two specialist hospitals in South India. Caregivers were interviewed at two distinct time points of the pandemic: during the national lockdown and 5 months after during later periods of the "cluster of cases" transmission phase. Participants were assessed via telephone utilizing validated instruments [neuropsychiatric inventory (NPI), clinical dementia rating (CDR) scale, and depression, anxiety and stress scale (DASS-21)] and a semistructured questionnaire. The questionnaire documented sociodemographic information, clinical history, infection measures adopted, changes in caregiving routines, involvement in functional rehabilitation activities, and access to medical and long-term care support services.

Result: The two-phase follow-up study found a significant worsening of behavior in dementia patients, demonstrated by a difference in the NPI sub-domain scores for anxiety [mean difference (standard deviation, SD) = −0.552 (1.993), t_{58} = −2.109, p = 0.039] and eating disturbances [mean difference (SD) = −1.121 (2.493), t_{59} = −3.424, p = 0.001]. A relatively high proportion of patients developed anxiety (cumulative incidence = 24.53%) and eating disturbances (cumulative incidence = 26.92%), without having these symptoms at baseline. There was a trend toward an increase in proportion of persons with severe dementia (19.7% vs. 39.4%) on follow-up. Caregiver distress reported was significantly associated with neuropsychiatric symptoms ($r = 0.712$, $p < 0.001$) and dementia severity ($p = 0.365$, $p = 0.004$). In addition, difficulties in accessing medical care persisted between the two assessments, and there were statistically significant differences between functional rehabilitation activities such as indoor activities ($p < 0.001$), outdoor activities ($p = 0.013$), and physical exercises ($p = 0.003$) between baseline and follow-up.

Conclusion: Findings suggest interruption of functional rehabilitation activities and disruption in medical care services are likely to have had an adverse impact on patients with dementia and contributed toward caregiver distress.

COMMENT

The COVID-19 isolation measures have caused significant negative impact on the cognitive and mental health of people with dementia across the world.[14] Understanding this impact of social and physical isolation on people with dementia is crucial to advance knowledge on risk factors for cognitive decline in elderly. This article seeks to investigate the relationship between COVID-19 isolation measures and the cognitive and behavioral symptoms, symptoms severity of dementia, and caregiver stress. The longitudinal study of a dementia cohort was conducted in two phases during the lockdown and cluster of transmission phase of COVID-19 pandemic in India and indicates that there was significant damage to cognition, behavior, and a worsening of clinical severity of dementia that was associated with an increase in caregiving stress during the pandemic. This was likely due to the concomitant association with the isolation, interruption of medical, social, and rehabilitative services care that occurred during the pandemic. The study brings to the forefront the need to develop protective mechanisms that safeguard needs of vulnerable populations like dementia in times-of societal crisis and emphasizes the crucial need for a multidisciplinary approach to dementia care that includes social engagement, physical activity, medical, and rehabilitative measures.

ARTICLE 11

A Randomized, Double-blind, Phase 2b Proof-of-concept Clinical Trial in Early Alzheimer's Disease with Lecanemab, an Anti-Aβ Protofibril Antibody

Swanson CJ, Zhang Y, Dhadda S. Wang J, Kaplow J, Lai RYK, et al. A randomized, double-blind, phase 2b proof-of-concept clinical trial in early Alzheimer's disease with lecanemab, an anti-Aβ protofibril antibody. *Alz Res Therapy. 2021;13:80.*

Abstract

Background: Lecanemab (BAN2401), an IgG1 monoclonal antibody, preferentially targets soluble aggregated amyloid beta (Aβ), with activity across oligomers, protofibrils, and insoluble fibrils. BAN2401-G000-201, a randomized double-blind clinical trial, utilized a Bayesian design with response-adaptive randomization to assess three doses across two regimens of lecanemab versus placebo in early Alzheimer's disease (AD), mild cognitive impairment due to AD and mild AD dementia.

Methods: BAN2401-G000-201 aimed to establish the effective dose 90% (ED90), defined as the simplest dose that achieves ≥90% of the maximum treatment effect. The primary endpoint was Bayesian analysis of 12-month clinical change on the Alzheimer's Disease Composite Score (ADCOMS) for the ED90 dose, which required an 80% probability of ≥25% clinical reduction in decline versus placebo. Key secondary endpoints included 18-month Bayesian and frequentist analyses of brain amyloid reduction using positron emission tomography; clinical decline on ADCOMS, Clinical Dementia Rating-Sum-of-Boxes (CDR-SB), and Alzheimer's Disease Assessment Scale-Cognitive Subscale (ADAS-Cog14); changes in cerebrospinal fluid (CSF) core biomarkers; and total hippocampal volume (HV) using volumetric magnetic resonance imaging.

Result: A total of 854 randomized subjects were treated (lecanemab, 609; placebo, 245). At 12 months, the 10-mg/kg biweekly ED90 dose showed a 64% probability to be better than placebo by 25% on ADCOMS, which missed the 80% threshold for the primary outcome. At 18 months, 10 mg/kg biweekly lecanemab reduced brain amyloid [−0.306 standardized uptake value ratio (SUVR) units] while showing a drug-placebo difference in favor of active treatment by 27% and 30% on ADCOMS, 56% and 47% on ADAS-Cog14, and 33% and 26% on CDR-SB versus placebo according to Bayesian and frequentist analyses, respectively. CSF biomarkers were supportive of a treatment effect. Lecanemab was well-tolerated with 9.9% incidence of amyloid-related imaging abnormalities-edema/effusion at 10 mg/kg biweekly.

Conclusion: BAN2401-G000-201 did not meet the 12-month primary endpoint. However, prespecified 18-month Bayesian and frequentist analyses demonstrated reduction in brain amyloid accompanied by a consistent reduction of clinical decline across several clinical and biomarker endpoints. A phase 3 study (Clarity AD) in early AD is underway.

COMMENT

With the global rise in dementia burden, there is an increasing need to develop therapies that target underlying pathophysiological mechanisms. This is a randomized double blind proof of concept trial for determining the effective dose 90% (ED90) for an antiamyloid beta (Aβ) protofibril antibody lecanemab. 10 mg/kg biweekly was determined as effective dose for lecanemab. Even though in the study, primary endpoint, i.e., 80% threshold for primary endpoint is not reached at 12 months but showed that is better than placebo in reducing clinical decline on Alzheimer's Disease Composite Score (ADCOMS). This study also demonstrated that lecanemab is better than placebo in reducing brain amyloid deposits in positron emission tomography (PET) standardized uptake value ratio (SUVR) and increasing cerebrospinal fluid (CSF) Aβ1–42 and reducing phosphorylated tau (pTau) which is consistent with previous reports of other amyloid therapies.[15] This study also showed that the antibody is well tolerated with only 9.9% incidence of ARI-E. This study provides early evidence of development of a possible therapeutic intervention that targets soluble aggregated Aβ to mitigate pathologic and potentially clinical effects of Alzheimer's disease.

REFERENCES (Dementia and Cognition)

1. Prince MJ, Wimo A, Guerchet MM, Ali GC, Wu YT, Prina M. World Alzheimer Report 2015-The Global Impact of Dementia: An analysis of prevalence, incidence, cost and trends.
2. Iyer G, Paplikar A, Alladi S, Dutt A, Sharma M, Mekala S, et al. Standardising Dementia Diagnosis Across Linguistic and Educational Diversity: Study Design of the Indian Council of Medical Research-Neurocognitive Tool Box (ICMR-NCTB). J Int Neuro Soc. 2020;26(2):172-86.
3. Ritchie C, Smailagic N, Noel-Storr AH, Ukoumunne O, Ladds EC, Martin S, et al. CSF tau and the CSF tau/Abeta ratio for the diagnosis of Alzheimer's disease dementia and other dementias in people with mild cognitive impairment (MCI). Cochrane Database Syst Rev. 2017;2017(3):CD010803.
4. Poos JM, Moore KM, Nicholas J, Russell LL, Peakman G, Convery RS, et al. Cognitive composites for genetic frontotemporal dementia: GENFI-Cog. Alzheimer's Res and Ther. 2022;14:10.
5. Lin FR, Yaffe K, Xia J, Xue QL, Harris TB, Purchase-Helzner E, et al; Health ABC Study Group. Hearing loss and cognitive decline in older adults. JAMA Intern Med. 2013;173(4):293-9.
6. Bruhn P, Dammeyer J. Assessment of Dementia in individuals with Dual Sensory Loss: Application of a Tactile Test Battery. Dement Geriatr Cogn Dis Extra. 2018;8(1):12-22.
7. Eissman JM, Dumitrescu L, Mahoney ER, Smith AN, Mukherjee S, Lee ML, et al. Sex differences in the genetic architecture of cognitive resilience to Alzheimer's disease. Brain. 2022;145(7)2541-54.
8. Groot C, Holstege H, Ossenkoppele R. Do genetic factors contribute to sex-specific differences in resilience to amyloid pathology? Brain. 2022;145(7):2239-41.
9. Ahlskog JE, Geda YE, Graff-Radford NR, Petersen RC. Physical Exercise as a Preventive or Disease-Modifying Treatment of Dementia and Brain Aging. Mayo Clin Proc. 2011;86(9):876-84.
10. Lin Y, Shan PY, Jiang WJ, Sheng C, Ma L. Subjective cognitive decline: preclinical manifestation of Alzheimer's disease. Neurol Sci. 2019;40(1):41-9.
11. Koran MEI, Wagener M, Hohman TJ, Alzheimer's Neuroimaging Initiative. Sex differences in the association between AD biomarkers and cognitive decline. Brain Imaging Behav. 2017;11(1):205-13.
12. Ou YN, Tan CC, Shen XN, Xu W, Hou XH, Dong Q, et al. Blood pressure and risks of cognitive impairment and dementia: A systematic review and meta-analysis of 209 prospective studies. Hypertension. 2020;76(1):217-25.
13. Evans RA, McAuley H, Harrison EM, Shikotra A, Singapuri A, Sereno M, et al. Physical, cognitive, and mental health impacts of COVID-19 after hospitalisation (PHOSP-COVID): a UK multicentre, prospective cohort study. Lancet Respir Med. 2021;9:1275-87.
14. Suárez-González A, Rajagopalan J, Livingston G, Alladi S. The effect of COVID-19 isolation measures on the cognition and mental health of people living with dementia: A rapid systematic review of one year of quantitative evidence. E Clin Med. 2021;39:101047.
15. Ostrowitzki S, Lasser RA, Dorflinger E, Scheltens P, Barkhof F, Nikolcheva T, et al. A phase III randomized trial of gantenerumab in prodromal Alzheimer's disease. Alzheimers Res Ther. 2017;9(1):95.

Section 8: Peripheral Neuropathy

Section Editor: Tapas Kumar Banerjee

Associate Editor: Joydeep Biswas

ARTICLE 1

Characterization of Mononeuropathy of the Lateral Cutaneous Nerve of the Calf

Oaklander AL, Van Houten T, Sabouri AS. Characterization of mononeuropathy of the lateral cutaneous nerve of the calf. *Muscle Nerve.* 2021;64(4):494-9.

Abstract

Introduction: Isolated injuries to the lateral cutaneous nerve of the calf (LCNC) branch of the common peroneal nerve can lead to obscure chronic posterolateral knee and result in upper calf pain and sensory symptoms. As the LCNC has no motor distribution and cannot be examined by a typical peroneal nerve conduction study, these remain undetected by routine examination and electrodiagnostic testing. Previous literature reveals only 10 prior cases, therefore, less physician awareness, which is a main reason why most LCNC injuries remain misdiagnosed or undiagnosed, thus hindering care.

Methods: We extracted medical records from seven patients who reported unexplained posterolateral knee/calf pain, six were labeled as complex regional pain syndrome, to investigate for mononeuropathies. Patients were asked to outline their skin area with abnormal responses to pin self-examination independently. Furthermore, three patients underwent an LCNC-specific electrodiagnostic study. Skin biopsy for epidermal innervation was performed for two patients. Cadaver dissection of the posterior knee nerves helped in identifying potential entrapment sites.

Results: Initiating events included knee surgery (3), bracing (1), extensive kneeling (1), and other knee trauma. All pin-outlines included the published LCNC-neurotome. Results of skin biopsies revealed significant LCNC neurotome denervation then reinnervation coexisting with symptom recovery. Cadaver dissection identified the LCNC traversing through the dense fascia of the proximolateral gastrocnemius muscle insertion.

Discussion: Isolated LCNC mononeuropathy can lead to unexplained posterolateral knee/calf pain syndromes. This study characterizes presentations and supports patient pin-mappings as a sensitive and cost-efficient diagnostic aid available worldwide. Enhanced recognition may result in a more rapid and accurate diagnosis, thus, optimizing management and improving outcomes.

COMMENT

The authors in this interesting study identified seven cases of lateral cutaneous nerve of calf (LCNC) mononeuropathy in those with unexplained chronic pain in the lateral knee and upper calf region. The nerve conduction study (NCS) has limited role in diagnosis since conventional NCS is normal and LCNC-specific tests are technically difficult.[1] The authors determined that the simple method of subjective pin-mapping could establish the diagnosis. Subjective pin mapping delineated the area of reduced sensation on the lateral side of knee and upper calf. In some, the affected area had reduced touch sensation or there were associated tactile allodynia. The usual entrapment site of LCNC is at the lateral head of gastrocnemius muscle where it traverses the popliteal fossa.[2] Proper diagnosis aids management through correction of associated metabolic disease and by avoidance of local compression. The prognosis of LCNC mononeuropathy is good with complete recovery in 5–15 years.

ARTICLE 2

Mononeuritis Multiplex: An Unexpectedly Frequent Feature of Severe COVID-19

Needham E, Newcombe V, Michell A, Thornton R, Grainger A, Anwar, et al. Mononeuritis multiplex: An unexpectedly frequent feature of severe COVID-19.
J Neurol. 2021:268(8):2685-9.

Abstract

A prolonged mechanical ventilation, which is often required by patients with severe SARS-CoV-2 virus infection, can result in significant intensive care unit-acquired weakness (ICU-AW) in many survivors. Furthermore, in our post-COVID-19 follow-up clinic, we found that, in addition to the anticipated global weakness caused by loss of muscle mass, most of these patients had disabling focal neurological deficits related to multiple axonal mononeuropathies. In a total sample of 69 patients with severe SARS-CoV-2 virus infection, who were discharged from the intensive care units in our hospital, 11 (16%) patients were reported with a mononeuritis multiplex. In many cases, the multifocal nature of the weakness in these patients was unrecognized at the beginning as the symptoms were wrongly diagnosed as simple "critical illness neuromyopathy". Although mononeuropathy is a well-recognized and occasional complication of intensive care, our experience suggests that these deficits are notably frequent and often disabling in patients who are recovering from severe SARS-CoV-2 virus infection.

COMMENT

This study identified mononeuritis multiplex (MM) in 11 post-COVID patients who were in intensive care units (ICUs) under prolonged ventilation. Among the ICU cases critical illness polyneuropathies or myopathies are often observed,[3,4] where there are usually symmetrical neurological deficits. The authors, however, demonstrated that those severely ill COVID cases who had asymmetric weakness, through elaborate neurophysiological investigations did reveal MM. The authors went on to postulate the underlying mechanisms for MM in the post-COVID cases.

My suggestion is that all critically ill patients of diverse etiologies who develop muscle weakness should be examined clinically and comprehensive neurophysiological investigations should be conducted upon them. It is quite possible that MM does occur in many acutely ill cases.

ARTICLE 3

Efficacy of a Fixed Combination of Palmitoylethanolamide and Acetyl-l-carnitine in the Treatment of Neuropathies Secondary to Rheumatic Diseases

Parisi S, Ditto MC, Borrelli R, Fusaro E. Efficacy of a fixed combination of palmitoylethanolamide and acetyl-l-carnitine (PEA+ALC FC) in the treatment of neuropathies secondary to rheumatic diseases.
Minerva Med. 2021;112(4):492-9.

Abstract

Background: Neurological complications of rheumatic diseases (RDs) are highly variable, and their manifestations are related to the pathogenesis and clinical phenotype of the specific RDs. For example, the peripheral nervous system is most commonly involved in rheumatoid arthritis (RA) and mononeuritis multiplex, nerve entrapment, and vasculitic sensorimotor neuropathies are not uncommon. The therapy for these disorders is not easy and involves use of different drugs. Palmitoylethanolamide (PEA) has been tested in a variety of animal models and has been examined in several clinical studies for nerve compression syndromes, showing that PEA acts as a safe and effective analgesic compound. Acetyl-l-carnitine (ALC) has also been shown to be an effective and safer treatment for painful peripheral neuropathy. In the past few years, synergistic effects between PEA and ALC have been studied. This study aimed to evaluate the efficacy of supplementation of standard therapy (STh) with Kalanit (Chelsea Italia Spa; Parma, Italy) in patients with peripheral neuropathy secondary to RDs.

Methods: At the time of enrollment, patients reported with RDs with neuropathy from <12 months as revealed by electromyography studies. The patients were treated with the STh selected on the basis of their RD [RA or spondyloarthritis (SpA)] and for their neuropathy (e.g., analgesic, nonsteroidal anti-inflammatory drugs, pregabalin, or gabapentin) as per clinical practice. Patients were divided into two groups. In group 1, the patients were treated with STh, along with a fixed combination of PEA (600 mg) and ALC (500 mg) (Kalanit) twice a day for 2 weeks and then once a day for 6 months. In group 2, the patients were treated only with STh. Clinical evaluations were performed for each patient and questionnaires were administered to examine their neuropathy and the efficacy of the therapy.

Results: Group 1 included 18 patients with sciatic pain, 16 patients with carpal tunnel syndrome, and 8 patients with peripheral neuropathy of the lower limbs. A fixed combination of PEA and ALC was added to the STh in group 1. These patients were compared with patients from group 2, who had the same demographic characteristics and a similar pathology: 20 patients with sciatic pain, 15 patients with carpal tunnel syndrome, and 5 patients with peripheral neuropathy of the lower limbs, respectively. This group was treated with STh only. Patients treated with a fixed combination of PEA and ALC showed significant improvement in pain visual analog scale compared with patients in group 2 for all the diseases analyzed (sciatic pain, $p = 0.032$; carpal tunnel syndrome, $p = 0.025$; and lower limbs neuropathy, $p = 0.041$). Patients in group 1 improved significantly compared with patients in group 2. Specifically, low back pain impact questionnaire (LBP-IQ) ($p = 0.031$) as well as Cochin hand functional disability (CHFD) ($p = 0.011$) and NPQ ($p = 0.025$) showed significant improvement in group 1.

Conclusion: Synergistic effects of PEA and ALC seem to provide a further advantage in the treatment of this type of pathology, including the anti-inflammatory effect and therapy optimization, and therefore of better adherence to treatments. Our study demonstrates that it is crucial to diagnose the type of pain to follow an accurate diagnostic algorithm, considering the clinical characteristics of the patient and carefully evaluating the indication, preferring a multimodal approach.

COMMENT

Preclinical data revealed anti-inflammatory, analgesic effects of palmitoylethanolamide (PEA)[5] and antiapoptotic, antinociceptive properties of acetyl-l-carnitine (ALC).[6,7] In this study, cases of active rheumatoid arthritis (RD)/spondyloarthropathy (SpA) complicated with wide range of neuropathies (mononeuropathy multiplex, vasculitic polyneuropathy, entrapment neuropathies) were recruited. They were categorized into two pathologically and demographically matched arms. Both arms received standard therapy (STh) for RD/SpA along with nonsteroidal anti-inflammatory drugs (NSAID), pregabalin, or gabapentin. In one arm, a fixed dose combination of PEA and ALC (PEA + ALC FC) was added to STh; this group showed statistically significant improvement in pain as determined through diverse parameters, namely, visual analog scale (VAS), low back pain impact questionnaire (LBP-IQ), Cochin hand functional disability (CHFD), and neuropathic pain questionnaire (NPQ).

The limitation of the study is the small sample size and nonrandomization of cohorts. Despite that the study is important as this indicates the efficacy and safety of PEA + ALC FC in neuropathic pain.

ARTICLE 4

Finger Drop Sign as a New Variant of Acute Motor Axonal Neuropathy

Yoon BA, Ha DH, Park HT, Kusunoki S, Kuwahara M, Lee JH, et al. Finger drop sign as a new variant of acute motor axonal neuropathy.
Muscle Nerve. 2021;63(3):336-43.

Abstract

We propose finger drop sign as a new clinical variant of acute motor axonal neuropathy (AMAN) as per the immunological and radiological evidence. A total of eight patients who had AMAN were identified. All of these patients developed prominent involvement of the finger extensors. Magnetic resonance imaging (MRI) of the extremity muscles and serological assays for antiganglioside antibodies and *Campylobacter jejuni* were performed. Patients with AMAN showed a characteristic and a markedly sustained weakness of the finger extensors with a peculiar pattern of the finger drop sign. MRI of the limb showed unevenly distributed abnormal signals in the muscles that were mainly innervated by the posterior interosseous nerve. All the patients who were tested were positive for the presence of immunoglobulin G antibody against ganglioside complex of GM1 and phosphatidic acid. A detailed pathophysiological understanding of this syndrome can help to gain insights into antiganglioside antibody-mediated axonal injury in Guillain–Barré syndrome.

COMMENT

The authors described in detail eight cases with unique presentation of acute onset selective weakness of the finger extensors preceded by infection. The electroneuromyographic study (ENMG) revealed acute motor axonal neuropathy (AMAN) affecting focally the posterior interosseous nerves. Axial magnetic resonance imaging (MRI) revealed fat-suppressed T2 hyperintensities in the forearm extensor muscles. Strong immunoglobulin G (IgG) antibody positivity is found in all cases against GM1:PA complex (ganglioside complex of GM1 and phosphatidic acid). These cases were clearly distinct from classical AMAN, multifocal motor neuropathy with conduction block (MMN-CB),[8] immune brachial plexopathy, and other focal neuropathies. The authors named this novel entity as finger drop variant (FDv) of Guillain–Barré syndrome.

ARTICLE 5

Small Fiber Neuropathy in the Cornea of COVID-19 Patients Associated with the Generation of Ocular Surface Disease

Barros A, Queiruga-Piñeiro J, Lozano-Sanroma J, Alcalde I, Gallar J, Cueto LFV, et al. Small fiber neuropathy in the cornea of Covid-19 patients associated with the generation of ocular surface disease.
Ocul Surf. 2022;23:40-8.

Abstract

Objective: This study aimed to analyze the association between SARS-CoV-2 infection and small fiber neuropathy in the cornea by in vivo corneal confocal microscopy.

Methods: This is an observational retrospective study, including 23 patients who recovered from SARS-CoV-2 infection. In addition, 46 uninfected volunteers were recruited as a control group. Images of corneal sub-basal nerve fibers of all participants were taken under in vivo confocal microscopy to observe the neuroma-like structures, axonal beadings, and dendritic cells. The Ocular Surface Disease Index (OSDI) questionnaire and Schirmer tear test were used as indicators of dry eye disease (DED) and ocular surface pathology.

Results: A total of 21 (91.3%) patients presented with alterations of the corneal sub-basal plexus and corneal tissue, which were consistent with small fiber neuropathy. Images from healthy participants did not reveal significant nerve fiber or corneal tissue damage. Furthermore, eight patients reported an increase in sensations of ocular dryness after SARS-CoV-2 infection and had positive DED indicators. Beaded axons were found in approximately 83% of the cases, mostly in patients presenting with ocular irritation symptoms. Neuroma-like images were found in 65% of the patients, more frequently in patients with OSDI scores >13. Dendritic cells were found in approximately 70% of the patients and were a frequent finding in younger patients who were asymptomatic. Presence of morphological changes in patients 10 months after recovering from SARS-CoV-2 infection implies to the chronic nature of the neuropathy.

Conclusion: To conclude, SARS-CoV-2 infection might be inducing small fiber neuropathy in the ocular surface, and thereby sharing symptoms and morphological landmarks with DED and diabetic neuropathy.

COMMENT

The study determined for the first time occurrence of corneal small fiber neuropathy in COVID-19 infection. 23 post-COVID patients (with no previous history of ocular pathology) were compared with 46 age- and gender-matched healthy controls. All were subjected to in vivo corneal confocal microscopy (IVCM); also they had Ocular Surface Disease Index (OSDI) and Schirmer tests to identify occurrence of dry eyes. With IVCM, the post-COVID cohorts were found to have reduced corneal nerve fiber density (CNFD), corneal nerve fiber length (CNFL), and corneal nerve fractal dimension (CNFrD) measurements. They also had high number of neuromas and beaded axons and high density of dendritic cells in the cornea indicative of small fiber neuropathy. Some developed symptoms of dry eyes with abnormalities in OSDI and Schirmer tests.

The corneal nerves have low number of angiotensin-converting enzyme 2 (ACE2) receptors but abundance of neuropilin-1 (NRP1) and NRP2 receptors. The authors postulated that in the COVID infected cases attachment of SARS-CoV-2 to the NRP1 and 2 receptors[9,10] leads to the development of corneal small fiber neuropathy.

ARTICLE 6

Antecedent Infections in Guillain–Barré Syndrome Patients from South India

Dutta D, Debnath M, Nagappa M, Das SK, Wahatule R, Sinha S, et al. Antecedent infections in Guillain–Barré syndrome patients from south India.
J Peripher Nerv Syst. 2021;26(3):298-306.

Abstract

Guillain–Barré syndrome (GBS) is the most common postinfectious inflammatory peripheral neuropathy with undiscerned etiology. The commonly reported antecedent infections implicated in India include *Campylobacter jejuni*, chikungunya, dengue, and Japanese encephalitis (JE). This study from south India aimed to investigate the role of these four agents as a trigger for GBS. This was a case–control study performed on 150 treatment-naïve patients with GBS and 150 age- and sex-matched controls from the same community. Enzyme-linked immunosorbent assay (ELISA) was used to detect immunoglobulin M (IgM) immunoreactivity for *C. jejuni*, chikungunya, and dengue in a serum sample of patients with GBS and control participants. Immunoreactivity against JE was detected in serum as well as cerebrospinal fluid (CSF) from patients ($n = 150$) and orthopedic control ($n = 45$) participants. The immunoreactivity against infections was compared between demyelinating and axonal subtypes of GBS. Overall, of the 150 patients with GBS, 149 had serological evidence of antecedent infection. Amongst those with evident antecedent infection, 24 (16%), 8 (5%), and 9 (6%) patients were exclusively immunoreactive to chikungunya, JE, and *C. jejuni*, respectively. Furthermore, in 78 patients, immunoreactivity to multiple pathogens was noted. Immunoreactivity to *C. jejuni* infection was reported in 32% of the patients with GBS compared with 2.7% of the control participants ($p < 0.001$), whereas immunoreactivity to chikungunya virus was reported in 66.7% of the patients with GBS compared with 44.7% of the control participants ($p = 0.006$). Antidengue immunoreactivity was significantly associated with the demyelinating subtypes of GBS. Patients positive for JE IgM (CSF) manifested demyelinating electrophysiology. In this large case–control study, immunoreactivity against multiple infectious agents was observed in a subset of patients. Chikungunya was the most common antecedent infection, followed by *C. jejuni*.

COMMENT

In this important case-control study, antecedent infection in Guillain-Barré syndrome (GBS) among the South Indian patients were analyzed. This is the largest such study in India. *Campylobacter jejuni*, chikungunya, dengue, and Japanese encephalitis (JE) viruses are the common infections identified; association of chikungunya with GBS has been observed for the first time. The only issue is that in some of the GBS cases, immunoglobulin M (IgM) serologies were positive for multiple organisms; in this situation it is not possible to determine the actual offending organism. The plaque reduction neutralization test (PRNT) might help in this situation but still would not be able to completely solve the problem of cross-reactivity among the pathogens.[11]

ARTICLE 7

Motor Demyelinating Tibial Neuropathy in COVID-19

Daia C, Toader C, Scheau C, Onose G. Motor demyelinating tibial neuropathy in COVID-19.
J Formos Med Assoc. 2021;120(11):2032-6.

Abstract

This study included 10 patients with residual symptoms manifesting as fatigue in the lower limbs after the resolution of SARS-CoV-2 infection. Nerve conduction studies were performed for these patients. Motor demyelinating neuropathy features mainly of the tibial nerves, but also involving peroneal, median, and ulnar nerves, were confirmed. The findings of this study might be considered as new neurological characteristics of the SARS-CoV-2 infection.

COMMENT

The SARS-COV-2-associated Guillain-Barré syndrome is a known entity.[12] The authors here described a unique form of neuropathy in COVID-19 cases. 10 post-COVID cases (6 females, 4 males) with the complaints of fatiguability and myalgia-like pain in the legs showed demyelinating neuropathies affecting the motor components of bilateral tibial nerves. Eight of them had additional bilateral peroneal and some also median or ulnar neuropathies, all demyelinating and selectively affecting the motor components. Peroneal neuropathies had secondary axonal degeneration. Paucity of sensory affection distinguishes this condition from classical Guillain-Barré syndrome. Demyelinating nature of neuropathy differentiates this entity from mononeuritis multiplex. Electrophysiologically, this condition is similar to multifocal motor neuropathy with conduction block (MMN-CB). SARS-CoV-2-induced immune dysregulation could be the underlying cause for this focal demyelinating motor neuropathy. Follow-up studies on these cases, however, were not available.

ARTICLE 8

Calprotectin in Chronic Inflammatory Demyelinating Polyneuropathy and Variants: A Potential Novel Biomarker of Disease Activity

Stascheit F, Hotter B, Klose S, Meisel C, Meisel A, Klehmet J. Calprotectin in chronic inflammatory demyelinating polyneuropathy and variants—A potential novel biomarker of disease activity.
Front Neurol. 2021;12:723009.

Abstract

Background: There is an urgent need for biomarkers to monitor ongoing disease activity in chronic inflammatory demyelinating polyneuropathy (CIDP). Serum calprotectin (CLP) induces signaling pathways that are involved in different inflammatory processes and has been shown to correlate with markers of disease activity in other autoimmune disorders. Therefore, this study was designed to examine the potential of CLP in comparison to serum neurofilament light chain (sNfL) in monitoring disease activity.

Material and Methods: This cross-sectional study included sera from 63 patients with typical and atypical CIDP and 6 patients with multifocal motoric neuropathy (MMN) with varying degrees of disease activity. These patients were compared with 40 healthy controls (HCs). Univariate and multivariate analysis were performed to investigate the association of CLP and sNfL levels with sociodemographics, disease duration, patient-reported outcome (PRO) parameters [SF-36 questionnaire, Beck's depression index (BDI), and fatigue severity scale (FSS)], and CIDP disease activity scale (CDAS) and impairment status [medical research council-sum score (MRC-SS), the inflammatory neuropathy cause and treatment disability score (INCAT-DS), grip strength, and maximum walking distance], as well as the treatment regimens.

Results: All patients with CIDP showed significantly high levels of CLP and sNfL as compared with the controls ($p = 0.0009$). Multivariate analysis adjusted for age and gender showed that CLP acts as an independent predictor of CIDP and MMN. CLP was significantly associated with active disease course according to CDAS and correlated with MRC-SS, whereas sNfL correlated with parameters of disease impairment. No correlation with PRO was revealed, except for sNfL and the mental health composite score. No differences were found between typical CIDP and atypical variants in the subgroup analysis.

Conclusion: To conclude, the study revealed that CLP levels were elevated in CIDP and variants and was associated with active disease course, whereas sNfL shows potential as a biomarker of axonal degeneration. Therefore, CLP might be an additive biomarker of choice to measure the ongoing inflammation, which is greatly required to aid better patient care in CIDP.

COMMENT

Serum neurofilament light chain (sNfL) correlates with axonal degeneration and disease duration of chronic inflammatory demyelinating polyneuropathy (CIDP),[13] but does not specifically indicate disease activity. In this study, the role of a novel calcium-binding protein calprotectin (CLP) was evaluated in CIDP. The serum CLP and sNfL levels of CIDP cohorts ($n = 60$) and healthy controls ($n = 40$) were compared in this cross-sectional case–control study. Several parameters were utilized for monitoring disease activity and impairment.

Elevation of CLP level strongly correlates with the ongoing inflammation of CIDP, which is essential in guiding clinical management. Being stable at room temperature CLP is also easy to measure. One shortcoming of sNfL is that it is an age-dependent biomarker but its age-specific cutoff values are not available.[14] On the contrary, CLP is age-independent and has been shown to be an important biomarker for monitoring active CIDP.

ARTICLE 9

Guillain–Barré Syndrome in Patients with SARS-CoV-2: A Multicentric Study from Maharashtra, India

Dhamne MC, Benny R, Singh R, Pande A, Agarwal P, Wagh S, et al. Guillian–Barré syndrome in patients with SARS-CoV-2: A multicentric study from Maharashtra, India.
Ann Indian Acad Neurol. 2021;24(3):339-46.

Abstract

Background: Previous studies have shown an association between Guillain–Barré syndrome (GBS) and severe acute respiratory syndrome coronavirus-2 (SARS-CoV-2) infection. This study aimed to assess the clinical profiles and outcomes of GBS in COVID-19 from the western region of India, the state of Maharashtra.

Methods: This was a retrospective, multicenter observational study from different hospitals in Maharashtra beginning from March, 2020 to November, 2020.

Results: The study included 42 patients with COVID-19 GBS. The mean age of participants was 59 years (range 24–85 years). Of the 42 patients, 31 (74%) were men. GBS was the presenting symptom in 14 of the 42 patients (33%), whereas 6 of them were asymptomatic for COVID-19 despite having a positive result for SARS-CoV-2 infection with a nasopharyngeal swab detected by reverse transcriptase polymerase chain reaction. The mean interval between COVID-19 and GBS was 14 [standard deviation (SD) 11] days, with minimum of 1 and maximum of 40 days. Clinical presentation was similar that of typical GBS. Electrophysiological studies showed a predominant demyelinating pattern in approximately 60% (25/42) of the patients. Inflammatory markers were elevated in 84% (35/42) of the patients and 91% (38/42) of the patients had an abnormal high-resolution computed tomography (HRCT) of chest. Furthermore, approximately 33% (14/42) of the patients required a ventilator, and nine deaths were reported. Intravenous immunoglobulin was the mainstay of treatment for GBS. Majority of the patients had good outcome and were walking independently or with minimal support at discharge. In a subgroup analysis, the postinfectious group reported a better outcome than the parainfectious group.

Conclusion: Guillain–Barré syndrome in COVID-19 occurs as both parainfectious and post-infectious GBS. Parainfectious GBS requires more rigorous monitoring and might benefit from COVID-19-specific treatment. Routine screening for SARS-CoV-2 virus should be performed in patients with GBS in view of the ongoing COVID-19 pandemic.

COMMENT

Since its first description from China,[15] there have been several case reports of SARS-COV-2-associated Guillain–Barré syndrome (GBS). The authors published one of the largest series of COVID-19 associated GBS. A total of 42 cases were collected from multiple centers in the state of Maharashtra, India between March, 2020 and November, 2020. "Parainfectious" GBS were those who had coexisting active COVID-19 infection with elevated inflammatory markers and supportive high-resolution computed tomography (HRCT) thorax. In contrast, those who recovered from COVID-19 infection and then developed GBS were the "postinfectious" GBS. The median interval between onset of COVID infection to GBS was 14 days (range, 1–40 days). Parainfectious GBS were more prevalent, comprising 61.9%; the rest 38.09% were postinfectious. Direct neurotoxic effect of virus as the cause was ruled out because of absence of SARS-CoV-2 in cerebrospinal fluid and because of the therapeutic benefit of intravenous immunoglobulin (IVIg). "Cytokine storm" associated with SARS-CoV-2 might be a possible explanation for parainfectious GBS.

Majority of the affected cases were elderly males. Six cases of GBS were asymptomatic for COVID-19. Based upon electrophysiology, demyelinating polyneuropathy (59.5%) was the most common subtype. In 34 patients, cerebrospinal fluid could be analyzed; 61.9% of them revealed elevated protein with albumin-cytological dissociation. IVIg was administered in 73.8% cases. The prognosis for recovery was better in the postinfectious than in the parainfectious GBS, since many of the latter succumbed to active COVID-related complications.

ARTICLE 10

Epidermal Neurite Density in Skin Biopsies from Patients with Juvenile Fibromyalgia

Boneparth A, Chen S, Horton DB, Moorthy LN, Farquhar I, Downs HM, et al. Epidermal neurite density in skin biopsies from patients with juvenile fibromyalgia.
J Rheumatol. 2021;48(4):575-8.

Abstract

Objective: Fibromyalgia (FM) is a chronic, idiopathic condition with a widespread stiffness and pain in the muscles, tendons, and joints. A meta-analysis of lower leg skin biopsy in adults with FM showed a 45% pooled prevalence of abnormally low epidermal neurite density (END). The diagnostic criteria for small fiber neuropathy is an END below the fifth centile of the normal distribution. However, clinical significance of these findings of abnormally low END in patients with FM is unclear. In this study, we assess the prevalence of small fiber neuropathy in juvenile patients with FM, which has not yet been elucidated by the prior studies.

Methods: We screened 21 patients with FM in the age groups of 13–20 years and diagnosed by pediatric rheumatologists. Of these, 15 patients who met the American College of Rheumatology criteria (modified for juvenile FM) proceeded for lower leg measurements of END. The participants completed the questionnaires assessing the symptoms of pain, functional disability, and dysautonomia. The primary outcome of the study was proportion of patients with FM with END below the fifth centile of age/sex/race-based laboratory norms. The cases were compared for the ethnicity, race, sex, and age with a previously biopsied control group of healthy adolescents. The selection was blinded to the results of biopsy. All 23 healthy controls who matched the demographic criteria were included in the study.

Results: Of the 15 biopsied juvenile patients with FM, 8 (53%) had END below the fifth centile as compared with the healthy controls (1/23, 4%; $p < 0.001$). Mean END for the patients was 273/mm^2 skin surface [95% confidence interval (CI) 198–389], whereas mean END for the control group was 413/mm^2 skin surface (95% CI 359–467; $p < 0.001$). As predicted, patients with FM reported a higher degree of pain, dysautonomia, and functional disability than the healthy controls.

Conclusion: The prevalence of abnormal END reduction is similar in both adolescents and adults with FM. However, further studies are required to comprehensively characterize the significance of low END in patients with FM and to elucidate the clinical indications of these findings.

COMMENT

In small-fiber neuropathy (SFN), the lower limb skin biopsy demonstrates epidermal neurite density (END) to be significantly low (less than fifth centile of normal distribution).[16] In this study, 53% of juvenile fibromyalgia (JFM) cohorts but only 4% of controls revealed END is less than fifth centile. Earlier literature on adult fibromyalgia cases also showed similar low END values.[17] SFN is phenotypically different from fibromyalgia, although chronic pain is a symptom for both. The explanation for the abnormal END findings in fibromyalgia is unclear. Some consider undiagnosed SFN to be cause for many cases of fibromyalgia. Others consider low END to be either just an incidental finding in fibromyalgia or an epiphenomenon of chronic central pain. Future study in this area is warranted.

REFERENCES (Peripheral Neuropathy)

1. Campagnolo DI, Romello MA, Park YI, Foye PM, Delisa JA. Technique for studying conduction in the lateral cutaneous nerve of calf. Muscle Nerve. 2000;23(8):1277-9.
2. Coert JH, Dellon AL. Clinical implications of the surgical anatomy of the sural nerve. Plast Reconstr Surg. 1994;94(6):850-5.
3. Shepherd S, Batra A, Lerner DP. Review of critical illness myopathy and neuropathy. Neurohospitalist. 2017;7(1):41-8.
4. Zhou C, Wu L, Ni F, Ji W, Wu J, Zhang H. Critical illness polyneuropathy and myopathy: a systematic review. Neural Regen Res. 2014;9:101-10.
5. Franklin A, Parmentier-Batteur S, Walter L, Greenberg DA, Stella N. Palmitoylethanolamide increases after focal cerebral ischemia and potentiates microglial cell motility. J Neurosci. 2003;23(21):7767-75.
6. Mansour HH. Protective role of carnitine ester against radiation-induced oxidative stress in rats. Pharmacol Res. 2006;54(3):165-71.
7. Chiechio S, Copani A, Gereau RW 4th, Nicoletti F. Acetyl-L-carnitine in neuropathic pain: experimental data. CNS Drugs. 2007;21(Suppl 1):31-8.
8. Galassi G, Girolami F. Acute-onset multifocal motor neuropathy (AMMN): how we meet the diagnosis. Int J Neurosci. 2012;122(8):413-22.
9. Daly JL, Simonetti B, Klein K, Chen KE, Williamson MK, Antón-Plágaro C, et al. Neuropilin-1 is a host factor for SARS-CoV-2 infection. Science. 2020;370(6518):861-5.
10. Canturi-Castelvetri L, Ojha R, Pedro LD, Djannatian M, Franz J, Kuivanen S, et al. Neuropilin-1 facilitates SARS-CoV-2 cell entry and infectivity. Science. 2020;370(6518):856-60.
11. Maeda A, Maeda J. Review of diagnostic plaque reduction neutralization tests for flavivirus infection. Vet J. 2013;195(1):33-40.
12. Filosto M, Piccinelli SC, Gazzina S, Foresti C, Frigeni B, Servalli MC, et al. Guillain-Barré syndrome and COVID-19: an observational multicentre study from two Italian hotspot regions. J Neurol Neurosurg Psychiatry. 2021;92(7):751-6.
13. van Lieverloo GGA, Wieske L, Verhamme C, Vrancken AFJ, van Doorn PA, Michalak Z, et al. Serum neurofilament light chain in chronic inflammatory demyelinating polyneuropathy. J Peripher Nerv Syst. 2019;24(2):187-94.
14. Khalil M, Pirpamer L, Hofer E, Voortman MM, Barro C, Leppert D, et al. Serum neurofilament light levels in normal aging and their association with morphologic brain changes. Nat Commun. 2020;11(1):812.
15. Zhao H, Shen D, Zhou H, Liu J, Chen S. Guillain-Barré syndrome associated with SARS-CoV-2 infection: causality or coincidence? Lancet Neurol. 2020;19(5):383-4.
16. Oaklander AL, Nolano M. Scientific advances in and clinical approaches to small-fiber polyneuropathy: A review. JAMA Neurol. 2019;76(10):1240-51.
17. Grayston R, Czanner G, Elhadd K, Goebel A, Frank B, Üçeyler N, et al. A systematic review and meta-analysis of the prevalence of small fiber pathology in fibromyalgia: Implications for a new paradigm in fibromyalgia etiopathogenesis. Semin Arthritis Rheum. 2019;48(5):933-40.

Section 9: Muscle Disorders

Section Editor: Satish Khadilkar
Associate Editor: Rakhil Yadav

ARTICLE 1

Clinical Practice with Steroid Therapy for Duchenne Muscular Dystrophy: An Expert Survey in Asia and Oceania

Takeuchi F, Nakamura H, Yonemoto N, Komaki H, Rosales RL, Kornberg AJ, et al. Clinical practice with steroid therapy for Duchenne muscular dystrophy: An expert survey in Asia and Oceania.
Brain Dev 2020;42(3):277-88.

Abstract

Background: There are many articles on beneficial and long-term effects of steroid in Duchenne muscular dystrophy (DMD) patients from western countries.

Objective: To evaluate the beneficial effects of steroids in before and after loss of ambulance state of DMD patients in Asian oceanic countries.

Method: Electronic response was collected from the clinic who had an experience of treating DMD patients. The questionnaire includes responders' background and his awareness and experience of steroids in clinical practice.

Results and Discussion: 89% clinicians had experience of steroid therapy. 52% clinicians believe that the ideal age for starting steroids is when the patient's motor development reached a plateau. Commonly used maintenance therapy is daily administration of prednisolone. Clinicians from Japan, Singapore, and South Korea tended to continue steroid treatment after the loss of ambulation. Usually after the loss of ambulation, clinicians reduce the dose of steroid. Most commonly observed side effects are obesity and behavior changes. Medications for bone protection were used commonly. Japan, China, and Hong Kong have detailed epidemiological and clinical information of their patients.

Conclusion: Most clinicians are aware of DMD care recommendations and prescribe steroids. Daily prednisolone was preferred by clinicians. Response to use of steroid in nonambulant patients and bone protection medications were inconsistent.

COMMENT

Corticosteroids have become a standard of care in Duchenne muscular dystrophy (DMD) and various regimen are used.[1,2] This survey sheds light on the current ground-level situation for the use of steroids in DMD in the Asia Oceania region. Most of clinicians are aware of the use of steroids and advise them, usually when the motor development reached a plateau. Daily administration is preferred in this region, instead of the on–off method. Infections are a particular concern in these regions of the world, in addition to the issues of obesity and osteoporosis outlined in this section. The concept that steroid are harmful are often expressed by families and it is a common experience in India that families do not opt for the therapy due to the perceived side effect profile. The instructions given to the families in order to avoid the side effects need to be more elaborate and in discussion with the pediatrician and endocrine consultant, depending upon the situation. Regular and rigorous monitoring schedules need to be put in place to minimize the unwanted effects. As the perspective of the therapy in the totality of this devastating disease is limited, reservations on part of the families, and practitioners are not surprising.

ARTICLE 2

Deflazacort versus Prednisone/Prednisolone for Maintaining Motor Function and Delaying Loss of Ambulation: A Post-HOC Analysis from the ACT DMD Trial

Shieh PB, Mcintosh J, Jin F, Souza M, Elfring G, Narayanan S, et al. THE ACT DMD STUDY GROUP. Deflazacort versus prednisone/prednisolone for maintaining motor function and delaying loss of ambulation: A post HOC analysis from the ACT DMD trial.
Muscle Nerve. 2018;58(5):639-45.

Abstract

Background: Corticosteroids slow down the decline in muscle strength and motor function. Commonly used corticosteroids are prednisone, prednisolone, or deflazacort.

Objective: To compare the efficacy and safety of deflazacort and prednisone/prednisolone.

Method: Post-hoc analysis of data from ACT DMD trial.

Primary endpoint: Ability to slow down the progression of disease measured by change from baseline to week 48 in 6-minute walk distance (6MWD).

Secondary endpoints: Improvement in proximal muscle function and functional ability.

Results and Discussion: 6MWD, four-stair climb, and other times function tests favored deflazacort. Both have comparable safety profiles. Deflazacort has less weight gain, behavior problems, and excessive hair growth. Post-hoc analysis has several limitations.

Conclusion: Deflazacort therapy may offer benefits as compared to prednisone/prednisolone. On a head-to-head comparison in future, this results may be more clarified.

COMMENT

This section is important because it discusses the various modes of steroid therapy in Duchenne muscular dystrophy.[3,4] This is post-hoc analysis of data from the ACT DMD trial. The primary endpoint of the trial was the ability to slow down the progression of the disease based on the results of the 6-minute walk test (6MWD). As it is well recognized, the 6MWD has limitations in performance that can be variable. The authors found that from the point of view of side effects, the safety profiles of prednisone, prednisolone, and deflazacort were compatible. However, the functional ability tests favors deflazacort. In clinical practice, the experiences are similar. Children who are on deflazacort have less weight gain endless issues of hair growth in behavioral problems. As the authors have pointed out, while this study favors deflazacort, it will be important to have a head-to-head comparison for the issues to be clarified further.

ARTICLE 3

Management of Adrenal Insufficiency Risk after Long-term Systemic Glucocorticoid Therapy in Duchenne Muscular Dystrophy: Clinical Practice Recommendations

Bowden SA, Connolly AM, Kinnett K, Zeitler PS. Management of adrenal insufficiency risk after long-term systemic glucocorticoid therapy in Duchenne muscular dystrophy: Clinical practice recommendations.
J Neuromuscul Dis. 2019;6(1):31-41.

Abstract

Background: At present, glucocorticoids (GCs) is an integral part of Duchenne muscular dystrophy (DMD) management though it has many side effects. It causes secondary adrenal insufficiency (AI). In the scenario of physiological stress, sudden discontinuation of long-term GC treatment, or gastrointestinal (GI) infection/emesis, chance of developing AI is high. AI is associated with high morbidity and mortality.

Important aspects of GC in relation to AI: GC potency is measured using hydrocortisone as a reference, with potency value of 1. Prednisolone dose (0.75 mg/kg/day) used in DMD patients is eight times the physiologic dose of hydrocortisone. Gradual tapering of GC rather than abrupt cessation helps the hypothalamic–pituitary–adrenal (HPA) axis to recover. During major stress, a patient needs an extra dose to cover deficiency. Manifestation of AI may be nonspecific like fatigue, nausea, vomiting, dizziness, or postural hypotension or life threatening like postural hypotension, dehydration, shock, or coma. Patients with AI should be treated with parenteral hydrocortisone depending on degree of stress. This stress dose should be tapered slowly. Patients on intermittent dose of GC than daily dose are at lower risk of AI. Endocrinologists should be a part of a team while planning to taper and later discontinue GC. Morning cortical value or adrenocorticotropic hormone (ACTH) stimulation test may guide for tapering of GC doses. HPA axis may take 1 year to recover fully after discontinuation of GC.

Conclusion: High index of suspicion and timely intervention by stress dose is an important part of DMD patient management who is on GC.

COMMENT

Patients on glucocorticoid therapy on long-term basis have many different aspects that need to be looked after by the treating physician. This section focuses on adrenal function and dysfunction in relation to long-term use of glucocorticoids.[5,6] The patient set is of Duchenne muscular dystrophy (DMD), who, at a very young age are put on long-term glucocorticoids, therefore, in some ways this set is unique. The article points out the need for gradual tapering of glucocorticoids in order to reduce the side effects and allow time for the hypothalamus pituitary adrenal axis to recover. The article also points out a very important aspect that often the manifestations of adrenal insufficiency are nonspecific and therefore, may not be picked up early by the clinician. They mention fatigue, nausea, vomiting, and dizziness which are so common in DMD children because their ambulation is limited, particularly when they become wheelchair-bound. In clinical practice, we observe, as has been mentioned by the authors, that a high index of suspicion on part of the clinician probably goes a long way in timely intervention of symptoms that arise out of glucocorticoid deficiency when used on long-term and then tapered abruptly.

ARTICLE 4

AdipoRon, A New Therapeutic Prospect for Duchenne Muscular Dystrophy

Abou-Samra M, Selvais CM, Boursereau R, Lecompte S, Noel L, Brichard SM. AdipoRon, a new therapeutic prospect for Duchenne muscular dystrophy.
J Cachexia Sarcopenia Muscle. 2020;11(2):518-33.

Abstract

Background: Adiponectin (ApN) is an adipocyte-secreted hormone with anti-inflammatory/oxidative actions through adiponectin receptor 1 (AdipoR1) and AMP-activated protein kinase (AMPK) pathway, which led to suppression of nuclear factor-kappa B (NF-κB) activity and upregulation of utrophin (a dystrophin analogue). Its effectiveness is proven in animal models. AdipoRon is an orally active synthetic small-molecule AdipoR agonist.

Objective: To prove its beneficial effects, discover mechanism of effectiveness and its effect on human myotubes.

Method: Young mdx mice treated with oral AdipoRon were compared with untreated mdx mice and wild type control mice. Changes in muscle strength and endurance were recorded in vivo while biochemical and molecular analyses were done ex vivo. Lastly, its effect on human myotubes were analyzed in vitro.

Results and Discussion: Hydroxynonenal (HNE), tumor necrosis factor-alpha (TNFα), interleukin-1 beta (IL-1β), and cluster of differentiation 68 (CD68)—markers of oxidative stress and inflammation—were decreased significantly with AdipoRon treatment while interleukin-10 (IL-10), anti-inflammation cytokine, was increased. Treated mice show positive results for markers of muscle proliferation, Myf5 and MyoD and muscle differentiation, MyoG and Mrf4. Adioren treatment increases more resistant fiber. Less sarcolemmal damage was reflected by decreases in plasma lactate dehydrogenase and creatine kinase. mdx-AR mice demonstrated enhancement of strength and endurance of muscles. It acts through both mechanisms—AMPK dependent and AMPK independent.

Limitation: It is unclear whether ApN level is less in Duchenne muscular dystrophy (DMD) patients.

Conclusion: Adiponectin could be a strong alternative to steroid due to its properties.

COMMENT

Duchenne muscular dystrophy (DMD) is its common condition seen in boys, throughout the world. While this is a genetically mediated condition, there are inflammatory components that are involved in progressive muscle damage.[7,8] It is very well known, that muscle biopsies from children with DMD often show an inflammatory response and in fact, corticosteroids have been used gainfully to slow down muscle degeneration and increase the duration of ambulation. As a result, corticosteroid therapy has become a standard of care in this condition.

On this background, this section is important because it deals with a way of reducing the inflammatory response seen in this condition. The experimental design is of treating the mice with an adipose-derived hormone that reduces inflammation. Various inflammatory markers of oxidative stress and inflammation were studied before and after the therapy and were found to be significantly decreased after therapy. The authors also assess the effects of this hormone on human Mayo tubes. On the whole, the results suggested that the treated fibers had less inflammation and were more resistant to ongoing damage. This strategy opens new avenues to reducing muscle damage seen in tuition muscular dystrophy and in this sense the section has its importance.

ARTICLE 5

Phase 1 Study of Edasalonexent (CAT-1004), an Oral NF-κB Inhibitor, in Pediatric Patients with Duchenne Muscular Dystrophy

Finanger E, Vandenborne K, Finkel RS, Lee Sweeney H, Tennekoon G, Yum S, et al. Phase 1 study of edasalonexent (CAT-1004), an oral NF-κB inhibitor, in pediatric patients with Duchenne muscular dystrophy. *J Neuromuscul Dis. 2019;6(1):43-54.*

Abstract

Background: Glucocorticoids are key anti-inflammatory agents in the management of Duchenne muscular dystrophy (DMD) patients but have many adverse effects. Long-term activation of nuclear factor-kappa B (NF-κB) is an important factor for muscle degeneration and suppression of muscle regeneration in DMD. Edasalonexent inhibits the transcription factor NF-κB. It shows positive results in mice and dog models and well tolerated in adult patients.

Objective: To assess safety and tolerability of edasalonexent. To assess pharmacokinetic properties of edasalonexent under different dietary conditions.

Method: Ambulatory, DMD patients with age between ≥4 and <8 years, who are immunized against chickenpox/influenza, and who are not on steroid treatment for 6 months were enrolled. A 1-week, open-label, multiple-dose study with three sequential ascending doses of edasalonexent under different dietary conditions were administered and various parameters of pharmacokinetics, safety and pharmacodynamic properties were calculated.

Results and Discussion: Edasalonexent is found to be safe though long duration study is needed. Edasalonexent exposure was greater at the higher dose and when administered with a high-fat meal. Short course of edasalonexent can directly reduce the levels of elevated NF-κB in circulating DMD mononuclear cells prior to any changes observable in muscle. Its effect is independent of the underlying dystrophin mutation so it is useful for all DMD patients.

Conclusion: Edasalonexent is safe, well tolerated, and NF-κB pathways inhibitor. Various dosing regimens will be tested in part 2 of study.

COMMENT

As we have seen before, inflammation is an important part of the cascade of muscle damage in Duchenne muscular dystrophy (DMD).[9,10] The cascade works through many inflammatory markers. Glucocorticoids have been traditionally used as anti-inflammatory agents and have been employed gainfully in this disease. However, as has been discussed earlier glucocorticoids, the key anti-inflammatory agents, have multiple side effects and need to be monitored very well. Hence it is important to develop other molecules which have anti-inflammatory action but do not have the side effects of glucocorticoids.

In this context this section is important because it assesses the safety and tolerability of a new molecule. This study recruited individuals who are between the age of 4 and 8 years and we are not treated with steroids for at least 6 months before being enrolled. Various inflammatory parameters were studied. The molecule is found to be safe and the article mentions that the short course of this molecule can directly reduce the levels of nuclear factor-kappa B (NF-kB) in circulating mononuclear cells. The importance of this section is in the fact that molecules such as the one studied here with better anti-inflammatory properties and lesser limiting side effects could be developed in the future and used in place of glucocorticoids in children with DMD in order to increase the duration of their ambulation and quality of life.

ARTICLE 6

Long-term Natural History Data in Duchenne Muscular Dystrophy Ambulant Patients with Mutations Amenable to Skip Exons 44, 45, 51, and 53

Brogna C, Coratti G, Pane M, Ricotti V, Messina S, D'Amico A, et al. on behalf of the International DMD group. Long-term natural history data in Duchenne muscular dystrophy ambulant patients with mutations amenable to skip exons 44, 45, 51 and 53.
PLoS One. 2019;14(6):e0218683.

Abstract

Background: Results of clinical trials using dystrophin restoration approaches become more obvious after the first year of treatment. Long-term natural history data of different genotypes become more important for evaluation of clinical trial results. 3 years follow-up data of patients amenable to skip exon 51 are available. Similar data about other genotypes will be helpful for future clinical trials.

Method: Multicentric study involving 14 tertiary neuromuscular centers with 7 years of recruitment period and 3 years of follow-up. Only ambulant patients with deletions amenable to skip exons 44, 45, 51, and 53 and without intellectual or behavior abnormalities were enrolled. 6 minute walk test (6MWT) and time to rise from the floor (TRF) were recorded.

Results and Discussion: Significant differences were noted at 24 months, not after 12 months, amongst different subgroups amenable to skip different exons. Mutations amenable to skip exon 53 and 51 had overall lower baseline values and more negative changes. Favorable results were seen in patients with deletions eligible to skip exon 44. Variable changes were noticed in patients with deletions amenable to skip for exon 45. Patients with a combination of TRF >6 seconds and

6MWT <350 m lost ambulation within 36 months, irrespective of the genotype. Though these combinations occur rarely, in older age and in patients amenable to skip exon 44.

Conclusion: Differences between different genotype subgroups becomes more obvious with longitudinal study. Patients amenable to skipping exon 53 have rapid progression and early loss of ambulance while patients amenable to skipping exon 45 have variable pattern of progression.

Limitation: Factors such as modifier genes were not studied. Variables like weight, height, and body mass index were not systematically noted.

COMMENT

This section deals with a rather important aspect of a small subgroup of children with Duchenne muscular dystrophy.[11,12] The authors have studied is the natural history of disease in patients who had deletions amenable to the skip exam 44, 45, 51, and 53. Since these deletions are amenable to the exon skipping strategies, it is important to know about the natural history and variations in the disease progression in these groups, to be able to judge the effects of therapy better. As the article points out, they noted significant differences at the end of 2 years in various deletions. Those with mutations amenable to skipping exon 53 and 51 did not do as well from the baseline as compared to the other mutations. Patients available to exon 45 skipping showed a variable pattern of progression. This study points out the much-needed information on how various mutations behave naturally so that the effects of treatment to be assessed and fine-tuned further.

ARTICLE 7

CRISPR Correction of Duchenne Muscular Dystrophy

Min YL, Bassel-Duby R, Olson EN. CRISPR correction of Duchenne muscular dystrophy. *Annu Rev Med. 2019;70:239-55.*

Abstract

Background: Duchenne muscular dystrophy (DMD) is a lethal disorder. Various treatment approaches show transient benefit. Gene edition using clustered regularly interspaced short palindromic repeats (CRISPRs) is a rapidly developing field of transformative therapy.

Genome Editing: Factors that favor genome editing in DMD are the modular structure of the rod domain of dystrophin allows deletion of mutant exons and restoration of open reading frame (ORF). Being X-linked recessive (XLR) disorder only one allele needs to be corrected. Minimum restoration of dystrophin protein expression is needed for therapeutic benefit. CRISPR/Cas9-mediated gene editing has been applied to correct a variety of DMD mutations found in human myoblasts and patient-derived-induced pluripotent stem cells (iPSCs) lines. Correction approaches for DMD include permanent exon removal, exon skipping, exon reframing, exon knock-in, and base editing. Functional dystrophin gene restoration has been demonstrated by CRISPR/Cas9 editing in iPSCs derived from DMD patients with exon deletions, exon duplications, and point mutations. The CRISPR technology has also evolved for gene regulation. The viral-based CRISPR delivery system uses lentivirus, adenovirus, and adeno-associated virus (AAV). Nonviral-based CRISPR delivery systems are electroporation and lipid or gold mediated nanoparticle delivery. This technology has an advantage over others as it eliminates disease responsible mutation, produces a normal form of dystrophin, and expression of dystrophin following gene editing originates from the endogenous dystrophin gene. Efficient body-wide delivery of gene editing components to all affected muscles and the heart is a major challenge. Longevity of dystrophin expression is unknown. Off-target mutagenesis and immunogenicity may be of concern.

Conclusion: CRISPR/Cas9 system technology has opened up new opportunities for correcting monogenic neuromuscular diseases.

COMMENT

This section is important as it discusses the much talked about clustered regularly interspaced short palindromic repeat (CRISPR) technology in the context of Duchenne muscular dystrophy. Amongst the various gene editing systems that have been employed for this disease CRISPR is a promising technology. As Duchenne muscular dystrophy is an X recessive disorder, only one allele of the X chromosome needs to be corrected.[13,14] The section discusses viral and nonviral-based CRISPR delivery systems. The advantage over other gene editing systems is, it eliminates disease-responsible mutation and results in the normal form of dystrophin. As the research is still in progress, the long-term achievements in terms of dystrophin expression are unclear, but it is evident that this technology opens new opportunities for correcting various genetic neuromuscular diseases.

ARTICLE 8

Emerging Strategies in the Treatment of Duchenne Muscular Dystrophy

Shieh PB. Emerging strategies in the treatment of Duchenne muscular dystrophy.
Neurotherapeutics. 2018;15(4):840-8.

Abstract

Duchenne muscular dystrophy (DMD) is a progressive X-linked degenerative muscle disease due to mutations in the DMD gene. Genetic confirmation has become standard in recent years. Improvements in the standard of care for DMD have led to improved survival. Novel treatments for DMD have focused on reducing the dystrophic mechanism of the muscle disease, modulating utrophin protein expression, and restoring dystrophin protein expression. Among the strategies to reduce the dystrophic mechanisms are: (1) inhibiting inflammation, (2) promoting muscle growth and regeneration, (3) reducing fibrosis, and (4) facilitating mitochondrial function. The agents under investigation include a novel steroid, myostatin inhibitors, idebenone, an anti-connective tissue growth factor (CTGF) antibody, a histone deacetylase inhibitor, and cardiosphere-derived cells. For utrophin modulation, adeno-associated virus (AAV)-mediated gene therapy with GALGT2 is currently being investigated to upregulate utrophin expression. Finally, the strategies for dystrophin protein restoration include (1) nonsense readthrough, (2) synthetic antisense oligonucleotides for exon skipping, and (3) AAV-mediated micro/minidystrophin gene delivery. With newer agents, we are witnessing the use of more advanced biotechnological methods. Although these potential breakthroughs provide significant promise, they may also raise new questions regarding treatment effect and safety.

COMMENT

This section summarizes the various current management strategies for Duchenne muscular dystrophy (DMD). As we know, DMD results from an abnormality of the dystrophin gene which alters the gene product that is dystrophin. It progressively leads to muscle degeneration and clinical weakness. Inflammation probably forms an important damaging pathway and this has been targeted with newer anti-inflammatory molecules which block or reduce the inflammatory response at various parts of the inflammatory cascade. Gene restoration is the second major strategy. The utrophin gene is located on the autosome and can perform some functions of dystrophin and therefore, upregulation of the utrophin has been one of the strategies that researchers have worked on. Exon skipping yes perhaps been the most explored technology and resulted in some genetic sequence abnormalities. More and more abnormalities of the single exons are coming under the purview of gene editing. There are other treatments which are also outlined in this section. This is a good section for the overview of current treatments of Duchenne muscular dystrophy.

There are various strategies that are under evaluation for DMD treatment: anti-inflammatory, myostatin inhibitors, utropin modulation, dystrophin protein restoration, and many others **(Table 1)**.[15,16]

TABLE 1: Treatment strategies of Duchenne muscular dystrophy.

Anti-inflammatory	Vamorolone	Membrane stabilizing and anti-inflammatory properties. No significant immunosuppressive or hormonal effects	NCT03439670
	Edasalonexent	NF-κB inhibitors	NCT02439216
Myostatin inhibitors	Domagrozumab	Humanized monoclonal antibody	Trial terminated due to lack of efficacy
	Talditercept alfa	Human IgG1(Fc)–adnectin fusion that binds myostatin	NCT03039686
Utrophin modulation	Ezutromid	Activate utrophin transcription	Lack of efficacy
	Adeno-associated virus (AAVrh74)-mediated gene delivery of the *GALGT2* gene	Overexpression of GALGT2 upregulate utrophin	NCT03333590
Dystrophin restoration	Ataluren	Nonsense suppression	NCT03648827
	Drisapersen	Exon 51 skipping	Not received FDA approval
	Eteplirsen	Exon 51 skipping	FDA approved
	Golodirsen	Exon 53 skipping	NCT02500381
	Casimersen	Exon 45 skipping	NCT02500381
	SRP-5051	Exon 51 skipping	NCT03375255
	NS-065	Exon 53 skipping	NCT02740972
	WVE-210201	Exon 51 skipping	NCT03508947
	DS-5141b	Exon 45 skipping	NCT02667483
	rAAVrh74.MHCK7.Micro-dystrophin	Gene restoration	NCT03375164
	SGT-001	Gene restoration	NCT03368742
	PF-06939926	Gene restoration	NCT03362502
Other	Idebenone	Facilitation of metabolic pathways	NCT02814019
	Givinostat	HDAC inhibitors having anti-inflammatory, antifibrotic, and proregenerative genes	NCT02851797
	Pamrevlumab	Antifibrotic properties	NCT02606136
	CAP-1002	Modulating the immune system, inhibiting fibrosis, and promoting regeneration	NCT03406780

(FDA: Food and Drug Administration; HDAC: histone deacetylase; Ig: immunoglobulin; NF-κB: nuclear factor-kappa B)

ARTICLE 9

Cardiac Management of the Patient with Duchenne Muscular Dystrophy

Buddhe S, Cripe L, Friedland-Little J, Kertesz N, Eghtesady P, Finder J, et al. Cardiac management of the patient with Duchenne muscular dystrophy.
Pediatrics. 2018;142(Suppl 2):S72-81.

Abstract

Duchenne muscular dystrophy (DMD) results in a progressive cardiomyopathy that produces significant morbidity and mortality. To improve the quality of life in patients with DMD, cardiac care is focused on surveillance and management, with the goal of slowing the onset and progression of heart failure complications. The current article is intended to be an expanded review on the cardiac management data used to inform the 2018 DMD Care Considerations recommendations as well as be a discussion on clinical controversies and future management directions. The new cardiac guidance includes changes regarding noninvasive imaging surveillance of cardiac function and pharmacologic therapy. Many emerging therapies lack sufficient evidence-based data to be recommended in the 2018 DMD Care Considerations. These are discussed in the present article as clinical controversies and future directions. Important emerging therapies include new heart failure medications, mechanical circulatory support with ventricular assist devices, heart transplantation, and internal cardiac defibrillators. Future research studies should be focused on the risks and benefits of these advanced therapies in patients with DMD. We conclude this review with a brief discussion on the relationship between the heart and the recently developed medications that are used to directly target the absence of dystrophin in DMD.

COMMENT

This article reviews important points for cardiac care as per 2018 Duchenne muscular dystrophy (DMD) Care Considerations. For a good quality of life in DMD patients, early diagnosis and treatment of cardiomyopathy is important.[17-19]

- Yearly cardiac screening should be started from the time of diagnosis.
- Cardiac magnetic resonance imaging (MRI) is preferred over echocardiography.
  - Less affected by body habitus
  - Superior for detecting ventricular dysfunction
  - It detects subepicardial myocardial fibrosis very early.
  - Time course and distribution of gadolinium enhancement within the myocardium is an important clinical biomarker.
  - Strain imaging has better correlation with left ventricular ejection fraction (LVEF).
  - Cost, availability, expertization, and patient positioning are major limitations.

- Myocardial t1 mapping and extracellular volume are emerging imaging techniques.
- *Medical management*:
  - First line therapy: Angiotensin-converting enzyme (ACE) inhibitors or angiotensin receptor blockers (ARBs)
  - Others: Eplerenone, β-adrenergic blockers, diuretics or digoxin
  - ACE inhibitors or ARBs should be started around 10 years of age in patients with normal cardiac function.
  - Newer medicines: Sacubitril/valsartan, ivabradine
- *Heart transplant and mechanical circulatory support (left ventricular assist device)*:
  - Emerging therapy
- Standard of care with refractory end stage heart failure
- It is a more realistic option when newer therapy will reduce noncardiac morbidity and mortality.
- *Arrhythmias and device therapy*:
  - Only predictor of mortality is LVEF, not arrhythmias.
  - Implanted cardioverter defibrillator effectiveness is not established for DMD patients.
  - For patients with sustained ventricular tachycardia (VT) or resuscitated sudden cardiac death, implantable cardioverter-defibrillator (ICD) implant is accepted class 1 indication.

ARTICLE 10

Respiratory Management of the Patient with Duchenne Muscular Dystrophy

Sheehan DW, Birnkrant DJ, Benditt JO, Eagle M, Finder JD, Kissel J, et al. Respiratory management of the patient with Duchenne muscular dystrophy.
Pediatrics. 2018;142(Suppl 2):S62-71.

Abstract

In 2010, Care Considerations for Duchenne muscular dystrophy (DMD), sponsored by the Centers for Disease Control and Prevention, was published in *Lancet Neurology*, and in 2018, these guidelines were updated. Since the publication of the first set of guidelines, survival of individuals with DMD has increased. With contemporary medical management, survival often extends into the fourth decade of life and beyond. Effective transition of respiratory care from pediatric to adult medicine is vital to optimize patient safety, prognosis, and quality of life. With genetic and other emerging drug therapies in development, standardization of care is necessary to accurately assess treatment effects in clinical trials. This revision of respiratory recommendations preserves a fundamental strength of the original guidelines: namely, reliance on a limited number of respiratory tests to guide patient assessment and management. A progressive therapeutic strategy is presented that includes lung volume recruitment, assisted coughing, and assisted ventilation (initially nocturnally, with the subsequent addition of daytime ventilation for progressive respiratory failure). This revision also stresses the need for serial monitoring of respiratory muscle strength to characterize an individual's respiratory phenotype of severity as well as provide baseline assessments for clinical trials. Clinical controversies and emerging areas are included.

COMMENT

Respiratory complications are major determinants of survival and quality of life.[20-22] All individuals should be immunized with inactivated influenza and pneumococcal vaccine.
- *Ambulatory stage*:
  - Yearly forced vital capacity (FVC) measurement and sleep study with capnography
- *Nonambulatory stage*:
  - Twice a year FVC, maximal inspiratory pressure (MIP)/maximal expiratory pressure (MEP), peak cough flow (PCF), SpO_2, Pet, CO_2/$PtcCO_2$
  - Lung volume recruitment when FVC ≤60% predicted.
  - Assisted coughing when FVC <50% predicted, PCF <270 L/min or MEP <60 cmH_2O.
  - Nocturnal-assisted ventilation with backup rate of breathing when there are sign or symptoms of sleep hypoventilation or other sleep-disordered breathing, abnormal sleep study, FVC <50% predicted, MIP <60 cmH_2O, or awake baseline SpO_2 <95% or pCO_2 >45 mm Hg.
  - Addition of assisted daytime ventilation when daytime SpO_2 <95%, pCO_2 >45 mm Hg, or symptoms of awake dyspnea.

ARTICLE 11

Making Sense of the Clinical Spectrum of Limb-girdle Muscular Dystrophies

Khadilkar SV, Patel BA, Lalkaka JA. Making sense of the clinical spectrum of limb-girdle muscular dystrophies. *Pract Neurol. 2018;18(3):201-10.*

Abstract

The expansion of the spectrum of limb-girdle muscular dystrophies (LGMDs) in recent years means that neurologists need to be familiar with the clinical clues that can help with their diagnosis. The LGMDs comprise a group of genetic myopathies that manifest as chronic progressive weakness of hip and shoulder girdles. Their inheritance is either autosomal dominant (LGMD1) or autosomal recessive (LGMD2). Their prevalence varies in different regions of the world; certain ethnic groups have documented founder mutations and this knowledge can facilitate the diagnosis. The clinical approach to LGMDs uses the age at onset, genetic transmission, and clinical patterns of muscular weakness. Helpful clinical features that help to differentiate the various subtypes include predominant upper girdle weakness, disproportionate respiratory muscle involvement, distal weakness, hip adductor weakness, "biceps lump" and "diamond on quadriceps" sign, calf hypertrophy, contractures and cardiac involvement. Almost half of patients with LGMD have such clinical clues. Investigations such as serum creatine kinase, electrophysiology, muscle biopsy, and genetic studies can complement the clinical examination. In this review, we discuss diagnostic clinical pointers and comment on the differential diagnosis and relevant investigations, using illustrative case studies.

COMMENT

The limb-girdle muscular dystrophies (LGMDs) compromise the group of genetic myopathies presented with progressive proximal muscle weakness.[23-26] They are divided into two types according to mode of inheritance: type 1 means autosomal dominant, while type 2 denotes to autosomal recessive inheritance. The further number is given according to chronology of identification. Sarcoglycanopathies and alpha-dystroglycanopathies present in early age, dysferlinopathies and calpainopathies present in the second decade, desminopathies and anoctaminopathies present later. Pattern of weakness—usually started in proximal lower limb muscles, sometimes in proximal upper limb, on progression there is involvement of semidistal muscles with mild asymmetry. Differential involvement of muscles and patchy areas of hypertrophy and atrophy within the same muscles points toward genetic nature **(Table 2)**.

TABLE 2: Patterns of limb-girdle muscular dystrophies.

Pattern	LGMDs
Prominent upper girdle involvement	Calpainopathy, sarcoglycanopathies, fukutin-related proteinopathy, and anoctaminopathy
Calf head on trophy sign	Dysferlinopathy
"Biceps lump" and "diamond on quadriceps" sign	Dysferlinopathy
Respiratory muscle weakness	Myotilinopathy, laminopathy, sarcoglycanopathies, and fukutin-related proteinopathy
Truncal muscle weakness	Calpainopathy, dysferlinopathy, sarcoglycanopathy, and LGMD 1F
Prominent distal weakness	Sarcoglycanopathies, calpainopathies
Prominent distal weakness	• *Anterior leg muscles*: Myotilinopathy, desminopathy, telethoninopathy, and titinopathy • *Posterior leg muscles*: Dysferlinopathy and anoctaminopathy

Continued

Continued

Pattern	LGMDs
Calf hypertrophy	Sarcoglycanopathy, fukutin-related proteinopathy, telethoninopathy, and caveolinopathy
Contractures	Calpainopathy, laminopathy, myotilinopathy, and sarcoglycanopathy
Bulbar muscle weakness	Myotilinopathy, HSP40 proteinopathy, and desminopathy
Muscle cramps, myalgia, and rippling muscles	Calpainopathy, dysferlinopathy, anoctaminopathy, fukutin-related proteinopathy, and caveolinopathy
Cardiac involvement	Sarcoglycanopathy, telethoninopathy, fukutin-related proteinopathy, myotilinopathy, and dystroglycanopathy

(LGMDs: limb-girdle muscular dystrophies)

ARTICLE 12

Plasmid-mediated Gene Therapy in Mouse Models of Limb-girdle Muscular Dystrophy

Guha TK, Pichavant C, Calos MP. Plasmid-mediated gene therapy in mouse models of limb girdle muscular dystrophy. *Mol Ther Methods Clin Dev. 2019;15:294-304.*

Abstract

Background: Large size of gene, delivery of multiple genes, immunogenicity, high-effective dose are the limitations of adeno-associated virus (AAV)-associated gene therapy for limb-girdle muscular dystrophy (LGMD). These limitations were overcome by use of plasmid-mediated therapy.

Method: Capn3 null mice injected with the therapeutic plasmid pgWIZCAPN3gl (CAPN3) in the gastrocnemius muscle of each leg. Electroporation was administered after injection of each left leg, while right legs received no electroporation. Similarly, gene delivery in the BL/AJ mouse model of LGMD2B was performed. Five mice were designated negative controls and received Hank's balanced salt solution (HBSS). Five mice received the pKLD-CAG-DSYF-CPL (DYSF-CPL) plasmid encoding human dysferlin, and five mice received pKLD-CAG-DYSF-CFL (DYSF-CFL) encoding both dysferlin and follistatin, injected in the quadriceps. Long-term effectiveness was also evaluated. Experiment was also done on Sgca-null mouse model of LGMD2D.

Results and Discussion: Long-term presence of therapeutic protein was detected. Plasmid DNA produces long-term expression of genes. Its vascular delivery is safe and effective and enhanced by electroporation. Follistatin stimulates muscle health when delivered with therapeutic genes.

Limitation: Electroporation is feasible for local gene delivery only.

COMMENT

Duchenne muscular dystrophy is one of the early dystrophies to be tackled by gene editing and gene restoration.[27,28] Limb-girdle muscular dystrophies are very common in India and there are many different types that have been documented. These are transmitted as autosomal dominant and autosomal recessive diseases and a plethora of genetic effects has been seen. On this background, this section discusses a plasmid-mediated gene therapy in a mouse model of lingerie muscular dystrophy. As the size of the gene is large adeno-associated virus (AAV)-associated gene therapy has limitations and therefore, the authors have used plasmid-mediated therapy and discussed it in this section. The disease under consideration is the calpain 3 abnormality. The results of the study showed that therapeutic protein was available and expressed on long-term basis. They also documented that vascular delivery is safe and effective. Thus, the article brings to the fore another strategy for the treatment of limb-girdle muscular dystrophy.

ARTICLE 13

The Limb-girdle Muscular Dystrophies: Is Treatment on the Horizon?

Chu ML, Moran E. The limb-girdle muscular dystrophies: Is treatment on the horizon?
Neurotherapeutics. 2018;15(4):849-62.

Abstract

There has been an ever-expanding list of the limb-girdle muscular dystrophies (LGMD). There are currently 8 subtypes of autosomal dominant (AD) and 26 subtypes of autosomal recessive (AR) LGMD. Despite continued research efforts to conquer this group of genetic neuromuscular disease, patients continue to be treated symptomatically with the aim of prevention or addressing complications. Mouse models have been helpful in clarifying disease pathogenesis as well as strategizing pathways for treatment. Discoveries in translational research as well as molecular therapeutic approaches have kept clinicians optimistic that more promising clinical trials will lead the way to finding the cure for these devastating disorders. It is well known that the challenge for these rare diseases is the ability to assemble adequate numbers of patients for a clinically meaningful trial, but current efforts in developing patient registries have been encouraging. Natural history studies will be essential in establishing and interpreting the appropriate outcome measures for clinical trials. Nevertheless, animal studies continue to be key in providing proof of concept that will be necessary in moving research along. This review will briefly discuss each type of LGMD, highlighting their distinguishing features, then focus on research efforts that have been published in the literature for the past few years, many of which are still in the preclinical trial stage.

COMMENT

Calpainopathies
- Bartoli et al. (2006) evaluated the safety and efficacy of adeno-associated virus (AAV)-mediated *Calpain 3* gene transfer in a mouse model of LGMD2A using rAAV2/1 pseudotyped vectors and muscle-specific promoters. They found it effective and safe.
- Roudaut et al. found it to be associated with cardiac toxicity due to upregulated proteolytic activity of overexpressed calplain 3 in the heart. So they developed new AAV vectors with skeletal muscle-specific promoters. Show the expression of the transgene is restricted to the skeletal muscles and reduction in other organs toxicity.
- Phram et al. experienced that daily low-dose injections with somatropin stabilize or improve muscle strength and walking capacity till treatment is continued.

Dysferlinopathies
- Walter et al. conducted a prospective randomized placebo-controlled crossover clinical trial in confirmed patients to determine the effect of deflazacort. But patients deteriorated rather than improving.
- Lee et al. evaluate the effect of blocking the myostatin pathway in dysferlin deficient mice. They found to have detrimental effects.
- Gushchina et al. proved that recombinant human MG53 protein to improve membrane repair in dysferlin deficient mouse model.
- Large size of dysferlin gene is a challenge for gene therapy. Wolff et al. investigated plasmid DNA as a vector to carry large dystrophin gene to the mdx mouse model and showed positive response.
- Gene editing using CRISPR/Cas9 technology is under trial.

Sarcoglycanopathies
- Herson et al. (2012) shows expression of γ-sarcoglycan protein by AAV serotype 1 gene transfer without serious adverse effects.
- Gao et al. (2015) exon skipping as a potential tool. They generate mini-Gama that removes four of the seven coding exons in γ-sarcoglycan.
- Mendell et al. (2010) showed long-term and sustainable gene expression of alpha sarcoglycan following AAV-mediated gene transfer.
- Carotti et al. (2018) used small molecules like cystic fibrosis transmembrane regulator (CFTR) correctors for proper relocalization of the whole sarcoglycan complex with consequent reduction of sarcolemma fragility.
- Poszgai et al. (2017) did preclinical study using AAV-mediated gene therapy with promising results.
- Qiao et al. (2014) evaluated gene transfer for α-dystroglycan.
- Thomas et al. (2016) demonstrate that GALGT2 overexpression can reduce the extent of muscle pathology in FKRP mutant muscles.
- Vannoy et al. (2017) showed AAV-mediated mini Agrin delivery was unable to improve dystrophic phenotype in vivo.

ARTICLE 14

The Effects of Resistance Exercise Training on Strength and Functional Tasks in Adults with Limb-girdle, Becker, and Facioscapulohumeral Dystrophies

Bostock EL, O'Dowd DN, Payton CJ, Smith D, Orme P, Edwards BT, et al. The effects of resistance exercise training on strength and functional tasks in adults with limb-girdle, becker, and facioscapulohumeral dystrophies. *Front Neurol. 2019;10:1216.*

Abstract

Background: Positive effect of exercise is well established in healthy as well other populations with muscle weakness. But it was discouraged in muscular dystrophy due to the historical fear of detrimental effects. A meta-analysis by Gianola et al. (2018) demonstrated no significant effect of exercise may be due to the small number of participants and continuous decline in strength due to illness.

Objective: The objective is to evaluate the effect of twice-weekly resistance training program of 12 weeks' duration on muscle strength and functional task in ambulatory adults with muscular dystrophy.

Method: Ambulatory adults with muscular dystrophy participated in three testing sessions at baseline, after 12 control periods and after 12-week resistance training periods. Each testing session includes (1) measurements of isometric knee extensor and knee flexor maximum voluntary contraction (MVC) torque and (2) functional tasks: sit-to-stand time, a four steps-stair ascent, and a four steps-stair descent.

Results and Discussion: Significant increase in knee flexor MVC torque was noticed after the resistance exercise program. There was no significant change in knee extensor MVC torque though the direction of change was positive. All functional tasks parameters show improvement.

Conclusion: A twice-weekly 12-week resistance training program improves muscle strength and performance in functional tasks. It should be included in management of muscular dystrophy patients.

COMMENT

In the management of muscular dystrophies of various types, exercises are very important and assume a major part of the rehabilitative process, in an attempt to maintain mobility and ambulation.[29-31] This section discusses the role of twice-weekly resistance training program of 3 months duration. At the end of 12 weeks, they measured the flexor maximum voluntary contraction (MVC) torque which had significantly increased after the twice-weekly resistance training program, but in the knee extensors there was no significant change. On functional parameters, most of the parameters showed improvement. The section concludes that its twice-weekly 12-week resistance program improves muscle strength and performance on functional tasks and it should be included in the management of muscular dystrophy patients.

ARTICLE 15

Genetic Determinants of Disease Severity in the Myotonic Dystrophy Type 1 OPTIMISTIC Cohort

Cumming SA, Jimenez-Moreno C, Okkersen K, Wenninger S, Daidj F, Hogarth F, et al. OPTIMISTIC Consortium. Genetic determinants of disease severity in the myotonic dystrophy type 1 OPTIMISTIC cohort.
Neurology. 2019;93(10):e995-e1009.

Abstract

Background: Myotonic dystrophy type 1 (DM1) is a trinucleotide repeat disorder caused by CTG repeat in the *DMPK* gene. Longer repeat size is associated with more severe disease and earlier onset. It is difficult to offer predictive phenotypic information based on the size of the CTG repeat.

Objective: To evaluate the role of genetic variation at the DMPK locus on symptomatic diversity in 250 adult, ambulant patients with DM1 recruited to the Observational Prolonged Trial in DM1 to Improve Quality of Life-Standards, a Target Identification Collaboration (OPTIMISTIC) clinical trial.

Method: Small-pool polymerase chain reaction (PCR) was used to correct age at sampling biases and estimate the progenitor allele CTG repeat length and somatic mutational dynamics, and AciI digests and repeat primed PCR to test for the presence of variant repeats.

Results and Discussion: Only moderately affected patients were involved in trial. Disease severity is influenced by progenitor allele length. It is modified by age but sex has little effect. Patients in whom CTG repeat expansion is more rapid in the soma have early manifestation than predicted. These variant repeats have an important role in reducing disease severity and delaying age at onset.

Conclusion: Knowledge of progenitor allele length and presence of variant in DMPK CTG repeat is important for understanding clinical variability. It also provides a genetic route for defining disease-specific outcome measures, and the basis of treatment response and stratification in DM1 trials.

COMMENT

Genotype phenotype correlation has always been an intriguing issue. In the context of myotonic dystrophy, this becomes more important because the triplet repeat sizes differ in different tissues of the body, explaining a plethora of phenotypic findings appearing in varying severities in given individuals.[32-34] This section tries to evaluate the role of genetic variations in the *DMPK* gene and correlating with symptomatic diversity. They conclude that the knowledge of progenitor allele length and the presence of the variant in the DMPK CTG repeat has furthered the understanding of clinical variability. Such information is very important from the point of view of the quality of life and predicting various issues during the lifetime of the individual and also to judge therapeutic responses and develop better therapies.

ARTICLE 16

Efficacy and Safety of Dichlorphenamide for Primary Periodic Paralysis in Adolescents Compared with Adults

Ciafaloni E, Cohen F, Griggs R. Efficacy and safety of dichlorphenamide for primary periodic paralysis in adolescents compared with adults.
Pediatr Neurol. 2019;101:43-6.

Abstract

Background: Primary periodic paralysis (PPP) are heterogeneous groups of skeletal muscle ion channelopathies which were usually prevented by lifestyle and diet modification. Attacks are more frequent in the younger age group and become less as age advanced. Dichlorphenamide (DCP) is the only Food and Drug Administration (FDA)-approved drug. Its efficacy and safety is well established in adults.

Objective: To establish efficacy and safety of DCP in adolescents.

Method: It is a randomized double-blind, controlled, crossover study. Adolescent (<18 years age) patients with more than one episode per week and less than three episodes per day were included. After 8 weeks of observation, patients were randomly assigned to receive DCP or placebo for 9 weeks, followed by a washout period of at least 9 weeks and crossover to the other treatment for 9 weeks. Attack rate and severity-weighted attack rate were calculated.

Results and Discussion: There is a significant reduction in attack rate and severity-weighted attack rate. Most common side effect noted in adolescents was skin rash while in adults, it was numbness.

Conclusion: DCP is safe and effective in adolescents with different side effect profiles than adults.

COMMENT

Periodic paralysis is encountered in clinical practice from time to time.[35,36] The quality of life of these patients suffers because of repeated events of weakness and sometimes these are unpredictable. While currently, some medications are available for this illness, they are not universally effective and the search for further medications is required.

In this randomized, double-blind, controlled, crossover study adolescent patients of periodic paralysis were observed for 8 weeks and then randomized to receive dichlorphenamide which is an Food and Drug Administration (FDA)-approved drug for the disease, or received a placebo. The results showed a significant reduction in the attack rate and severity-weighted attack frequency; showing that the drug was more effective than the placebo. Thus, as the section mentions dichlorphenamide is a safe and effective drug in the armamentarium of the neurologist.

ARTICLE 17

The PRINTO Evidence-based Proposal for Glucocorticoids Tapering/Discontinuation in New Onset Juvenile Dermatomyositis Patients

Giancane G, Lavarello C, Pistorio A, Oliveira SK, Zulian F, Cuttica R, et al. Paediatric Rheumatology International Trials Organisation (PRINTO). The PRINTO evidence-based proposal for glucocorticoids tapering/discontinuation in new onset juvenile dermatomyositis patients.
Pediatr Rheumatol Online J. 2019;17(1):24.

Abstract

Background: Juvenile dermatomyositis (JDM) is rare. Its management in adults is not standardized while those for children are essentially based on consensus and literature revision.

Objective: To provide guidelines for glucocorticoid (GC) tapering or discontinuation and identify predictors of clinical remission and GC discontinuation in patients with new onset JDM.

Method: Data was analyzed from Paediatric Rheumatology International Trials Organisation (PRINTO) trial. Patients were randomized to three groups: GC alone, GC with cyclosporine (CSA), and GC with methotrexate (MTX). Trial has 2 months of induction phase, 22 months of maintenance phase followed by 3 years of extension phase.

Prednisolone was given as per the schedule given in **Table 3**.

TABLE 3: Schedule for prednisolone.

Duration of treatment	Core set measurement (CSM) decreased by	Prednisolone dose
First month		2 mg/kg/day
Second month	50–94%	Tapering 0.25 mg/kg/day
3–6 months	8–60%	Reach up to 0.2 mg/kg/day
6–12 months		Reach up to 0.1 mg/kg/day
12–24 months		Alternate day 0.1 mg/kg/day
24–36 months		Observation

Responses were recorded in three groups: Reference group [clinical remission with no major therapeutic changes (MTCs)], not achieve remission without MTC, and not achieve remission with MTC.

Results and Discussion: Trial provides large prospective data on rare condition. GC with MTX is the best treatment option from a safety and efficacy point. Group 1 and 2 showed a similar trend of decrease in disease activities while patients in group 3 had the worst outcome since just one-third was able to discontinue GCs.

Conclusion: It provides a clear guideline for how to use steroids and when and how to taper it. Earlier and more aggressive treatment may lead to better results.

COMMENT

Inflammatory myopathies form that group of myopathies which a clinician never wants to miss.[37,38] Within the inflammatory myopathies, children are often affected with dermatomyositis where the skin as well as the muscles are affected. The condition is rare and therefore, large data is not available on the therapeutic parameters of this disease. The role of corticosteroids and the other steroid sparing agents, either single or in combinations has been a point of interest and various clinicians are known to follow various strategies based on their comfort zone and literature review. In this context, this section is important because it provides large data from three groups of patients. It gives important information about steroids alone versus steroids in combination with other agents such as methotrexate. The methotrexate and steroid group fared the best in this study. This section is also important as it provides guidelines as to how to use steroids, when to taper them and when to add the second agents. This information is important for the treatment and management perspective of these conditions occurring in childhood.

ARTICLE 18

A Randomized, Double-blind, Placebo-controlled Trial of Infliximab in Refractory Polymyositis and Dermatomyositis

Schiffenbauer A, Garg M, Castro C, Pokrovnichka A, Joe G, Shrader J, et al. A randomized, double-blind, placebo-controlled trial of infliximab in refractory polymyositis and dermatomyositis.
Semin Arthritis Rheum. 2018;47(6):858-64.

Abstract

Background: Polymyositis (PM) and dermatomyositis (DM) are chronic, progressive, and lethal inflammatory muscle disorders. Available therapies show suboptimal response and/or high toxicities. Pathological role of tumor necrosis factor-alpha (TNF-α) in PM and DM is well established.

Objective: To assess the safety and efficacy as well to determine the effective dose of infliximab in patients with DM and PM.

Method: It is a randomized, double-blind, placebo-controlled crossover study. Adult patient with probable or definite PM or DM, proximal manual muscle test (MMT) scores between 80 and 120 out of 160, no signs of distal muscle weakness, active myositis, and at least 4 weeks of a stable dose of prednisone + immunosuppressive agents were enrolled. Study was conducted in two phases. In phase 1, patients were randomized to the placebo or infliximab group. Both groups were analyzed at 16 week by using MMT. In phase 2, nonresponder patients in the placebo group as well infliximab group, received a higher dose of infliximab while responder groups continued to receive the same dose. Final evaluation was done by using MMT at 40 weeks.

Results and Discussion: Out of 14 randomized patients, only one patient from the infliximab group was able to achieve expected MMT score improvement at the end of phase 1. In phase 2, two out of six placebo patients who received 5 mg/kg of infliximab, one out of one patient who continue on 5 mg/kg of infliximab and one out of three patients who received 7.5 mg/kg of infliximab met the improvement criteria. Minor adverse events noted with infliximab were back pain, fatigue, myalgia, edema, and infusion-related reaction.

Conclusion: Infliximab therapy is well tolerated and partially effective. As study has a limitation of a small number of patients, study with more number of patients may give more information about effectiveness.

COMMENT

Polymyositis and dermatomyositis are potentially modifiable diseases as they have immunological basis for the muscle damage.[39-41] While a certain number of individuals suffering from this category of diseases improve with therapy, there are others in whom standard treatment does not yield good results. For such patients who are refractory to treatment, various second and third-line agents need to be tried.

This small study discusses the use of a monoclonal antibody-infliximab, in such resistant inflammatory myopathies. The study is small and consists of 14 randomized patients. The improvement was judged by the manual muscle test (MMT) scores and the section clearly shows that a certain degree of improvement achieved in a good number of patients who were termed as refractory to standard therapy. Infliximab thus forms another option in patients who do not respond to standard therapy.

REFERENCES (Muscle Disorders)

1. Fenichel GM, Mendell JR, Moxley RT, Griggs RC, Brooke MH, Miller JP, et al. Comparison of daily and alternate-day prednisone therapy in the treatment of Duchenne muscular dystrophy. Arch Neurol. 1991;48:575-9.
2. Angelini C, Pegoraro E, Turella E, Intino MT, Pini A, Costa C. Deflazacort in Duchenne dystrophy: study of long-term effect. Muscle Nerve. 1994;17:386-91.
3. Griggs RC, Miller JP, Greenberg CR, Fehlings DL, Pestronk A, Mendell JR, et al. Efficacy and safety of deflazacort vs prednisone and placebo for Duchenne muscular dystrophy. Neurology. 2016;87(20):2123-31.
4. Moxley RT III, Ashwal S, Pandya S, Connolly A, Florence J, Mathews K, et al. Practice parameter: corticosteroid treatment of Duchenne dystrophy: Report of the Quality Standards Subcommittee of the American Academy of Neurology and the Practice Committee of the Child Neurology Society. Neurology. 2005;64(1):13-20.
5. Kinnett K, Noritz G. The PJ Nicholoff Steroid Protocol for Duchenne and Becker Muscular Dystrophy and Adrenal Suppression. PLoS Currents. 2017;9.
6. Shulman DI, Palmert MR, Kemp SF. Adrenal insufficiency: still a cause of morbidity and death in childhood. Pediatrics. 2007;119(2):e484-94.
7. Chen YW, Nagaraju K, Bakay M, McIntyre O, Rawat R, Shi R, et al. Early onset of inflammation and later involvement of TGFβ in Duchenne muscular dystrophy. Neurology. 2005;65:826-34.
8. De Paepe B, Creus KK, Martin JJ, De Bleecker JL. Upregulation of chemokines and their receptors in Duchenne muscular dystrophy: Potential for attenuation of myofiber necrosis. Muscle Nerve. 2012;46:917-25.
9. Delfín DA, Xu Y, Peterson JM, Guttridge DC, Rafael-Fortney JA, Janssen PM. Improvement of cardiac contractile function by peptide-based inhibition of NF-κB in the utrophin/dystrophin-deficient murine model of muscular dystrophy. J Transl Med. 2011;9:68.
10. Peterson JM, Kline W, Canan BD, Ricca DJ, Kaspar B, Delfín DA, et al. Peptide-based inhibition of NF-κB rescues diaphragm muscle contractile dysfunction in a murine model of Duchenne muscular dystrophy. Mol Med. 2011;17(5-6):508-15.
11. Pane M, Mazzone ES, Sivo S, Sormani MP, Messina S, D'Amico A, et al. Long term natural history data in ambulant boys with Duchenne muscular dystrophy: 36-month changes. PLoS One. 2014;9(10):e10820510.
12. Wang RT, Barthelemy F, Martin AS, Douine ED, Eskin A, Lucas A, et al. DMD genotype correlations from the Duchenne Registry: Endogenous exon skipping is a factor in prolonged ambulation for individuals with a defined mutation subtype. Hum Mutat. 2018;39(9):1193-202.
13. Hoffman EP, Brown RH, Jr, Kunkel LM. Dystrophin: The protein product of the Duchenne muscular dystrophy locus. Cell. 1987;51:919-28.
14. Abbs S, Tuffery-Giraud S, Bakker E, Ferlini A, Sejersen T, Mueller CR. Best practice guidelines on molecular diagnostics in duchenne/becker muscular dystrophies. Neuromuscul Disord. 2010;20:422-7.
15. Eagle M, Baudouin S, Chandler C, Giddings DR, Bullock R, Bushby K. Survival in Duchenne muscular dystrophy: improvements in life expectancy since 1967 and the impact of home nocturnal ventilation. Neuromuscul Disord. 2002;12:926-9.
16. Manzur AY, Kuntzer T, Pike M, Swan A. Glucocorticoid corticosteroids for Duchenne muscular dystrophy (Review) Cochrane Database Syst Rev. 2004;(2):CD003725.
17. Gilroy J, Cahalan JL, Berman R, Newman M. Cardiac and pulmonary complications in Duchenne's progressive muscular dystrophy. Circulation. 1963;27(4, pt 1):484-93.
18. Viollet L, Thrush PT, Flanigan KM, Mendell JR, Allen HD. Effects of angiotensin-converting enzyme inhibitors and/or beta blockers on the cardiomyopathy in Duchenne muscular dystrophy. Am J Cardiol. 2012;110(1):98-102.
19. van Bockel EA, Lind JS, Zijlstra JG, Wijkstra PJ, Meijer PM, van den Berg MP, et al. Cardiac assessment of patients with late stage Duchenne muscular dystrophy. Neth Heart J. 2009;17(6):232-7.

20. Gomez-Merino E, Bach JR. Duchenne muscular dystrophy: prolongation of life by noninvasive ventilation and mechanically assisted coughing. Am J Phys Med Rehabil. 2002;81(6):411-5.
21. Finder JD, Birnkrant D, Carl J, Farber HJ, Gozal D, Iannaccone ST, et al. Respiratory care of the patient with Duchenne muscular dystrophy: ATS consensus statement. Am J Respir Crit Care Med. 2004;170(4):456-65.
22. Birnkrant DJ, Bushby KM, Amin RS, Bach JR, Benditt JO, Eagle M, et al. The respiratory management of patients with Duchenne muscular dystrophy: A DMD care considerations working group specialty article. Pediatr Pulmonol. 2010;45(8):739-48.
23. Angelini C, Nardetto L, Borsato C, Padoan R, Fanin M, Nascimbeni AC, et al. The clinical course of calpainopathy (LGMD2A) and dysferlinopathy (LGMD2B). Neurol Res. 2010;32:41-6.
24. Blázquez L, Aiastui A, Goicoechea M, Martins de Araujo M, Avril A, Beley C, et al. In vitro correction of a pseudoexon-generating deep intronic mutation in LGMD2A by antisense oligonucleotides and modified small nuclear RNAs. Hum Mutat. 2013;34:1387-95.
25. Bushby K. Diagnosis and management of the limb girdle muscular dystrophies. Pract Neurol. 2009;9:314-23.
26. Dadali EL, Shagina OA, Ryzhkova OP, Rudenskaia GE, Fedotov VP, Poliakov AV. Clinical-genetic characteristics of limb girdle-muscular dystrophy type 2A. Zh Nevrol Psikhiatr Im S S Korsakova. 2010;110:79-83.
27. Bartoli M, Roudaut C, Martin S, Fougerousse F, Suel L, Poupiot J, et al. Safety and efficacy of AAV-mediated calpain 3 gene transfer in a mouse model of limb-girdle muscular dystrophy type 2A. Mol Ther. 2006;13:250-9.
28. Lostal W, Bartoli M, Bourg N, Roudaut C, Bentaïb A, Miyake K, et al. Efficient recovery of dysferlin deficiency by dual adeno-associated vector-mediated gene transfer. Hum Mol Genet. 2010;19:1897-907.
29. Morse CI, Bostock EL, Twiss HM, Kapp LH, Orme P, Jacques MF. The cardiorespiratory response and physiological determinants of the assisted 6-minute handbike cycle test in adult males with muscular dystrophy. Muscle Nerve. 2018;58:427-33.
30. Beenakker EA, Maurits NM, Fock JM, Brouwer OF, van der Hoeven JH. Functional ability and muscle force in healthy children and ambulant Duchenne muscular dystrophy patients. Eur J Paediatr Neurol. 2005;9:387-93.
31. Gianola S, Pecoraro V, Lambiase S, Gatti R, Banfi G, Moja L. Efficacy of muscle exercise in patients with muscular dystrophy: a systematic review showing a missed opportunity to improve outcomes. PLoS One. 2013;8:e65414.
32. Mahadevan M, Tsilfidis C, Sabourin L, Shutler G, Amemiya C, Jansen G, et al. Myotonic dystrophy mutation: an unstable CTG repeat in the 3' untranslated region of the gene. Science. 1992;255:1253-5.
33. Harley HG, Rundle SA, MacMillan JC, Myring J, Brook JD, Crow S, et al. Size of the unstable CTG repeat sequence in relation to phenotype and parental transmission in myotonic dystrophy. Am J Hum Genet. 1993;52:1164-74.
34. Salehi LB, Bonifazi E, Stasio ED, Gennarelli M, Botta A, Vallo L, et al. Risk prediction for clinical phenotype in myotonic dystrophy type 1: data from 2,650 patients. Genet Test. 2007;11:84-90.
35. Tawil R, McDermott MP, Brown R Jr, Shapiro BC, Ptacek LJ, McManis PG, et al. Randomized trials of dichlorphenamide in the periodic paralyses. Ann Neurol. 2000;47(1):46-53.
36. Sansone VA, Burge J, McDermott MP, Smith PC, Herr B, Tawil R, et al. Randomized, placebo-controlled trials of dichlorphenamide in periodic paralysis. Neurology. 2016;86(15):1408-16.
37. Enders FB, Bader-Meunier B, Baildam E, Constantin T, Dolezalova P, Feldman BM, et al. Consensus-based recommendations for the management of juvenile dermatomyositis. Ann Rheum Dis. 2017;76(2):329-40.
38. Stringer E, Bohnsack J, Bowyer SL, Griffin TA, Huber AM, Lang B, et al. Treatment approaches to juvenile dermatomyositis (JDM) across North America: the childhood arthritis and rheumatology research Alliance (CARRA) JDM treatment survey. J Rheumatol. 2010;37(9):1953-61.
39. Efthimiou P. Tumor necrosis factor-alpha in inflammatory myopathies: pathophysiology and therapeutic implications. Seminars Arthritis Rheum. 2006;36:168-72.
40. Li YP, Reid MB. Effect of tumor necrosis factor-alpha on skeletal muscle metabolism. Curr Opin Rheumatol. 2001;13:483-7.
41. Albayda J, Christopher-Stine L. Novel approaches in the treatment of myositis and myopathies. Ther Adv Musculoskelet Dis. 2012;4:369-77.

Section 10: Sleep Medicine

Section Editor: Manjari Tripathi

Associate Editor: Kamalesh Chakravarty

ARTICLE 1

High-risk Characteristics for Recurrent Cardiovascular Events among Patients with Obstructive Sleep Aponea in the SAVE Study

Quan W, Zheng D, McEvoy RD, Barbe F, Chen R, Liu Z, et al.; SAVE Investigators. High risk characteristics for recurrent cardiovascular events among patients with obstructive sleep apnoea in the SAVE study.
E Clinical Medicine. 2018;2-3:59-65.

Abstract

Objective: To identify the specific obstructive sleep apnea (OSA) clinical phenotypes relating to risks of serious cardiovascular (CV) events and response to continuous positive airway pressure (CPAP) treatment.

Methods: This was a post-hoc analyses of the SAVE (Sleep Apnea Cardiovascular Endpoints) study. The participants with moderate-to-severe OSA and coronary artery disease (CAD) and/or cerebrovascular disease (CeVD) were randomized to CPAP with usual care or usual care alone. Latent class analysis (LCA) was done to identify the OSA clinical phenotypes in 2,649 patients with 19 patient-centered variables, supported by Bayesian information criteria and clinical interpretability. Cox regression analysis were used to evaluate the risk of composite cardiac and stroke outcomes. Response to CPAP treatment was evaluated using interaction terms and chi-square test.

Results: Four OSA clinical phenotypes were identified by LCA: CAD alone and with diabetes mellitus (CAD + DM), and CeVD alone and with DM (CeVD + DM), in 39, 15, 37, and 9% of participants, respectively. Highest rate of composite CV events were noted in CAD + DM phenotype [hazard ratio (HR) 2.08; 95% confidence interval (CI) 1.57–2.76], while highest risk of stroke were observed in CeVD + DM phenotype (HR 6.84; 95% CI 3.77–12.42). Adherence to CPAP treatment (nil or <4 hours vs. ≥4 hours in the first 2 years of the study) was found to influence the risk of composite CV outcome (p-interaction = –0.04). Lowest risk of CV outcome was noted in CPAP adherent patients of the CeVD + DM phenotype (p = 0.02).

Conclusion: High-risk clinical phenotypes for CV events were identified and response to CPAP therapy was assessed. This might allow targeted therapies in the OSA patients.

COMMENT

Risk stratification for recurrent cardiovascular (CV) events are essential for deciding optimal management and secondary preventive measures. This secondary analysis of the SAVE (Sleep Apnea Cardiovascular Endpoints) clinical trial defines different clinical phenotypes for the purpose of risk stratification. The authors describe that prior history of cardiovascular disease (CVD) and diabetes were the strongest factors for distinguishing different phenotypes. Patients with obstructive sleep apnea (OSA) were found to have the highest risk for CV events. Intensive continuous positive airway pressure (CPAP) treatment and ensuring high level of adherence among these patients might offer benefits to these patients. Some previous studies had also demonstrated benefits of CPAP on CV risk.[1,2] However, in this study the effect of CPAP was not uniform. Hence, the authors suggest stratification of different clinical phenotypes with OSA to provide tailored CPAP therapy while ensuring high adherence in those with comorbidities like diabetes, vascular events, and OSA.

ARTICLE 2

Effects of Continuous Positive Airway Pressure on Depression and Anxiety Symptoms in Patients with Obstructive Sleep Apnoea: Results from the Sleep Apnoea Cardiovascular Endpoint Randomized Trial and Meta-analysis

Zheng D, Xu Y, You S, Hackett ML, Woodman RJ, Li Q, et al. Effects of continuous positive airway pressure on depression and anxiety symptoms in patients with obstructive sleep apnoea: Results from the sleep apnoea cardiovascular Endpoint randomised trial and meta-analysis.
E Clinical Medicine. 2019;11:89-96.

Abstract

Objective: To evaluate whether continuous positive airway pressure (CPAP) treatment can improve depression or anxiety symptoms in obstructive sleep apnea (OSA) patients.

Methods: Secondary analysis of the SAVE (Sleep Apnea Cardiovascular Endpoints) trial, combined with a systematic review of randomized evidence was conducted. The SAVE secondary analyses included 2,110 patients with moderate-to-severe OSA and established cardiovascular disease (CVD), who were randomly allocated to CPAP treatment plus usual care or usual care alone. Mean follow-up was 3.7 [standard deviation (SD) 1.6] years. Anxiety and depression were assessed at baseline and at 6, 24, 48, 72, and 84-month visits, using the Hospital Anxiety and Depression Scale (HADS). Effect of CPAP treatment was evaluated on depression and anxiety caseness (defined as score ≥8 on the HADS subscales) for OSA patients.

Results: Continuous positive airway pressure treatment was associated with a reduced odd of depression caseness [adjusted odds ratio (OR) 0.80; 95% confidence interval (CI) 0.65–0.98; $p = 0.031$] in comparison to usual care and the treatment effect was greater in patients with preexisting depression. Systematic review of 20 randomized trial including 4,255 patients demonstrated a reduction in depression in OSA patients with CPAP therapy. The overall effect (standardized mean difference) was –0.18 (95% CI –0.24 to –0.12). However, no significant effect of CPAP therapy was noted on anxiety caseness both in the patients of SAVE study (adjusted OR 0.98; 95% CI 0.78–1.24; $p = 0.89$) and the systematic review.

Conclusion: Continuous positive airway pressure treatment reduces depressive symptoms in patients with OSA and CVD independently of improvement in sleepiness.

COMMENT

The association between sleep disturbances and abnormal mood has been found to be robust and bidirectional.[3,4] Mood disorders, especially depression has been associated with higher risk of cardiovascular (CV) disease. It contributes greatly to the morbidity and premature mortality.[5] This study is a secondary analyses and meta-analysis of previous studies on the effect of continuous positive airway pressure (CPAP) therapy on anxiety and depression. The authors report a significant reduction in clinically significant depression, but not in anxiety with CPAP treatment. The effect of CPAP treatment on depression was independent of the improvement noted in daytime sleepiness. Depression is often missed and undertreated, it needs to be emphasized that for mental health obstructive sleep apnea (OSA) treatment with CPAP trumps managing both apneas and improving depression.

ARTICLE 3

Sleep Duration and Risk of Cardiovascular Events: The SAVE Study

Li J, Zheng D, Loffler KA, Wang X, McEvoy RD, Woodman RJ, et al.; SAVE Investigators. Sleep duration and risk of cardiovascular events: The SAVE study.
Int J Stroke. 2020;15(8):858-65.

Abstract

Objective: To assess the relationship of sleep duration and major recurrent cardiovascular (CV) events in patients with obstructive sleep apnea (OSA) and established CV disease.

Methods: This was secondary analyses of the international, multicenter SAVE (Sleep Apnea Cardiovascular Endpoint) trial. Sleep duration was assessed from the overnight home oximeter used for OSA diagnosis and were categorized to <6 hours, 6–8 hours (reference), and >8 hours. Cox proportional hazard models were used to determine associations of sleep durations and major CV outcomes. The CV outcomes were primary composite of CV death, nonfatal myocardial infraction (MI), nonfatal stroke, and any hospitalization for unstable angina, heart failure, or transient ischemic attack (TIA); secondary composite of cardiac and cerebral (stroke or TIA) events.

Results: Sleep duration derived from pulse oximetry was available in 2,687 patients. The mean age was 61.2 years and 80.9% were males. A total of 436 CV events were recorded over a mean follow-up of 3.7 years. In comparison to reference category, sleep duration was not associated with risk of primary composite CV outcomes [adjusted hazard ratio (HR) 1.00; 95% confidence interval (CI) 0.76–1.33 for sleep duration <6 hours and HR 1.22; 95% CI 0.98–1.52 for sleep duration >8 hours). However, longer sleep duration was found to be associated with increased cerebral events and stroke alone (HR 1.67; 95% CI 1.17–2.39; $p = 0.0005$ and HR 1.79; 95% CI 1.11–2.63; $p = 0.0003$, respectively).

Conclusion: Longer sleep duration was associated with increased risk of stroke but not cardiac events in OSA patients with established CV disease.

COMMENT

Association between sleep duration and risk of cardiovascular event has been a matter of debate for long. Previous studies have reported that both short (<7 h/day) and long sleep duration (≥9 h/day), has been associated with increased risk of developing coronary heart diseases (CHD) and stroke.[6] However, short sleep duration has not been found to be associated with no increased risk of stroke.[7] This study is the secondary analysis of the SAVE (Sleep Apnea Cardiovascular Endpoint) study, with a long follow-up which evaluates the sleep duration with risk of cardiovascular events. The authors report no association of sleep duration with composite serious cardiovascular events. However, long sleep duration, defined as >8 hours, was found to be associated with higher risk of stroke and transient ischemic attack (TIA). This points toward a possibility of acute or long-term intermittent hypoxia effecting the brain and heart vasculature differently.[8] The physiological disturbances associated with longer sleep duration may have greater adverse effect on the cerebral endothelium. In association with obstructive sleep apnea (OSA), increased sleep duration might contribute to atherosclerotic process thereby contributing to the increased risk of cerebrovascular events. Hence, it is essential that an appropriate duration of 6–7 hours of sleep in a person with OSA is safer in terms of avoiding cerebrovascular risk.

ARTICLE 4

Sleep Abnormalities and Polysomnographic Profile in Children with Drug-resistant Epilepsy

Manokaran RK, Tripathi M, Chakrabarty B, Pandey RM, Gulati S. Sleep abnormalities and polysomnographic profile in children with drug-resistant epilepsy.
Seizure. 2020;82:59-64.

Abstract

Objective: To assess the prevalence of sleep abnormalities in children with drug-resistant epilepsy (DRE) and to compare their polysomnographic profile with well-controlled epilepsy (WCE) and age matched typically developing children (TDC).

Methods: This cross-sectional study consisted of 40 participants in each group (DRE, WCE, and TDC). The CSHQ (Children's Sleep Habits Questionnaire) and MPEDSS (Modified Pediatric Epworth Daytime Sleepiness Scale) were administered to assess prevalence of sleep abnormalities. 35 children each in the DRE and WCE group and 17 in TDC group underwent single night polysomnography (PSG).

Result: The prevalence of sleep abnormalities determined by CSHQ in DRE group was 72.5% [95% confidence interval (CI) 58.7–86.3%; mean score 47.5 ± 7.1] compared to 32.5% (42.4 ± 6.2) in WCE group, and 15% (37.3 ± 5) in TDC group ($p = 0.01$). Excessive daytime sleepiness assessed by MPEDSS was noted in 52.5% of children in DRE, 12.5% in WCE, and 5% in TDC group ($p = 0.03$). Overnight PSG revealed significant reduction in sleep efficiency and rapid eye movement (REM) sleep duration, and significantly increased N2 duration, REM latency, arousal, and apnea-hypopnea index in the DRE group in comparison to WCE and TDC groups.

Conclusion: Sleep abnormalities were found to be a major comorbidity in up to 75% of children with DRE and sleep architecture was significantly altered in them.

COMMENT

Person with epilepsy suffer from sleep-related issues which are mostly overlooked,[9] this effects their overall quality of life and has a deleterious effect on their cognitive parameters.[10,11] This study evaluates the prevalence of sleep abnormalities in children with drug-resistant epilepsy (DRE). The assessment was done by CSHQ (Children's Sleep Habits Questionnaire), and overnight polysomnography (PSG). The prevalence of sleep abnormalities was about 75% in the study population. The cognitive impairment was also more marked in patients with drug refractory epilepsy in comparison to well-controlled epilepsy. Poor sleep efficiency, decreased rapid eye movement (REM), and N3 suggests an overall poor quality of sleep in children with DRE. Underlying brain abnormality, antiseizure medications also contribute to the sleep issues. This study highlights the need to recognize sleep abnormalities with children with epilepsy. Targeted interventions to improve sleep in DRE will improve seizure outcomes and a modifiable factor.

ARTICLE 5

Guidelines of the Indian Society for Sleep Research (ISSR) for Practice of Sleep Medicine during COVID-19

Gupta R, Kumar VM, Tripathi M, Datta K, Narayana M, Sarmah KR, et al. Guidelines of the Indian Society for Sleep Research (ISSR) for practice of sleep medicine during COVID-19.
Sleep Vigil. 2020;4(2):61-72.

Abstract

Objective: Sleep services are assigned a nonessential status during the COVID-19 pandemic. However, the importance of sleep in one's health and well-being cannot be ignored. Therefore, to protect the health of the population, it is essential to find ways and means to continue the practice of sleep medicine during the COVID-19 pandemic.

Methods: The sleep environment and work ethics varies in different countries. Under the circumstance of COVID-19 pandemic, the Indian Society for Sleep Research (ISSR) created a task force to develop guidelines for practice of sleep medicine in India and in other countries affected by the COVID-19 pandemic. Documents regarding practice of sleep medicine and associated specialties during COVID-19 by various government authorities and professional organizations were examined by the task force. The recommendations were examined for their applicability. Consensus was reached based on available evidences, wherever gaps were identified.

Results and Recommendations: The emphasis of the guidelines is to avoid doctor to patient contact during the pandemic period. Tele consultation and other audio–visual modes can be considered as modes of medical practice during this period. Presence of a family member or reliable informant in addition to patient is recommended. The ISSR guidelines also provide a list of medications allowed to be prescribed in the teleconsultations. The recommendations stress up on the need to reduce contact with COVID-19 patients and follow personal protection guidelines and also discusses the strategies for safe conduct of level 1 sleep studies. Home sleep testing was suggested to be given more attention. On opening up of the sleep laboratories, safety of patients and staff should be given priority. ISSR recommends to postpone and reschedule in-laboratory positive pressure therapy, however, it mentions the special considerations to be followed in emergency situations. High clinical risk patients may be diagnosed on basis of clinical findings without performing polysomnography or home sleep testing. Regular assessment of the COVID-19 situation in the community along with periodic review of the situation with local public health and state health department is advised.

COMMENT

The COVID-19 pandemic has forced a transformation in the neurological practice worldwide. Of all the neurological specialties, sleep medicine has been probably more affected than others. This article is about the recommendations and guidelines of the task force formed Indian Society for Sleep Research (ISSR) for practice of sleep medicine during COVID-19 pandemic. Use of teleconsultations was encouraged. Guidelines for conducting sleep study was issued in lines of those of American Academy of Sleep Medicine (AASM) and European guidelines.[12,13] All the recommendations followed the regular advisories of Ministry of Health and Family Welfare, Government of India and was aimed at ensuring the public safety of public, patients, healthcare professionals, and reducing the COVID-19 spread in community. Anxiety and uncertainty in COVID times makes the need to improve sleep to safely counter the effects and improve quality of life (QOL).

ARTICLE 6

Cognitive and Behavioral Therapy for Insomnia Increases the Use of Continuous Positive Airway Pressure Therapy in Obstructive Sleep Apnea Participants with Comorbid Insomnia: A Randomized Clinical Trial

Sweetman A, Lack L, Catcheside PG, Antic NA, Smith S, Chai-Coetzer CL, et al. Cognitive and behavioral therapy for insomnia increases the use of continuous positive airway pressure therapy in obstructive sleep apnea participants with comorbid insomnia: A randomized clinical trial.
Sleep. 2019;42(12):zsz178.

Abstract

Objective: Insomnia and obstructive sleep apnea (OSA) often coexist, making it difficult to treat OSA with continuous positive airway pressure (CPAP). This study aimed to test the hypothesis that initial treatment with cognitive and behavioral therapy for insomnia (CBT-i) versus treatment as usual (TAU) would improve insomnia symptoms and increase subsequent acceptance and use of CPAP.

Methods: One hundred and forty-five patients with OSA (apnea-hypopnea index ≥15) and comorbid insomnia were randomized to either four sessions of CBT-i, or TAU before commencing CPAP therapy until 6 months postrandomization. Primary outcome included objective CPAP adherence and changes in objective sleep efficiency by 6 months between the groups. Secondary outcomes included rates of immediate CPAP acceptance or rejection, and changes in sleep parameters, insomnia severity, and day time impairments by 6 months between the groups.

Results: In comparison to TAU, participants in the CBT-i group had 61 minutes greater adherence to CPAP during night time [95% confidence interval (CI) 9–113; $p = 0.023$, $d = 0.38$] and higher acceptance to initial CPAP treatment (99% vs. 89%, $p = 0.034$). Greater improvement of global insomnia severity and dysfunctional sleep-related cognition at 6 months (both $p < 0.001$) were observed in CBT-i group. Greater improvement in sleep impairment measures were noted immediately following CBT-i. However, no difference in sleep outcomes and day time impairments were noted between the groups at 6 months.

Conclusion: CBT-i treatment prior to initiating CPAP in OSA patients with comorbid insomnia, improves CPAP use and insomnia symptoms compared to starting CPAP without CBT-i.

COMMENT

Obstructive sleep apnea (OSA) and insomnia often coexist, with population prevalence varying from 27 to 85%.[14] Although continuous positive airway pressure (CPAP) treatment remains the mainstay of treatment for moderate-to-severe OSA, patient acceptance and adherence to CPAP remains a big hurdle to satisfactory outcome. This randomized clinical trial compares the efficacy of initial cognitive and behavioral therapy of insomnia (CBT-i) in comparison to "treatment as usual" in ensuring the acceptance and adherence of CPAP therapy and improvement in sleep quality. The authors report 87% lower rate of immediate rejection of CPAP therapy among patients receiving four sessions of CBT-i prior to initiation of CPAP therapy. However, no improvement in polysomnography (PSG) or diary measured sleep efficiency or other sleep parameters were noted. This study findings are similar to another study where investigators reported therapist delivered integrated CBT-i had increased the CPAP adherence.[15] In view of growing evidences, use of CBT prior to CPAP therapy may be beneficial. It can improve both short- and long-term treatment objectives in patients with comorbid insomnia. Adapting to CPAP and the mask is not easy and CBT helps in adapting to these.

ARTICLE 7

Association of Obstructive Sleep Apnea and Cerebral Small Vessel Disease: A Systematic Review and Meta-analysis

Huang Y, Yang C, Yuan R, Liu M, Hao Z. Association of obstructive sleep apnea and cerebral small vessel disease: A systematic review and meta-analysis.
Sleep. 2020;43(4):zsz264.

Abstract

Objective: To investigate the association between obstructive sleep apnea (OSA) and presence of neuroimaging markers of cerebral small vessel disease (CSVD).

Methods: Systematic search in online databases like PubMed, Embase, Web of Sciences, Scopus, and Cochrane library were done from inception to May 2019 for studies evaluating the association between OSA and CSVD. The markers for CSVD included were white matter hyperintensities (WMH), silent brain infarction (SBI), cerebral microbleeds (CMBs), and perivascular spaces (PVS). Random effect meta-analysis was used to estimate pooled odds ratios (ORs) with 95% confidence interval (CI).

Results: Out of 7,290 publications screened, 20 studies involving 6,036 subjects were included in the meta-analysis. Sample size ranges from 27 to 1,763 (median 158, interquartile range; 67–393). Moderate-to-severe OSA was positively associated with WMH (13 studies, $n = 4,412$; OR 2.23; 95% CI 1.53–3.25; $I^2 = 80.3\%$) and SBI (12 studies, $n = 3,353$; OR 1.54; 95% CI 1.06–2.23; $I^2 = 52\%$). However, no association was noted with CMBs (three studies, $n = 342$; OR 2.17; 95% CI 0.61–7.73; $I^2 = 60.2\%$) or PVS (two studies, $n = 267$; OR 1.56; 95% CI 0.28–8.57; $I^2 = 69.5\%$). No relationship was noted between mild OSA and CSVD.

Conclusion: Current evidence suggests that moderate-to-severe sleep apnea is positively related to WMH and SBI but not CMBs or PVS. The findings indicate that OSA may contribute to the pathogenesis of CSVD.

COMMENT

Cerebral small vessel disease (CSVD) has been increasingly associated with increased risk of stroke, cognitive impairment, and dementia.[16,17] Traditional risk factors like age, hypertension, diabetes, and smoking though has been attributed for CSVD, they do not explain the pathogenesis CSVD. Obstructive sleep apnea (OSA) has been associated with all these established vascular risk factors, however, its association with CVSD is unexplored. This study is a systematic review and meta-analysis evaluating the association between the two entities. The authors report an association of moderate-to-severe OSA with white matter hyperintensities (WMH) and silent brain infarction (SBI). A possible hypothesis is that effects of nocturnal apnea associated with OSA, usually induces changes in cerebrovascular hemodynamic, which in turn may lead to endothelial dysfunction. In addition OSA often results in systemic inflammation with increase in inflammatory biomarkers like C-reactive protein and tumor necrosis factor.[18] Endothelial dysfunction along with systematic inflammation might lead to development of CSVD. OSA is often undetected and not thought of risk factor in persons with white matter changes. Larger cohort studies might be prioritized to evaluate the association of OSA with CSVD.

ARTICLE 8

Long-term Efficacy and Safety of Phrenic Nerve Stimulation for the Treatment of Central Sleep Apnea

Fox H, Oldenburg O, Javaheri S, Ponikowski P, Augostini R, Goldberg LR, et al. Long-term efficacy and safety of phrenic nerve stimulation for the treatment of central sleep apnea.
Sleep. 2019;42(11):zsz158.

Abstract

Objective: To assess long-term efficacy and safety of phrenic nerve stimulation (PNS) in patients with moderate-to-severe central sleep apnea (CSA) through 3 years of therapy.

Methods: Patients enrolled in the previously conducted remedē System Pivotal Trial (transvenous PNS) were observed every 3 months after implants until US Food and Drugs Administration approval in October 2017. All patients completed 24 months of follow-up. Sleep metrics (polysomnography) and echocardiographic parameters were reported at baseline, 12, 18, and 24 months in addition to available 36-month sleep results from polygraphy. Safety was assessed through 36 months.

Results: 109 and 60 patients were assessed at 24 and 36 months, respectively. The mean age was 64 years, 91% were male and mean apnea-hypopnea index (AHI) was 47 per hour. Sleep metrics namely AHI, central apnea index, arousal index, oxygen desaturation index, and rapid eye movement sleep remained improved in the 24 and 36 months with continuous use of PNS therapy. At least 60% of patients achieved at least 50% reduction in AHI through 24 months. Serious adverse events (SAEs) related to the remedē System implant procedure, device, or therapy were reported in 10% patients at 24 months. No unanticipated adverse effect or deaths were reported. No additional SAEs were reported between 24 and 36 months.

Conclusion: These data suggest beneficial effects of long-term PNS in patients with CSA appear to persist at 36 months without any additional adverse events.

COMMENT

Central sleep apnea (CSA) is frequent among patients with cardiovascular disease and heart failure.[19] It also affects the sleep and quality of life in nonheart failure patients. CSA is characterized neurophysiologically by central breathing instability with transient inhibition of ventilator motor function.[20] Treatment options depends on the underlying cause, and varies from positive pressure devices, pharmacological therapy to phrenic nerve stimulation (PNS). Mask-based therapies are associated with mask and pressure intolerance leading to poor adherence. Recently, adaptive seroventilation has been shown to increase mortality among patients with reduced ejection fraction with CSA.[21] Hence, novel therapeutic like PNS is being actively evaluated. This study explores the long term, safety, and efficacy of PNS. Investigators of the study reported a consistent therapeutic effectiveness at 36 months of follow-up. Serious side effects were mainly related to implant procedure, device, and delivered therapy and were noted in first year of therapy. Improved safety profile and long-term beneficial effect of PNS may a viable therapeutic option in CSA.

ARTICLE 9

Multiple Treatment Comparison in Narcolepsy: A Network Meta-analysis

Lehert P, Falissard B. Multiple treatment comparison in narcolepsy: A network meta-analysis. *Sleep. 2018;41(12):zsy185.*

Abstract

Objective: Multiple randomized controlled trials (RCTs) that compared the safety and efficacy of medical treatments for narcolepsy were analyzed using network meta-analysis.

Methods: The RCTs evaluating the medical treatment for narcolepsy were searched. The included studies provided at least one of the following selected outcomes for both efficacy and safety: the Epworth Sleepiness Score (ESS), the maintenance of wakefulness test (MWT), number of cataplexy (CTP) attacks during treatment and adverse effects. The network meta-analysis compared efficacy and safety of various treatments. Multiarm studies and multicriteria treatment decisions, based on a random model that assumed heterogeneity between studies with corrections for multiarm studies.

Results: Fourteen RCTs, three-drug treatments, and six doses were identified: sodium oxybate (6 and 9 g/day), modafinil (between 200 and 400 mg/day), and pitolisant (up to 20 and up to 40 mg/day). Significant heterogeneity (>50%) was noted between studies for almost all endpoints, however between-design consistency was present. For ESS and MWT, sodium oxybate 9 g/day, modafinil, and pitolisant up to 40 mg/day reported similar efficacy. For reducing CTP, pitolisant 40 mg/day, and sodium oxybate 9 g/day in two nightly doses were found to have similar efficacy. Overall good safety profile characterized by a treatment emergent adverse effect (TEAE) incidence risk ratio (IRR) <1.5 was noted for all compared treatments except for sodium oxybate 9 g/day. Pitolisant 40 mg was shown with best *P* scores for the benefit/risk (BR) ratio, however, it was not statistically significant.

Conclusion: Modafinil (200–400 mg/day), sodium oxybate 9 g/day, and pitolisant up to 40 mg/day had similar efficacy for reducing excessive day time sleepiness. Only sodium oxybate 9 g/day and pitolisant up to 40 mg/day had similar efficacy on CTP. Overall Pitolisant had best *P* score on BR ratio.

COMMENT

Currently, there is no equivocal recommendations for pharmacological agents for treatment of narcolepsy.[22] Only few comparative studies are available on medical therapy and optimal dosage in patients with narcolepsy. This study is a network metadata analysis of 14 randomized controlled trials to compare the efficacy, safety of different drugs used in management of narcolepsy. Modafinil was the most investigated drug and resulted in significant improvement in excessive day time sleepiness (EDS), but had no significant effect on cataplexy. Pitolisant,[23] a new histamine H3 receptor antagonist, was studied in three studies. It had good efficacy in reducing EDS and cataplexy. Among the available agents, Pitolisant had the best benefit/risk (BR) ratio. Newer and novel medications are required for cataplexy while sodium oxybate is a restricted and controlled substance not available in India. Pitolisant awaits its presence in India.

ARTICLE 10

Clinical and Video-polysomnographic Analysis of Rapid Eye Movement Sleep Behavior Disorder and Other Sleep Disturbances in Dementia with Lewy Bodies

Fernández-Arcos A, Morenas-Rodríguez E, Santamaria J, Sánchez-Valle R, Lladó A, Gaig C, et al. Clinical and video-polysomnographic analysis of rapid eye movement sleep behavior disorder and other sleep disturbances in dementia with Lewy bodies.
Sleep. 2019;42(7):zsz086.

Abstract

Objective: To study rapid eye movement (REM) sleep behavior disorder (RBD) and other sleep disorders in patients with dementia with Lewy bodies (DLB).

Methods: Consecutive patients with DLB and mild dementia were recruited irrespective of sleep complaints. They underwent clinical interview, assessment of sleep scales [Pittsburgh sleep quality index (PSQI)] for overall sleep quality, Epworth Sleepiness Scale (ESS) for excessive daytime sleepiness, Mayo sleep questionnaires (MSQ) for screening for RBD followed by video-polysomnography (V-PSG). RBD was diagnosed with V-PSG based on electromyographic and audio–visual analysis.

Results: Thirty-five patients were enrolled in the study. Mean age was 77.7 ± 6.1 years, 65.7% were men. Poor sleep quality, hypersomnia, snoring, and abnormal nocturnal behaviors were reported in 54.3, 37.1, 60, and 77.1% of patients, respectively. Sleep wake architecture abnormality was noted in 75% patients. On electroencephalography (EEG) occipital slowing on awake was noted in 34.4%, absence of sleep spindles and K complexes in 12.9%, slow frequency sleep spindles in 12.9%, delta activity in REM sleep in 19.2%, and REM sleep without atonia in 44% of patients. Three patients had hallucinatory-like behavior and 10 patients had abnormal behaviors during arousal mimicking RBD. RBD was diagnosed in 50% of patients among whom sufficient REM sleep was attained. Out of them, 72.7% were not aware of displaying dream enacting behaviors and in 63.7% onset of RBD preceded the onset of cognitive impairments. MSQ had a sensitivity of 50%, and specificity of 66.7%, positive predictive value of 83.3%, and negative predictive value of 28% for diagnosing RBD. Occipital EEG frequency while awake and rate of electromyographic activity in REM sleep were negatively correlated, pointing toward a common subcortical origin.

Conclusion: Rapid eye movement sleep behavior disorder, sleep wake disorders are common and very complex in patients of DLB. Their identification is challenging in without V-PSG.

COMMENT

Sleep disturbances like insomnia, hyper somnolence, and rapid eye movement (REM) sleep behavior disorders are quite frequent in dementia with Lewy bodies (DLB). The sleep disturbances adversely affect the overall quality of life and pose a significant challenge in their management.[24,25] In this study, the authors aim to describe the sleep disturbances in patients with DLB with use of clinical and video-polysomnography (V-PSG). High prevalence of sleep abnormalities and varied pattern of REM sleep behavior disorders (RBDs) were reported in the study cohort. The questionnaires like Mayo sleep questionnaires (MSQ) were found to have low sensitivity and specificity for diagnosing RBD. This highlights the fact that diagnosis of RBD in DLB patient is not straightforward. V-PSG may be required to characterize the complex behavior associated with RBDs. Abnormal sleep parameters, altered sleep stages in PSG further points toward a complex pathophysiology of RBD and sleep abnormalities among these patients. Intervening specific sleep disturbances and rectifying them may be an exciting new therapeutic option in degenerative dementias and further studies are needed as we decipher their basic pathophysiology.

ARTICLE 11

Insomnia with Objective Short Sleep Duration and Risk of Incident Cardiovascular Disease and All-cause Mortality: Sleep Heart Health Study

Bertisch SM, Pollock BD, Mittleman MA, Buysse DJ, Bazzano LA, Gottlieb DJ, et al. Insomnia with objective short sleep duration and risk of incident cardiovascular disease and all-cause mortality: Sleep Heart Health Study. *Sleep. 2018;41(6):zsy047.*

Abstract

Objective: To evaluate the association between insomnia or poor sleep with objective short sleep duration and incident cardiovascular disease (CVD) and mortality in general population.

Methods: This was a time-to-event analysis of Sleep Heart Health Study data. Questionnaire and at-home polysomnography (PSG) were conducted between 1994 and 1998. Median follow-up of the participants was 11.4 years [interquartile range (IQR) 8.8–12.4 years]. The primary exposure was insomnia or poor sleep with short sleep defined as: difficulty in falling asleep, difficulty in returning to sleep, early morning awakenings or sleeping pill use, 16–30 nights per month; and total sleep of <6 hours on PSG. Proportional hazard models were used to estimate the association between insomnia or poor sleep with short sleep and CVD and all-cause mortality.

Results: A total of 4,994 participants were enrolled. Mean age was 64.0 ± 11.1 years. Insomnia or poor sleep was reported in 14.1%, of which 50.3% had a sleep duration <6 hours. Out of 4,437 CVD-free patients at baseline, 818 incident CVD events were observed. After propensity adjustment, a 29% higher risk of incident CVD was noted in the insomnia or poor sleep with short sleep group in comparison to reference group [hazard ratio (HR) 1.29; 95% confidence interval (CI) 1.00–1.66], but neither the insomnia or poor sleep only nor short sleep only groups were associated with higher incident CVD. Insomnia or poor sleep with objective short sleep was not associated with all-cause mortality (HR 1.07; 95% CI 0.86–1.33).

Conclusion: Insomnia with poor sleep with short sleep was associated with a higher risk of incident CVD.

COMMENT

Insomnia and short sleep duration has been associated with prevalent and incident cardiovascular disease (CVD).[26,27] Some researchers have suggested that co-occurrence of insomnia with objective short sleep duration represent a sever phenotype and is associated with increased burden of CVD risk factors.[28,29] In this study, that authors used the data from Sleep Heart Health Study (SHHS), a multicenter community-based prospective cohort study. Persons with insomnia and short sleep (<6 hours) were followed for a median of 11.4 years to evaluate the risk of CVD and all-cause mortality. There was a 29% higher risk of incident CVD among patients with insomnia and short sleep duration. This study indicates that patients with insomnia and objective short sleep duration identified and intervened early to prevent cardiovascular events. This study also highlights the need to characterize both insomnia symptoms and objective sleep duration while undertaking the risk assessments. Further studies are warranted to evaluate the pathophysiological basis of increased CVD risk in these patients.

ARTICLE 12

Sleep Disturbances and Sleep Disorders in Adults Living with Chronic Pain: A Meta-analysis

Mathias JL, Cant ML, Burke ALJ. Sleep disturbances and sleep disorders in adults living with chronic pain: A meta-analysis.
Sleep Med. 2018;52:198-210.

Abstract

Objective: Chronic pain (CP) with or without an identifiable cause is widespread and is commonly associated with sleep disturbances. However, poor quality measures of sleep used in different researches have limited their reliability and applicability in wider CP patients. This meta-analysis aimed at analyzing the findings from studies that used objective polysomnography (PSG) parameters or examined diagnosed sleep disorders in people with CP.

Methods: Electronic databases (PubMed, PsychInfo, Embase) were searched from inception to June 2017. Case-controlled PSG studies and studies that reported the prevalence of diagnosed sleep disorders in adults with CP were included. Hedge's g effect sizes and prevalence rates were calculated using the data from included studies.

Results: Total of 37 studies were included in the meta-analysis. Of the included studies, 22 were PSG studies (total of 674 patients of CP, 536 healthy control) and 15 ($n = 5,769$) were sleep disorder studies. PSG measures of sleep onset latency, sleep efficiency, time awake after sleep onset, and awakenings were all significantly worse in patients with CP in comparison to healthy controls (large effects). Total sleep time, light sleep duration, number of stage shifts, respiratory-related events, and periodic limb-movements were worse in patients of CP (small to medium effects). The pooled prevalence of sleep disorders in CP was found to be 44%. Among specific sleep disorders, insomnia was found in 72%, restless leg syndrome in 32%, and obstructive sleep apnea in 32% of patients.

Conclusion: Objective PSG parameters demonstrates that individual with CP have significant sleep disturbances in sleep architecture, particularly in sleep initiation and maintenance. Clinically diagnosed sleep disorders are very prevalent among patients with CP.

COMMENT

About 10–25% of adults suffer from chronic pain (CP).[30] Many have clear medical cause of pain like arthritis, neuropathy cancer, etc., while many other have no identifiable cause.[31] Studies have reported poor sleep quality in patients with CP.[32]

In this meta-analysis involving 37 studies, authors concluded that sleep quality was significantly poorer in patients with CP with greater time for sleep onset, greater time awake after falling asleep, and more sleep fragmentations. However, sleep architecture was less affected with mild prolongation of nonrapid eye movement 1 (NREM1) and no changes in NERM3. The relationship of pain and its effect on sleep pathology needs more research. Greater knowledge on this association will further help to tailor the pain management which can improve the sleep quality and overall quality of life in adult population with CP.

ARTICLE 13

Long-term Effects of an Unguided Online Cognitive Behavioral Therapy for Chronic Insomnia

Vedaa Ø, Hagatun S, Kallestad H, Pallesen S, Smith ORF, Thorndike FP, et al. Long-term effects of an unguided online cognitive behavioral therapy for chronic insomnia.
J Clin Sleep Med. 2019;15(1):101-10.

Abstract

Objective: To test the efficacy of fully automated internet delivered cognitive behavioral therapy for insomnia (CBT-i) 18 months after the intervention period on sleep, daytime functioning and beliefs about sleep for adults with chronic insomnia.

Methods: Participants of this study were previously enrolled in a randomized controlled trial to compare the efficacy of unguided internet CBT-i with web-based patient education. Those who had received internet CBT-i ($n = 95$) completed online questionnaire and online sleep diaries 18 months after the intervention period. Linear mixed models were used to study changes from baseline to postassessment and to 18-month follow-up. A separate mixed-model analysis was used to study changes from postassessment to 18-month follow-up.

Results: Mean age of the participants was 45.5 ± 12.6 years, 64% were females. 66 participants (70%) completed the follow-up at 18 months. Significant improvement was noted from baseline to 18-month follow-up on the insomnia severity index (ISI) [Cohen $d = 2.04$; 95% confidence interval (CI) 1.66–2.42] and the Bergan insomnia scale (BIS) ($d = 1.64$; 95% CI 1.30–1.98), day time fatigue ($d = 0.85$; 95% CI 0.59–1.11), psychological distress ($d = 0.51$; 95% CI 0.29–0.73), and beliefs about sleep ($d = 1.44$; 95% CI 1.15–1.73). Diary-derived sleep variables also demonstrated moderate to large effect improvements. All the improvements from baseline to postassessment were maintained at the 18-month follow-up.

Conclusion: Unguided internet-based CBT-i seems to have a sustained effect on sleep, day time functioning, and beliefs about sleep up to 18 months postintervention.

COMMENT

Both guided and unguided internet-delivered cognitive behavioral therapy for insomnia (CBT-i) has been shown to be beneficial in chronic insomnia patients.[33] However, their long-term efficacy was not evaluated. This study evaluates the efficacy of unguided internet-based CBT-i at 18 months. This was a follow-up study of a randomized control trial which established superiority of internet delivered CBT-i over patient education.[34] The authors reported a sustained benefit on sleep, day time functioning. Long-term effects of unguided CBT-i has the potential for a cost-effective method for management of chronic insomnia at a population level. Nonavailability of therapists who deliver CBT can be circumvented by alternate distant modes of delivery very pertinent in COVID times.

ARTICLE 14

Effect of CPAP Treatment of Sleep Apnea on Clinical Prognosis after Ischemic Stroke: An Observational Study

Haba-Rubio J, Vujica J, Franc Y, Michel P, Heinzer R. Effect of CPAP treatment of sleep apnea on clinical prognosis after ischemic stroke: An observational study.
J Clin Sleep Med. 2019;15(6):839-47.

Abstract

Objective: To evaluate the effect of continuous positive airway pressure (CPAP) treatment in patients with moderate-to-severe sleep-disordered breathing (SDB) after an ischemic stroke.

Methods: Patients were selected from those included in Acute STroke Registry and Analysis of Lausanne (ASTRAL), who underwent polysomnography after an acute ischemic stroke. Patients without significant SDB [apnea-hypopnea index (AHI) <15 events/h: SDB –ve] with AHI ≥15 events/h who refused CPAP or with poor CPAP adherence (SDB+, CPAP–), and patients with SDB effectively treated by CPAP (SDB+, CPAP+).

Results: Data form 101 patients were analyzed. The mean age was 68.5 ± 11.1 years, and 84.15 were men. In multivariate analysis, the SDB+ CPAP+ group was found to have a significant reduction in stroke recurrence and mortality [odds ratio (OR) 0.13; 95% confidence interval (CI) 0.00–0.86; $p = 0.031$], while atrial fibrillation was independently found to have a higher risk (OR 4.32; 95% CI 1.51–12.33; $p = 0.006$). Event-free survival analysis (for stroke recurrence and death) after 2-year follow-up showed significantly higher cardiovascular survival for the SDB+ CPAP+ group and cox proportion hazard model demonstrated CPAP treatment to be significantly associated with survival time ($p = 0.025$). AHI and the National Institute of Health Stroke Scale subacute score were independently associated with CPAP adherence among patients with SDB.

Conclusion: Continuous positive airway pressure treatment in stroke patients with moderate-to-severe SDB was found to be associated with lower rates of stroke recurrence and death in this observational study.

COMMENT

Sleep-disordered breathing (SBD) has been considered as a risk factor for stroke[35] and it has been found to be more severe in the acute phase of stroke.[36] In this observational study authors aimed to evaluate the effect of continuous positive airway pressure (CPAP) therapy in patients with moderate-to-severe SBD after an ischemic stroke. Significant reduction in stroke recurrence and mortality was noted among patients with CPAP at 2 years of follow-up. The CPAP therapy was started after the acute phase of stroke. This might have contributed to the better adherence to CPAP therapy and moreover, CPAP therapy in acute phase of stroke might be challenging. This study highlights that in addition to management of traditional risk factors, SBD should also be actively evaluated and treated with patients with stroke. Early diagnosis of obstructive SDB with use of clinical questionnaires and polysomnography and swift management with CPAP can reduce the morbidity and mortality in stroke patients.

ARTICLE 15

Effectiveness of an Intensive Weight-loss Program for Severe OSA in Patients Undergoing CPAP Treatment: A Randomized Controlled Trial

López-Padrós C, Salord N, Alves C, Vilarrasa N, Gasa M, Planas R, et al. Effectiveness of an intensive weight-loss program for severe OSA in patients undergoing CPAP treatment: A randomized controlled trial.
J Clin Sleep Med. 2020;16(4):503-14.

Abstract

Objective: To determine the effectiveness of an intensive weight-loss program (IWLP) for reducing weight, the severity of the obstructive sleep apnea (OSA) and metabolic variables in patients with obesity and severe OSA undergoing continuous positive airway pressure (CPAP) treatment.

Methods: Forty-two patients were enrolled in the study. They were randomized to the [control group (CG), $n = 20$] or the [intervention group (IG), $n = 22$] who followed a 12-month IWLP. Primary outcome was reduction in the apnea-hypopnea index (AHI) as measured by full polysomnography (PSG) at 3 and 12 months. Metabolic variables, blood pressure, body fat composition by bioimpedance, carotid intima media thickness, and visceral fat by computed tomography was also measured.

Results: The over all mean age was 49 ± 6.7 years, body mass index was 35 ± 2.7 kg/m^2 and AHI 69 ± 20 events/h. The baseline characteristics in both the groups were similar. Weight reduction was higher in the IG than the CG at 3 months [−10.5 vs. −2.3 kg ($p < 0.001$)] and 12 months [−8.2 vs. −0.1 kg ($p < 0.001$)]. Visceral fat reduction was more in IG in comparison to CG at 12 months. AHI decreased more in the IG at 3 months (−23.72 vs. −9 events/h), however, the difference was not significant at 12 months. 28% of patients from the IG had an AHI <30 events/h compared to none in CG ($p = 0.046$). Among the metabolic profile. The IG showed a reduction in C-reactive protein ($p = 0.013$), glycated hemoglobin ($p = 0.031$), and an increase in high-density lipoprotein cholesterol ($p = 0.027$) at 12 months.

Conclusion: An IWLP in patients with obesity and severe OSA is effective in reducing weight and OSA severity. Improvement in lipid profile, glycemic control and inflammatory markers were noted with the IWLP.

COMMENT

While continuous positive airway pressure (CPAP) has been gold standard therapy for obstructive sleep apnea (OSA), weight loss has been considered as an adjuvant treatment.[37] Although it is desirable for patients on CPAP therapy to lose weight, a meta-analysis has reported an increase in body mass index (BMI).[38] This randomized controlled trial evaluates the efficacy of an intensive weight-loss program (IWLP) in OSA patients on CPAP therapy. The authors report a significant reduction in weight and OSA severity at 12 months among patients who received the intervention. The program included a low-calorie diet, physical activity, and behavioral therapy. The reduction in weight thus noted had a direct effect on central obesity with marked visceral fat. The weight reduction was also associated with improvement in other metabolic parameters like lipid profiles, glycemic status, and inflammatory markers. Although the finding is encouraging, its long-term effect remains to be seen. Weight loss works great provided it can be implemented and maintained both for OSA and metabolic syndromes.

ARTICLE 16

Effects of a 12-week Yoga versus a 12-week Educational Film Intervention on Symptoms of Restless Legs Syndrome and Related Outcomes: An Exploratory Randomized Controlled Trial

Innes KE, Selfe TK, Montgomery C, Hollinshead N, Huysmans Z, Srinivasan R, et al. Effects of a 12-week yoga versus a 12-week educational film intervention on symptoms of restless legs syndrome and related outcomes: An exploratory randomized controlled trial.
J Clin Sleep Med. 2020;16(1):107-19.

Abstract

Objective: To assess the effects of yoga versus educational film (EF) program on restless legs syndrome (RLS) symptoms and related outcomes in adults with RLS.

Methods: Forty-one community-dwelling, ambulatory nonpregnant adults with moderate-to-severe RLS were enrolled. The participants were randomized to a 12-week yoga ($n = 19$) and EF program group ($n = 22$). In addition to attending classes, the participants of both groups completed practice/treatment logs. Yoga group participants were asked to practice yoga for 30 min/day on nonclass days, while the EF participants were instructed to record any RLS treatments used by them in their daily logs. Outcomes measured pretreatment and posttreatment were RLS symptoms and symptoms severity [International RLS Study Group Scale (IRLS) and RLS ordinal scale], sleep quality, mood, perceived stress, and quality of life (QOL).

Results: 30 participants (13 in yoga group, 17 in EF group) completed the 12-week study period. The overall mean age was 50.4 ± 2.4 years, and 78% were female. At the end of 12 weeks, both groups showed significant improvement in RLS symptoms and severity, perceived stress, mood, and QOL-mental health ($p \leq 0.04$). In comparison to EF group, yoga group had a significantly greater reductions in RLS symptoms and severity ($p \leq 0.01$) and greater improvements in perceived stress and mood ($p \leq 0.04$), sleep quality ($p = 0.09$). Among the yoga participants, RLS symptoms decreased to minimal/mild in 77%, none scored in severe range at the end of 12 weeks. However, in the EF group, 24% had minimal/mild and 12% had scores in severe range at the end of 12 weeks. In the yoga group, IRLS and RLS severity scores declined with increasing minutes of homework practice ($r = 0.7$, $p = 0.009$, and $r = 0.6$, $p = 0.03$), indicating a possible dose-response relationship.

Conclusion: This exploratory randomized controlled trial (RCT) indicates that yoga may be an effective tool in reducing the RLS symptoms and severity, decreasing in perceived stress, and improving mood and sleep in adults with RLS.

COMMENT

Nonpharmacological measures, relaxation are often recommended for management of restless leg syndrome, however, properly designed studies are lacking to establish their effectiveness.[39] This is an exploratory randomized controlled trial (RCT) assessing the effect of 12-week yoga versus educational film program on restless legs syndrome (RLS) symptoms among patients with moderate-to-severe RLS. The people on yoga arm reported a significant reduction in RLS symptoms and severity at 12 weeks. Although the mechanism underlying the improvement remains unknown, possible explanations like decreased sympathoadrenal and hypothalamic–pituitary–adrenal axis activation, restoration of parasympathetic/sympathetic balance has been proposed.[40] Neurophysiological and neuroimaging studies have also suggested at selective activation of specific neurochemical systems with yoga might promote beneficial changes in autonomic, neuroendocrine, and metabolic functions thereby alleviating the RLS symptoms.[41] This exploratory study shows yoga to be a safe and effective intervention for RLS. However, more larger RCTs are needed to confirm these benefits.

ARTICLE 17

Sleepiness and Sleepiness Perception in Patients with Parkinson's Disease: A Clinical and Electrophysiological Study

Bargiotas P, Lachenmayer ML, Schreier DR, Mathis J, Bassetti CL. Sleepiness and sleepiness perception in patients with Parkinson's disease: A clinical and electrophysiological study.
Sleep. 2019;42(4):zsz004.

Abstract

Objective: To assess the prevalence, the severity and the daytime course of excessive daytime sleepiness (EDS) in advanced Parkinson's disease (PD) and to investigate how people with PD perceive the degree and onset of their sleepiness objective sleep tests. Occurrence of early onset rapid eye movement (REM) periods [sleep-onset REM periods (SOREMPs)] in PD was also assessed.

Methods: In this single-center retrospective study, data from patients with advanced PD who underwent routine clinical workup, sleep–wake measurements, and video-polysomnography (v-PSG) before undergoing deep brain stimulation were analyzed. The sleep–wake measurements included Epworth Sleepiness Scale (ESS), Karolinska Sleepiness Scale (KSS), and objective [PSG, multiple sleep latency test (MSLT)], and maintenance of wakefulness tests (MWTs) measures.

Results: 46 patients were included, out of which 26 were male. The mean age was 63.5% and mean Unified Parkinson's Disease Rating Scale (UPDRS)-III-OFF was 34.7. Subjective (ESS >10) and objective (mean sleep latency, MSL <5 minutes in MSLT) EDS were present in 43 and

41% patients, respectively. The MSL in MSLT and MWT remained unchanged throughout the day and significantly correlated with KSS during the trial but not with KSS shortly before it. In MWT, about 25% of patients failed to signal their sleepiness before falling asleep. SOREMPs were recorded in 24% of the patients and it was found to be arising from nonrapid eye movement 1 (NREM1) or wake in 83% patients. People with SOREMPs had significantly lower MSL in MSLT and MWT and higher apnea-hypopnea index (AHI) in comparison to those without SOREMPs.

Conclusion: Patients with PD manifest daylong increased EDS but they underestimate its degree and often fail to recognize the onset. SOREMPs in PD have a narcoleptic character in sleep-stage sequencing and are associated with the presence of sleep-disturbed breathing.

COMMENT

The spectrum of sleep disturbances in patients with Parkinson's disease (PD) can be diverse and can have a negative impact on the overall quality of life.[42] Excessive daytime sleepiness (EDS) has been reported to be the most prevalent and disabling sleep symptom, which can also be a premotor manifestation of PD.[43] In this study the authors evaluated the EDS with objective measurement of multiple sleep latency test (MSLT) and maintenance of wakefulness (MWT). Almost half of the patients with advanced PD had increased likelihood of falling asleep while about 40% had severe situational sleep propensity as measured by MSLT. The perception of sleepiness were underestimated by the patients ion this study. The finding of this study points that rapid onset sleep and sleep-onset rapid eye movement period (SOREMP) are underrecognized in PD and is an important nonmotor symptom. Most neurologists depend on the self-reported daytime sleepiness and perception to assess sleep problem among patients with PD, however, this approach may underestimate the sleep abnormality. Detailed sleep evaluation with MSLT may be needed for diagnosis in select patients.

ARTICLE 18

The Associations of Long-time Mobile Phone Use with Sleep Disturbances and Mental Distress in Technical College Students: A Prospective Cohort Study

Liu S, Wing YK, Hao Y, Li W, Zhang J, Zhang B. The associations of long-time mobile phone use with sleep disturbances and mental distress in technical college students: A prospective cohort study.
Sleep. 2019;42(2).

Abstract

Objective: To determine the longitudinal associations of long-time mobile phone use (LTMPU) with sleep disturbances and mental distress in a prospective cohort of technical college students.

Methods: In this prospective cohort study, a total of 4,333 (response rate: 91.5%) and 3,396 (response rate: 78.4%) participants were recruited at baseline and 8-month follow-up, respectively. Data collected included sociodemographic profiles, lifestyle practice, duration of mobile phone use per day, sleep patterns on weekdays and weekends. The questionnaires used to evaluate sleep complaints were insomnia severity index, Epworth Sleepiness Scale, reduced morningness–eveningness questionnaire. Beck depression inventory was used for evaluating depression and Zung self-rating anxiety scale was used to assess anxiety. LTMPU was defined as using mobile phone ≥4 h/day.

Results: At baseline, 23.5% (n = 1,020) of the participants were found to be using mobile phones ≥4 h/day. LTMPU at baseline was associated with new incidences (adjusted odds ratio 1.31–1.53) of a series of sleep disturbances and mental stresses at follow-up. The discontinuation of LTMPU was associated with amelioration of most of these complaints. Bidirectional associations of duration of mobile phone use with poor sleep and mental health outcomes were noted in cross-lagged analyses.

Conclusion: Long-time mobile phone use predicts the new incidences of most sleep disturbances and mental stress, while discontinuation of LTMPU is associated with reversal of these problems. There are bidirectional associations between the duration of mobile phone use and various sleep and mental outcomes.

COMMENT

Excessive use of electronic media particularly use of mobile phones has raised concerns about their potential impact on mental and sleep health. They have been associated with reduced sleep duration, poor sleep quality, and sleep efficiency.[44,45] This is a prospective school-based cohort study which evaluated the long-term mobile phone use and its long-term effect on the sleep quality and mental health. Mobile phone use >4 h/day was associated with increased daytime sleepiness, short weekday sleep duration (<7 h), long weekend sleep compensation (>2 h), and higher incidence of eveningness chronotype. There was higher incidence of anxiety and depressive symptoms among these students. However, discontinuation of long-term mobile phone use was associated with reversal of these symptoms, thereby highlighting the need for early recognition and use of preventive strategies among students.

REFERENCES (Sleep Medicine)

1. Peker Y, Glantz H, Eulenburg C, Wegscheider K, Herlitz J, Thunström E. Effect of positive airway pressure on cardiovascular outcomes in coronary artery disease patients with nonsleepy obstructive sleep apnea. The RICCADSA randomized controlled trial. Am J Respir Crit Care Med. 2016;194(5):613-20.
2. Campos-Rodriguez F, Martinez-Garcia MA, Reyes-Nuñez N, Caballero-Martinez I, Catalan-Serra P, Almeida-Gonzalez CV. Role of sleep apnea and continuous positive airway pressure therapy in the incidence of stroke or coronary heart disease in women. Am J Respir Crit Care Med. 2014;189(12):1544-50.
3. Lyall LM, Wyse CA, Graham N, Ferguson A, Lyall DM, Cullen B, et al. Association of disrupted circadian rhythmicity with mood disorders, subjective wellbeing, and cognitive function: A cross-sectional study of 91 105 participants from the UK Biobank. Lancet Psychiatry. 2018;5(6):507-14.
4. Kahn M, Sheppes G, Sadeh A. Sleep and emotions: Bidirectional links and underlying mechanisms. Int J Psychophysiol. 2013;89(2):218-28.
5. Drudi LM, Ades M, Turkdogan S, Huynh C, Lauck S, Webb JG, et al. Association of depression with mortality in older adults undergoing transcatheter or surgical aortic valve replacement. JAMA Cardiol. 2018;3(3):191-7.
6. St-Onge MP, Grandner MA, Brown D, Conroy MB, Jean-Louis G, Coons M, et al.; American Heart Association Obesity, Behavior Change, Diabetes, and Nutrition Committees of the Council on Lifestyle and Cardiometabolic Health, Council on Cardiovascular Disease in the Young, Council on Clinical Cardiology, and Stroke Council. Sleep duration and quality: Impact on lifestyle behaviors and cardiometabolic health: A scientific statement from the American Heart Association. Circulation. 2016;134(18):e367-e386.
7. Cappuccio FP, Cooper D, D'Elia L, Strazzullo P, Miller MA. Sleep duration predicts cardiovascular outcomes: A systematic review and meta-analysis of prospective studies. Eur Heart J. 2011;32(12):1484-92.
8. Steiner S, Schueller PO, Schulze V, Strauer BE. Occurrence of coronary collateral vessels in patients with sleep apnea and total coronary occlusion. Chest. 2010;137(3):516-20.
9. Baxter P. Epilepsy and sleep. Dev Med Child Neurol. 2005;47(11):723.
10. Chakravarty K, Shukla G, Poornima S, Agarwal P, Gupta A, Mohammed A, et al. Effect of sleep quality on memory, executive function, and language performance in patients with refractory focal epilepsy and controlled epilepsy versus healthy controls - A prospective study. Epilepsy Behav. 2019;92:176-83.
11. Pereira AM, Bruni O, Ferri R, Nunes ML. Sleep instability and cognitive status in drug-resistant epilepsies. Sleep Med. 2012;13(5):536-41.
12. American Academy of Sleep Medicine. 2021. Summary of CDC recommendations relevant for sleep practices during COVID-19. [online] Available from https://aasm.org/covid-19-resources/covid-19-mitigation-strategies-sleep-clinics-labs [Last accessed October, 2022].
13. Altena E, Baglioni C, Espie CA, Ellis J, Gavriloff D, Holzinger B, et al. Dealing with sleep problems during home confinement due to the COVID-19 outbreak: Practical recommendations from a task force of the European CBT-I Academy. J Sleep Res. 2020;29(4):e13052.
14. Sweetman AM, Lack LC, Catcheside PG, Antic NA, Chai-Coetzer CL, Smith SS, et al. Developing a successful treatment for co-morbid insomnia and sleep apnoea. Sleep Med Rev. 2017;33:28-38.
15. Alessi C, Martin JL, Fung CH, Dzierzewski JM, Fiorentino L, Stepnowsky C, et al. 0407 Randomized controlled trial of an integrated behavioral treatment in veterans with obstructive sleep apnea and coexisting insomnia. Sleep. 2018;41(Suppl_1):A155.
16. Rensma SP, van Sloten TT, Launer LJ, Stehouwer CDA. Cerebral small vessel disease and risk of incident stroke, dementia and depression, and all-cause mortality: A systematic review and meta-analysis. Neurosci Biobehav Rev. 2018;90:164-73.
17. Bos D, Wolters FJ, Darweesh SKL, Vernooij MW, de Wolf F, Ikram MA, et al. Cerebral small vessel disease and the risk of dementia: A systematic review and meta-analysis of population-based evidence. Alzheimers Dement. 2018;14(11):1482-92.
18. Gozal D, Serpero LD, Kheirandish-Gozal L, Capdevila OS, Khalyfa A, Tauman R. Sleep measures and morning plasma TNF-alpha levels in children with sleep-disordered breathing. Sleep. 2010;33(3):319-25.
19. Arzt M, Oldenburg O, Graml A, Erdmann E, Teschler H, Wegscheider K, et al.; SchlaHF Investigators. Phenotyping of sleep-disordered breathing in patients with chronic heart failure with reduced ejection fraction-the SchlaHF Registry. J Am Heart Assoc. 2017;6(12):e005899.
20. Javaheri S, Barbe F, Campos-Rodriguez F, Dempsey JA, Khayat R, Javaheri S, et al. Sleep apnea: Types, mechanisms, and clinical cardiovascular consequences. J Am Coll Cardiol. 2017;69(7):841-58.
21. Cowie MR, Woehrle H, Wegscheider K, Angermann C, d'Ortho MP, Erdmann E, et al. Adaptive servo-ventilation for central sleep apnea in systolic heart failure. N Engl J Med. 2015;373(12):1095-105.
22. Kallweit U, Bassetti CL. Pharmacological management of narcolepsy with and without cataplexy. Expert Opin Pharmacother. 2017;18(8):809-17.
23. Kollb-Sielecka M, Demolis P, Emmerich J, Markey G, Salmonson T, Haas M. The European Medicines Agency review of pitolisant for treatment of narcolepsy: Summary

of the scientific assessment by the Committee for Medicinal Products for Human Use. Sleep Med. 2017;33:125-9.
24. Chwiszczuk L, Breitve M, Hynninen M, Gjerstad MD, Aarsland D, Rongve A. Higher frequency and complexity of sleep disturbances in dementia with Lewy bodies as compared to Alzheimer's disease. Neurodegener Dis. 2016;16(3-4):152-60.
25. Bliwise DL, Mercaldo ND, Avidan AY, Boeve BF, Greer SA, Kukull WA. Sleep disturbance in dementia with Lewy bodies and Alzheimer's disease: A multicenter analysis. Dement Geriatr Cogn Disord. 2011;31(3):239-46.
26. Javaheri S, Redline S. Insomnia and risk of cardiovascular disease. Chest. 2017;152(2):435-44.
27. Liu Y, Wheaton AG, Chapman DP, Croft JB. Sleep duration and chronic diseases among U.S. adults age 45 years and older: Evidence from the 2010 Behavioral Risk Factor Surveillance System. Sleep. 2013;36(10):1421-7.
28. Vgontzas AN, Fernandez-Mendoza J, Liao D, Bixler EO. Insomnia with objective short sleep duration: The most biologically severe phenotype of the disorder. Sleep Med Rev. 2013;17(4):241-54.
29. Fernandez-Mendoza J. The insomnia with short sleep duration phenotype: An update on it's importance for health and prevention. Curr Opin Psychiatry. 2017;30(1):56-63.
30. Goldberg DS, McGee SJ. Pain as a global public health priority. BMC Public Health. 2011;11:770.
31. Blyth FM, March LM, Cousins MJ. Chronic pain-related disability and use of analgesia and health services in a Sydney community. Med J Aust. 2003;179(2):84-7.
32. Finan PH, Goodin BR, Smith MT. The association of sleep and pain: An update and a path forward. J Pain. 2013;14(12):1539-52.
33. Zachariae R, Lyby MS, Ritterband LM, O'Toole MS. Efficacy of internet-delivered cognitive-behavioral therapy for insomnia - A systematic review and meta-analysis of randomized controlled trials. Sleep Med Rev. 2016;30:1-10.
34. Hagatun S, Vedaa Ø, Nordgreen T, Smith ORF, Pallesen S, Havik OE, et al. The short-term efficacy of an unguided internet-based cognitive-behavioral therapy for insomnia: A randomized controlled trial with a six-month nonrandomized follow-up. Behav Sleep Med. 2019;17(2):137-55.
35. Loke YK, Brown JW, Kwok CS, Niruban A, Myint PK. Association of obstructive sleep apnea with risk of serious cardiovascular events: A systematic review and meta-analysis. Circ Cardiovasc Qual Outcomes. 2012;5(5):720-8.
36. Johnson KG, Johnson DC. Frequency of sleep apnea in stroke and TIA patients: A meta-analysis. J Clin Sleep Med. 2010;6(2):131-7.
37. Veasey SC, Guilleminault C, Strohl KP, Sanders MH, Ballard RD, Magalang UJ. Medical therapy for obstructive sleep apnea: A review by the medical therapy for obstructive sleep apnea task force of the standards of Practice Committee of the American Academy of Sleep Medicine. Sleep. 2006;29(8):1036-44.
38. Drager LF, Brunoni AR, Jenner R, Lorenzi-Filho G, Bensenõr IM, Lotufo PA. Effects of CPAP on body weight in patients with obstructive sleep apnoea: A meta-analysis of randomised trials. Thorax. 2015;70(3):258-64.
39. Garcia-Borreguero D, Kohnen R, Silber MH, Winkelman JW, Earley CJ, Högl B, et al. The long-term treatment of restless legs syndrome/Willis-Ekbom disease: Evidence-based guidelines and clinical consensus best practice guidance: a report from the International Restless Legs Syndrome Study Group. Sleep Med. 2013;14(7):675-84.
40. Innes KE, Selfe TK. The effects of a gentle yoga program on sleep, mood, and blood pressure in older women with restless legs syndrome (RLS): A preliminary randomized controlled trial. Evid Based Complement Alternat Med. 2012;2012:294058.
41. Streeter CC, Whitfield TH, Owen L, Rein T, Karri SK, Yakhkind A, et al. Effects of yoga versus walking on mood, anxiety, and brain GABA levels: A randomized controlled MRS study. J Altern Complement Med. 2010;16(11):1145-52.
42. Bargiotas P, Schuepbach MW, Bassetti CL. Sleep-wake disturbances in the premotor and early stage of Parkinson's disease. Curr Opin Neurol. 2016;29(6):763-72.
43. Pont-Sunyer C, Hotter A, Gaig C, Seppi K, Compta Y, Katzenschlager R, et al. The onset of nonmotor symptoms in Parkinson's disease (the ONSET PD study). Mov Disord. 2015;30(2):229-37.
44. Dube N, Khan K, Loehr S, Chu Y, Veugelers P. The use of entertainment and communication technologies before sleep could affect sleep and weight status: A population-based study among children. Int J Behav Nutr Phys Act. 2017;14(1):97.
45. Arora T, Broglia E, Thomas GN, Taheri S. Associations between specific technologies and adolescent sleep quantity, sleep quality, and parasomnias. Sleep Med. 2014;15(2):240-7.

Section 11: Neuro-ophthalmology

Section Editor: Vivek Lal

Associate Editors: Aastha Takkar Kapila, Karthik Vinay Mahesh, Surbhi Mahajan, Karthik Harisankar

ARTICLE 1

Incidentally Detected MRI Signs of Increased Intracranial Pressure

Chen BS, Meyer BI, Saindane AM, Bruce BB, Newman NJ, Biousse V. Prevalence of incidentally detected signs of intracranial hypertension on magnetic resonance imaging and their association with papilledema. *JAMA Neurol. 2021;78(6):718-25.*

Abstract

In this prospective, cross sectional study; 296 patients undergoing brain magnetic resonance imaging (MRI) for any clinical indication were recruited. Prevalence of MRI signs of intracranial hypertension (IH) among consecutive patients was noted and fundus images were recorded. Radiographic signs of IH included empty sella, optic nerve head protrusion, posterior scleral flattening, increased perioptic cerebrospinal fluid (CSF), vertical tortuosity of intraorbital optic nerve, enlarged Meckel's caves, encephaloceles, cerebellar tonsillar ectopia, presence of bilateral transverse sinus stenosis with at least 50% narrowing, and optic nerve enhancement. Radiographic signs were found to be common, with almost one half of patients having at least one sign. Only five patients (1.7%) had papilledema and patients with papilledema had two or more signs of IH. The prevalence of papilledema increased from 2.8% among patients with at least one MRI sign of idiopathic intracranial hypertension (IIH) to 40.0% among patients with four or more MRI signs of IH. Authors concluded that MRI features of raised intracranial pressure were very common in patients undergoing MRI for varied indications but was rarely associated with presence of papilledema.

The study portends to challenge the practice of performing systemic investigations among all patients with incidentally detected IH. The effect of the underlying disease may itself lead to papilledema. Hence, MRI evaluation and subanalysis on the basis of underlying etiology needs to be taken into consideration.

COMMENT

In this well-designed prospective study authors report an increased prevalence of incidentally detected signs of increased intracranial pressure on magnetic resonance imaging (MRI) amongst patients undergoing neuroimaging for unrelated clinical indications. While imaging signs are commonly detected they are rarely associated with papilledema underscoring the importance of an adequate and detailed clinical examination.[1] While some studies in literature have commented upon the role of combination of MRI findings to identify patients who may have idiopathic intracranial hypertension (IIH) without papilledema, invasive investigations like lumbar puncture should be based upon clinical suggestion in combination with MRI signs. Given the increased prevalence of incidentally detected signs in normal population, a physician should be careful in interpreting these signs in isolation.

ARTICLE 2

Statistical Significance of Neuroimaging Signs in Idiopathic Intracranial Hypertension

Prabhat N, Chandel S, Takkar A, Ahuja C, Singh R, Kathirvel S, et al. Sensitivity and specificity of neuroimaging signs in patients with idiopathic intracranial hypertension.
Neuroradiol J. 2021;34(5):421-7.

Abstract

Diagnosis of idiopathic intracranial hypertension (IIH) involves the presence of raised intracranial pressure (ICP), a normal cerebrospinal fluid (CSF) composition along with normal brain imaging. Although they cannot be considered diagnostic, there are various imaging patterns that might suggest raised ICP. This study assessed the prevalence of these signs in IIH, their correlation with the clinical findings, and analysis of their sensitivity/specificity for diagnostic purposes. 80 patients fulfilling the diagnostic criteria for IIH were enrolled and compared with 30 healthy controls. The most common abnormality noted on magnetic resonance imaging (MRI) was optic nerve tortuosity (82.5%) followed by posterior scleral flattening in 80%, perioptic subarachnoid space (SAS) dilatation in 73.8%, optic nerve hyperintensity in 20%, and partial empty sella in 68.8%. 88% of the patients had presence of more than one MRI signs and 61.3% had more than three MRI signs of IIH. Highest specificity for diagnosis of IIH was seen for posterior scleral flattening and perioptic SAS dilatation. Significant correlation of MRI signs with the severity of vision loss and visual outcome was noted. The presence of tortuous optic nerves was found to have significant correlation with the presence of diplopia, tinnitus, vision loss, and papilledema.

The study highlighted the utility of MRI in diagnosing and prognosticating visual outcome in patients with IIH.

COMMENT

The latest diagnostic criteria for idiopathic intracranial hypertension (IIH) suggest a paramount role of recognizing features suggestive of increased intracranial pressure (ICP).[2] Neuroimaging is undoubtedly a valuable tool for diagnosing IIH. It is not uncommon to find isolated magnetic resonance imaging (MRI) findings of increased ICP without clinical suggestion.[3] On the other hand, neuroimaging may be normal in patients with other clinical symptoms of increased ICP. This study describes the sensitivity and specificity of these neuroimaging signs in IIH. It also highlights the role of neuroimaging in prognosticating visual outcome in these patients. While the presence of these signs should alert a physician to suspect increased ICP, they have to be considered under relevant clinical scenarios only.

ARTICLE 3

More Guts than Brains

Berkowitz E, Kopelman Y, Kadosh D, Carasso S, Tiosano B, Kesler A, et al. "More Guts Than Brains?"–The role of gut microbiota in idiopathic intracranial hypertension.
J Neuroophthalmol. 2022;42(1):e70-e77.

Abstract

Idiopathic intracranial hypertension (IIH) is a syndrome of raised intracranial pressure (ICP) with normal imaging and cerebrospinal fluid (CSF) composition. Among others, obesity is a predominant risk factor underlying this disease. It has been increasingly implicated that gut microbiota, along with environmental and genetic factors have a role to play in genesis of obesity and thereby, also in IIH. There is an interplay of various factors by vast number of microorganisms present in the obese persons presumed to cause IIH by modulation of "gut–brain axis". This study investigated the role of gut microbiome in 25 patients with IIH and compared with 20 healthy controls using shotgun metagenomic sequencing. A list of bacterial species was produced along with species diversity and significant variation between IIH patients and healthy controls was noted. In addition effect of acetazolamide treatment on their gut microbiome was analyzed. Lower diversity of bacterial species was noted in IIH as compared to healthy individuals. The study suggested the role of methanogenic archaea and anaerobic microbacteria predominantly in patients with IIH. High alpha diversity was noted among the controls suggestive of more diverse population of bacteria. The microbiota predominantly found in healthy controls including *Lactobacillus ruminis* had potential immunomodulatory effects beneficial to the host. The patients treated with acetazolamide had the increased prevalence of *Lactobacillus brevis* which harbors probiotic properties, and thereby influences bowel microenvironment. It seems fairly reasonable to find the gut microbial populations predisposing to obesity in IIH patients but the implications are yet far sighted. Linking IIH with gut microbiota may pave the way for another pathophysiologic mechanism and further enhancement of new treatment modalities by virtue of gut–brain axis.

COMMENT

Idiopathic intracranial hypertension (IIH) is considered to be the new neurological "metabolic syndrome".[4] While obesity is considered to be a prominent risk factor, there are various unanswered queries with regards to the disease etiology.[1] This study revealed a novel association of the gut microbiota an IIH and has introduced role of microbiota–gut–brain axis in IIH. While the given evidence does not support targeting the gut microbiome in IIH at present, but this is an interesting research area paving path for future research in this field.

ARTICLE 4

Papilledema – 'True' or 'Pseudo'!

Flowers AM, Longmuir RA, Liu Y, Chen Q, Donahue SP. Variability within optic nerve optical coherence tomography measurements distinguishes papilledema from pseudopapilledema.
J Neuroophthalmol. 2021;41(4):496-503.

Abstract

This retrospective review studied the role of variability in clock-hour measurements of optical coherence tomography (OCT) in distinguishing pseudopapilledema from papilledema. 44 eyes with papilledema [predominantly idiopathic intracranial hypertension (IIH) related] and 72 eyes with pseudopapilledema (36 with optic nerve drusen) were included. The absolute consecutive difference in retinal nerve fiber layer (RNFL) thickness, between adjacent clock hours and the mean magnitude of thickness for clock hours 1–12 were compared between the two groups. The average RNFL thickness for papilledema group was found to be higher than pseudopapilledema group. The papilledema group also had higher variability, with overlap present over the two groups. Linear score with outcome metric, optic disc edema index (ODEI) was calculated to mark the differences between the two groups more clearly. On combining the average values of covariates, the RNFL thickness and the mean absolute consecutive difference between clock-hour segments, area under the curve (AUC) of 98.4% was achieved. Nearly all the papilledema eyes had a value >14.8 and all the pseudopapilledema eyes had a linear combination values of 13.2. Hence, both RNFL thickness and absolute clock-hour variability did not differentiate the two variables significantly but ODEI >14.8 was associated with papilledema. Authors concluded that patients with papilledema had higher intrinsic variability and magnitude in RNFL thickness on OCT, and this finding can reliably differentiate them from patients with pseudopapilledema.

COMMENT

Differentiating papilledema from pseudopapilledema has been a constant conundrum for neurologists.[5] While misclassifying pseudopapilledema can lead on to unnecessary invasive investigations, failure to recognize true papilledema may have fatal consequences. Optical coherence tomography (OCT) is a comparatively user-friendly investigation with high sensitivity to detect disc edema.[6] This study highlights the variability of the clock-hour disc elevation in patients with true papilledema. While the average retinal nerve fiber layer (RNFL) thickness is higher in the papilledema group, the high intrinsic variability and magnitude within their OCT may prove to be a highly reliable differentiating clue.

ARTICLE 5

Diplopia: Causes and Outcomes

Kumar N, Kaur S, Raj S, Lal V, Sukhija J. Causes and outcomes of patients presenting with diplopia: A hospital-based study.
Neuroophthalmology. 2021;45(4):238-45.

Abstract

This prospective observational study evaluated the etiologies and outcomes in 160 patients presenting with diplopia over a period of 1 year. Data regarding age at presentation, mode of onset, type of diplopia, inciting cause, history of any treatment along with the course of disease were noted. Most patients (37.5%) were young, belonging to 20–40 years age group {mean [standard deviation (SD)] 40.34 (16.98)}. The mean (SD) duration of diplopia was 2.87 (1.2) years. About 94% patients presented with diplopia on binocular gaze. The most common overall cause of binocular diplopia was found to be vasculopathy (28.66%) secondary to diabetes, hypertension, migraine, etc. Other causes were traumatic, decompensating heterophorias, inflammatory, neoplastic, etc. Decompensating heterophorias and trauma were most common in 20–40 years age group and vasculopathic causes were frequent in patients above the age of 40 years. In this cohort, 95.6% patients were managed medically and 4.3% surgically. On 3 months follow-up, decompensating heterophorias resolved in 82.3% of cases and sixth nerve palsies resolved in 41.5% patients. Multiple cranial nerve palsies, fourth nerve and supranuclear palsies did not tend to improve significantly. Out of all diagnoses, third nerve palsy showed the least recovery. The study reported myriad of diseases with diplopia as presenting complaint with description of the course and outcome accordingly. The description of presentation of binocular as well as monocular diplopia with different etiologies and treatment patterns, provided insights into the variability of the disease, and this understanding may help in early diagnosis and proper management in these patients.

COMMENT

Diplopia is a common disabling condition encountered by a neurologist/neuro-ophthalmologist. While myriad of etiologies have been described, it is important to differentiate ophthalmic causes from neurological and neurosurgical causes. Mono-ocular diplopia are primarily caused by ophthalmic causes as against binocular diplopia which can be caused by primary ophthalmic or neurological causes. Vasculopathic causes are far more common when isolated/single ocular–cranial nerve involvement is present.[7]

Surprisingly, only a small subset of patients in this study was diagnosed with etiologies like idiopathic intracranial hypertension, myasthenia gravis, and other infectious causes which commonly present to neurologists and should be considered in differential diagnosis. This prospective study of 160 patients with diplopia focused on important etiological and diagnostic considerations and also provides an orderly description of how to approach a patient with diplopia based upon clinical findings.

ARTICLE 6

Pregnancy and Neuromyelitis Optica Spectrum Disorder: Important Considerations

Collongues N, Do Rego CA, Bourre B, Biotti D, Marignier R, da Silva AM, et al. Pregnancy in patients with AQP4-Ab, MOG-Ab, or double-negative neuromyelitis optica disorder.
Neurology. 2021;96(15):e2006-e2015.

Abstract

Pregnancy represents a unique challenge in management of patients with neuromyelitis optica spectrum disorder (NMOSD). This retrospective multicentric study analyzed the effects of pregnancy on patients (89 pregnancies in 58 patients) with NMOSD according to their serostatus [aquaporin-4 (AQP4)-Ab, MOG-Ab, or double-negative]. The study showed a decrease in the annualized relapse rate (ARR) during the pregnancy as compared to the prepregnancy period, followed by a rebound during the postpartum state irrespective of the serogroup. Further the ARR was significantly lower in the group which received preconception immunosuppressive therapy (IST) during pregnancy and 1 year postpartum when compared to the untreated patients (26% vs. 53%, $p = 0.04$). This effect was pronounced in the antibody positive group. 73 relapses occurred in 89 pregnancies and 11% of these were inaugural of NMOSD. 45% relapses occurred during the first trimester postpartum and 18% occurred in the second trimester postpartum period. 40% relapses occurred in pregnancies occurring after the disease onset, of which 70% pregnancies occurred in patients who did not receive IST. 10 miscarriages (11%) were noted, mainly in patients with AQP4-antibodies (with or without IST). Pre-eclampsia was noted in two (2%) patients, both with AQP-4 antibody disease. AQP-4 antibody positive serostatus, history of previous miscarriages, high maternal age, higher age at NMOSD onset, coexisting autoimmunity, and higher ARR before pregnancy were associated with increased rate of miscarriages in these patients. Effects of pregnancy in NMOSD needs to be described and understood in great details considering its propensity in women in reproductive age group.

COMMENT

Pregnancy has been considered as a relative immune privileged state and the relapses of most autoimmune diseases decrease during pregnancy.[8] It is also common to see the postpregnancy or postpartum rebound of relapses.[9] Similar to the pattern observed in multiple sclerosis, in this cohort of patients of NMOSD also reduction in the risk of relapse during pregnancy (especially during the third trimester) followed by a rebound during the postpartum period was noted. The dose-dependent effect of estrogens on immune cells, with low estrogen levels facilitating cell-mediated immunity has been considered the basis of this response. The authors also talk about the role of prepregnancy immunosuppressive therapies and their role in reducing the risk of relapses during pregnancy and even postpartum state. It seems essential to supervise the pregnancy and also the preconception period in patients with seropositive NMOSD in order to ensure optimal clinical outcome.

ARTICLE 7

Newer Treatment Regimens in Neuromyelitis Optica-associated Optic Neuritis

Zhao S, Zhou H, Xu Q, Dai H, Wei S. Efficacy of low-dose rituximab on neuromyelitis optica-associated optic neuritis. *Front Neurol. 2021;12:637932.*

Abstract

This study prospectively investigated the efficacy and tolerance of low-dose rituximab (RTX) for the treatment of neuromyelitis optica-associated optic neuritis (NMO-ON). Intravenous RTX, as an empirical immunotherapy in treating neuromyelitis optica spectrum disorder (NMOSD) has been listed as the first-line treatment in the remission phase. Regimens of RTX treatments in NMO have been based on the use of RTX by patients with lymphoma which were high-cost, off-label therapies, and might have a high risk of adverse reactions. This study administered low-dose RTX (20% of conventional dose; 100 mg × 4 infusions) to 43 patients (75 involved eyes) with NMO-ON [aquaporin-4 (AQP4)-antibody seropositive]. Patients were closely followed monthly for a minimum duration of 3 months and reinfusion of 100 mg RTX was given when CD19 + B lymphocytes were elevated to above 1%. After the induction therapy a significant decrease in AQP-4 antibody concentration along with CD19 + B-cell clearance in peripheral blood was noted in 97.7% patients. B-cell clearance was maintained up to 5.2 ± 2.25 months. Significant reduction in the annualized relapse rate (ARR) was noted and the relapse-free rate was 92.3% in patients followed up for over a year. Up to 96.2% of patients had stable or improved vision and a decrease in the average expanded disability status scale (EDSS) score was found. No major adverse effects were noted, and rates of infusion-related reactions and long-term adverse events were noted in 18.6% and 23.1% patients, respectively. Over all the authors concluded that low-dose RTX is an efficient and well-tolerated option in patients with NMO-ON.

COMMENT

Regimens to manage remission in neuromyelitis optica-associated optic neuritis (NMO-ON) are one of paramount importance to control clinical relapses and hence offering a favorable prognosis. The current era has been one of monoclonal antibodies in practically all neuroimmunological disorders. While the role of conventional-dose rituximab (RTX) for neuromyelitis optica spectrum disorder (NMOSD) cannot be challenged, it is associated with its own share of logistic problems, lack of patient tolerance, increased risk of infections like tuberculosis, and adverse drug reactions.[10] This prospective study proposes a novel low-dose regimen of RTX in NMO-ON and demonstrates that it is not only well tolerated but is also efficient. While the conventional dose has not been compared to comment upon superiority of either treatment regimens, this study opens the avenues to further and probably safer management regimens in NMOSD. Multicentric, randomized, and controlled trials in future comparing various regimens with long-term follow-up may further clarify many queries with regards to management in NMOSD.

ARTICLE 8

The Epidemic of Idiopathic Intracranial Hypertension

Miah L, Strafford H, Fonferko-Shadrach B, Hollinghurst J, Sawhney IM, Hadjikoutis S, et al. Incidence, prevalence, and healthcare outcomes in idiopathic intracranial hypertension: A population study.
Neurology. 2021;96(8):e1251-e1261.

Abstract

The epidemic of overnutrition is growing in the more developed parts of the world coupled with the relative less energy expenditure due to sophisticated technologies. Obesity is growing globally. Idiopathic intracranial hypertension (IIH) is now increasingly being recognized as an extension of metabolic syndrome. This retrospective cohort study analyzed 35 million patient-years of data and looked into the temporal trends of IIH incidence and prevalence and healthcare utilization in Wales. 1,765 patients of IIH were identified in 2017 (85% females). The prevalence and incidence of IIH was noted to have increased greatly from 12/100,000 (2.3/100,000/y) in 2003 to 76/100,000 (7.8/100,000/y) in 2017 ($p < 0.001$). The proportion of obese individuals [body mass index (BMI > 30 kg/m^2] in Wales measured using primary care data was also noted to have increased significantly from 29 to 40% during this time period. Increasing deprivation was further linked to increasing prevalence of IIH in the cohort under consideration. While the causation of IIH is multifactorial, a steady increase in obesity epidemic and increased awareness of symptoms are prominent causes of increasing incidence and prevalence of IIH. Interestingly in this study, 9% of IIH patients had cerebrospinal fluid (CSF) shunts with <0.2% undergoing bariatric surgery. Healthcare utilization trends were noted by the authors and it was noted that the patients with IIH had higher proportion of unscheduled hospital admissions as compared to controls. These admissions were further higher in the subgroup which underwent CSF diversion procedure. The prominent implications of this IIH epidemic on the overall health system cannot be underrated.

COMMENT

The sedentary lifestyle and the increasing obesity rates explain the advent of recent epidemic of idiopathic intracranial hypertension (IIH).[4] Despite the obviously increasing incidence of IIH, there has been a paucity of large scale epidemiological studies. While IIH is considered to be multifactorial, the authors noted strong association with higher body mass index (BMI), and increasing deprivation. An increased prevalence in women was noted which further increased with increasing BMI and deprivation.[1] Higher awareness amongst public and improvement of diagnostic infrastructure may be other factors contributing toward increased diagnosis of the condition. The pattern of healthcare utilization in these patients suggested increased unscheduled hospital visits, up to 2 years after their diagnosis underscoring the importance of early and adequate treatment of these patients. Though the data was a routinely collected one and suspectable to bias, it gives massive insight into various important implications of oncoming IIH epidemic over patients, physicians, and the healthcare systems.

ARTICLE 9

Diagnosing Idiopathic Intracranial Hypertension without Lumbar Puncture

Vosoughi AR, Margolin EA, Micieli JA. Can lumbar puncture be safely deferred in patients with mild presumed idiopathic intracranial hypertension?
J Neuroophthalmol. 2021.

Abstract

Lumbar puncture (LP), documentation of cerebrospinal fluid (CSF) pressure, and demonstration of normal CSF composition are an essential part of the diagnostic criteria for idiopathic intracranial hypertension (IIH). Confirmation of an elevated opening pressure and exclusion of other causes like meningeal inflammation and in rare circumstances neoplastic diseases have been considered essential before a diagnosis of "idiopathic" IH can be made. This retrospective analyses of a total of 132 eyes (68 patients) looked into the clinical characteristics, final visual outcome, and diagnosis of patients with presumed IIH and papilledema without subjecting them to LP. Adequate attention was given to rule out secondary causes of increased intracranial pressure (ICP). The mean [standard deviation (SD)] age of the patients was 31.4 (10.2) years and mean (SD) body mass index (BMI) was 35.1 (6.8) kg/m^2. Other clinical details were noted and patients were followed for a mean (SD) duration of 63.3 (78.3) weeks. Significant improvement in the automated mean deviation (−1.73 ± 1.74 dB; $p < 0.001$) and optical coherence tomography (OCT) retinal nerve fiber layer (RNFL) thickness (128.1 ± 38.6 µm; $p < 0.001$) was noted post-treatment at final follow-up. No patient in the study underwent any worsening of visual status after managing without LP. 38 patients (76 eyes) were noted to have resolution of papilledema at the final follow-up.

COMMENT

Even though it is very useful to get a lumbar puncture (LP) in all cases of idiopathic intracranial hypertension (IIH), it has its own set of practical challenges. LP can be a technically challenging procedure in obese patients and difficult to obtain in certain geographic areas, may require inpatient hospital admission and may induce significant patient anxiety.[11] Potential medicolegal issues due to risk of complications from the procedure and limited reliability of results (as the opening pressure obtained through LP can also be variable depending on the time of the day hydration status, etc.), are other factors in consideration while ordering LP.[12] This study identifies the role of diagnosing IIH (mild IIH) without LP. While factors like patient refusal, nonavailability of expertise, failed LP were prime indications of avoiding LP, the authors conclude that in a subset of patients with typical demographic and clinical suggestion, LP may be avoided. The findings of this study should not be generalized and be judiciously applied. In patients with atypical clinical features, visual loss, marked disc edema it is important to make a definitive diagnosis and to assess the status by doing cerebrospinal fluid (CSF) tap. Moreover, the role of therapeutic LP as an important temporizing measure to protect the optic nerves cannot be totally ignored.

ARTICLE 10

Optic Nerve Drusen and Pseudotumor Cerebri: Dual Pathology?

Genizi J, Meiselles D, Arnowitz E, Segal I, Cohen R, Goldenberg-Cohen N. Optic nerve drusen is highly prevalent among children with pseudotumor cerebri syndrome.
Front Neurol. 2021;12:789673.

Abstract

Optic disc drusen, an acellular calcified deposit buried in the surface of the optic disc is an important cause of pseudopapilledema. Genizi et al. studied medical records of 34 children evaluated for pseudotumor cerebri syndrome (PTCS) between 2008 and 2020. Ophthalmic B-mode ultrasonography was carried out in these patients. Mean age of patients was 10.1 years (50% boys). Five patients (14.7%) were diagnosed to be having optic nerve drusen via B-mode ultrasonography despite fulfilling the clinical diagnostic criteria for PTCS. There was no statistically significant difference in patients' age, clinical onset, complaints, gender, weight, or cerebrospinal fluid (CSF) opening pressure between the group with optic nerve drusen and the rest of the patients. Interestingly even in patients with optic disc drusen improvement in disc swelling was noted after treatment with intracranial pressure (ICP) lowering agents. The authors concluded that optic nerve drusen are a common finding in pediatric age group and their presence should not rule out diagnosis of increased ICP in suggestive clinical scenarios.

COMMENT

An increased incidence of drusen in patients with pseudotumor cerebri syndrome (PTCS) compared to general population has been reported across PTCS in adults. Papilledema and related disruption of axonal transport in optic nerve are the presumed reasons for this phenomenon.[13] This retrospective cohort study of 34 patients with PTCS suggested that optic nerve drusen were common among pediatric patients with PTCS. Hence, a physician should not put down his guards and should adequately rule out increased intracranial pressure (ICP) where ever clinically suggestive. The response to treatment (with ICP lowering agents) in patients with optic disc drusen further underscores the need of considering dual pathology in a subset of these patients. While a prospective, multicentric trial with a well-matched control group would be ideal to answer, whether optic drusen is more prevalent in patients with PTCS as compared to general population,[14] this study caters to a common dilemma in routine neuro-ophthalmology clinics.

REFERENCES (Neuro-ophthalmology)

1. Takkar A, Lal V. Idiopathic intracranial hypertension: The monster within. Ann Indian Acad Neurol. 2020;23(2):159-66.
2. Mollan SP, Markey KA, Benzimra JD, Jacks A, Matthews TD, Burdon MA, et al. A practical approach to, diagnosis, assessment and management of idiopathic intracranial hypertension. Pract Neurol. 2014;14(6):380-90.
3. Digre KB, Nakamoto BK, Warner JE, Langeberg WJ, Baggaley SK, Katz BJ. A comparison of idiopathic intracranial hypertension with and without papilledema. Headache. 2009;49(2):185-93.
4. Westgate CS, Botfield HF, Alimajstorovic Z, Yiangou A, Walsh M, Smith G, et al. Systemic and adipocyte transcriptional and metabolic dysregulation in idiopathic intracranial hypertension. JCI Insight. 2021;6(10):e145346.
5. Freund P, Margolin E. (2022). Pseudopapilledema. [online] In: StatPearls [Internet]. Treasure Island (FL): StatPearls Publishing. Available from https://www.ncbi.nlm.nih.gov/books/NBK538291/ [Last accessed September, 2022].
6. Bassi ST, Mohana KP. Optical coherence tomography in papilledema and pseudopapilledema with and without optic nerve head drusen. Indian J Ophthalmol. 2014;62(12):1146-51.
7. Tamhankar MA, Biousse V, Ying GS, Prasad S, Subramanian PS, Lee MS, et al. Isolated third, fourth, and sixth cranial nerve palsies from presumed microvascular versus other causes: a prospective study. Ophthalmology. 2013;120(11):2264-9.
8. Davoudi V, Keyhanian K, Bove RM, Chitnis T. Immunology of neuromyelitis optica during pregnancy. Neurol Neuroimmunol Neuroinflamm. 2016;3(6):e288.
9. D'Souza R, Wuebbolt D, Andrejevic K, Ashraf R, Nguyen V, Zaffar N, et al. Pregnancy and neuromyelitis optica spectrum disorder-reciprocal effects and practical recommendations: a systematic review. Front Neurol. 2020;11:544434.
10. Kasi PM, Tawbi HA, Oddis CV, Kulkarni HS. Clinical review: serious adverse events associated with the use of rituximab-a critical care perspective. Crit Care. 2012;16(4):231.
11. Edwards C, Leira EC, Gonzalez-Alegre P. Residency training: a failed lumbar puncture is more about obesity than lack of ability. Neurology. 2015;84(10):e69-72.
12. Evans RW. Complications of lumbar puncture. Neurol Clin. 1998;16(1):83-105.
13. Birnbaum FA, Johnson GM, Johnson LN, Jun B, Machan JT. Increased prevalence of optic disc drusen after papilloedema from idiopathic intracranial hypertension: on the possible formation of optic disc drusen. Neuroophthalmology. 2016;40(4):171-80.
14. Rossiter JD, Lockwood AJ, Evans AR. Coexistence of optic disc drusen idiopathic intracranial hypertension in a child. Eye. 2005;19(2):234-5.

Section 12: Autoimmune Disorders

Section Editors: Bijoy Jose, Jino Vincent, Sudheeran Kannoth

Associate Editors: Thomas Mathew, Raghunandan Nadig

ARTICLE 1

Updated Diagnostic Criteria for Paraneoplastic Neurologic Syndromes

Graus F, Vogrig A, Muñiz-Castrillo S, Antoine JCG, Desestret V, Dubey D, et al. Updated diagnostic criteria for paraneoplastic neurologic syndromes.
Neurol Neuroimmunol Neuroinflamm. 2021;8(4):e1014.

Abstract

Summary: The purpose of this article was to update the 2004 paraneoplastic neurologic syndromes (PNSs) diagnostic criteria, which have become partially outdated due to recent breakthroughs in PNS research that resulted in the discovery of new phenotypes and antibodies. A modified criteria was developed by a panel of experts in this field through consensus, which would be helpful in clinical decision-making and research purposes. In light of new information on PNS acquired from published and unpublished data provided by the many laboratories involved in the project, the panel reevaluated the 2004 criteria. The panel advocated replacing the term "classical syndromes" with "high-risk phenotypes" for cancer and introducing the idea of "intermediate-risk phenotypes". "High risk" (> 70% associated with cancer) and "intermediate risk" (30–70% associated with cancer) antibodies have replaced the term "onconeural antibody". The panel divided PNS evidence into three categories: definite, probable, and possible. The PNS-Care Score, which considers clinical phenotype, antibody type, cancer presence or absence, and follow-up time, can help you reach each level. The proposed criteria and guidelines will aid in improving clinical care for PNS patients and encouraging uniformity of PNS research projects.

COMMENT

It was after 16 years that Professor Graus and the team of autoimmune neurologists came up with an updated version of the diagnostic criteria for paraneoplastic neurological syndromes. This new criterion is more precise as it is based on the scoring system—PNS-Care Score ≥ 8 is definite PNS, 6–7 is probable PNS, 4–5 is possible PNS, and <3 is non-paraneoplastic. This has taken into account newer antibodies and disease mechanisms, emphasizing the causal role of antibodies in the disease rather than associations. Its strength is the accuracy, and the limitation is that it is too restrictive. This may result in the noninclusion of many newer syndromes. These new criteria have given due importance to immune checkpoint inhibitor-related PNS and made recommendations. They have also made recommendations regarding gold standard testing methods emphasizing the need for serum and cerebrospinal fluid (CSF) testing and confirming the diagnosis with research laboratories.

ARTICLE 2

Difference in the Source of Antiaquaporin-4-immunoglobulin G and Antimyelin Oligodendrocyte Glycoprotein-immunoglobulin G Antibodies in Cerebrospinal Fluid in Patients with Neuromyelitis Optica Spectrum Disorder

Akaishi T, Takahashi T, Misu T, Kaneko K, Takai Y, Nishiyama S, et al. Difference in the source of anti-AQP4-IgG and anti-MOG-IgG antibodies in CSF in patients with neuromyelitis optica spectrum disorder.
Neurology. 2021;97(1):e1-e12.

Abstract

Summary: In the study, the authors investigate the differences in the source and level of intrathecal synthesis between antiaquaporin-4-immunoglobulin G (AQP4-IgG) antibodies and antimyelin oligodendrocyte glycoprotein (MOG)-IgG antibodies. The antibody titers in the sera and cerebrospinal fluid (CSF) of 38 patients with MOG-IgG-associated disease and 36 patients with AQP4-IgG-positive neuromyelitis optica spectrum disorders (NMOSDs) were investigated in acute attacks. The quotients between albumin, total IgG, and each disease-specific antibody level in CSF and serum were determined. The antibody index was calculated using these quotients to determine the intrathecal production level of each disease-specific antibody. 11 of the 38 patients with MOG-IgG were positive for antibody only in the CSF. There were no patients in the AQP4-IgG group who solely had AQP4-IgG positivity in their CSF. The blood–brain barrier was compromised in 75% of MOG-IgG-positive subjects and 43.8% of AQP4-IgG-positive cases, as evidenced by higher albumin quotients. MOG-IgG quotients were also more than 10 times greater than AQP4-IgG quotients. With MOG-IgG, an elevated antibody index (>4.0) was confirmed in 12 of 21 cases, whereas with AQP4-IgG, it was only detected in 1 of 16 cases. The CSF MOG-IgG titers (0.519, $p = 0.001$) and MOG-IgG antibody indexes (0.472, $p = 0.036$) were proportional to CSF cell counts but not to clinical severity.

COMMENT

Neuromyelitis optica spectrum disorder (NMOSD) antibodies consist of aquaporin-4-immunoglobulin G (AQP4-IgG), and myelin oligodendrocyte glycoprotein (MOG)-IgG. As per the existing studies, it is believed that pathogenic antibodies are produced outside the central nervous system (CNS) and transported to the CNS by a breach in the blood–brain barrier or by other mechanisms. In multiple sclerosis, unlike this, there is intrathecal antibody synthesis. In this study by the Japanese group, it was found that 11 out of 38 patients were MOG-IgG positive in CSF alone, while in AQP4-IgG, none were positive in CSF alone. In AQP4-IgG group, there is a correlation between serum and CSF levels. 80% of the cases of MOG-IgG had more CSF levels than serum levels. CSF levels of MOG-IgG correlate with CSF cell count. This study opens up a new disease mechanism in MOG antibody disease. From the transfer of MOG antibodies across the blood–brain barrier, evidence is building up for intrathecal antibody synthesis. The take-home lesson for a practitioner is that paired testing of serum and CSF samples should be done for the best results. It has an implication in the therapy also—drugs targeting the intrathecal antibody-producing cells may yield a better result.

ARTICLE 3

Rituximab Treatment and Long-term Outcome of Patients with Autoimmune Encephalitis: Real-world Evidence from the GENERATE Registry

Thaler FS, Zimmermann L, Kammermeier S, Strippel C, Ringelstein M, Kraft A, et al. Rituximab treatment and long-term outcome of patients with autoimmune encephalitis: Real-world evidence from the GENERATE registry. *Neurol Neuroimmunol Neuroinflamm. 2021;8(6):e1088.*

Abstract

Summary: The goal of this study was to see how rituximab was used in the real world in autoimmune encephalitis (AE) and to see if there was a link between rituximab treatment and long-term outcomes. The study population consisted of patients with N-methyl-D-aspartate receptor (NMDAR)-AE, leucine-rich glioma-inactivated-1 (LGI1)-AE, contactin-associated protein-like-2 (CASPR2)-AE, or glutamic acid decarboxylase 65 (GAD65) disease from the GENERATE (GErman Network for Research on Autoimmune Encephalitis) who had received at least one rituximab dose. A retrospective analysis was done with a control cohort of nonrituximab-treated patients. 163 (46%) of the 358 patients were given rituximab (NMDAR-AE: 57%, CASPR2-AE: 44%, LGI1-AE: 43%, and GAD65 disease: 37%). When compared to CASPR2-AE or GAD65 disease (median: 632 and 1,209 days), rituximab treatment was started much earlier in NMDAR- and LGI1-AE (median: 54 and 155 days after disease onset). The modified

Rankin Scale (mRS) scores of patients with NMDAR-AE improved considerably with and without rituximab treatment. Despite being more seriously impaired at the beginning, rituximab-treated NMDAR-AE patients were found to achieve independent living more frequently (mRS score ≤ 2) (94% vs. 88%). Both rituximab-treated and nontreated patients improved considerably in LGI1-AE, whereas only rituximab-treated patients improved significantly in CASPR2-AE. Patients with GAD65 illness did not show any improvement. In rituximab-treated patients, the relapse rate was significantly reduced (5% vs. 13%). The presence of NMDAR antibodies was linked to a substantial improvement in mRS score. Early therapy commencement was also associated with a positive outcome.

COMMENT

GENERATE (GErman Network for Research on Autoimmune Encephalitis) registry is the German registry on autoimmune encephalitis (AE). The current paper is on the effect of rituximab on AE. Less than half of these patients received rituximab, and most of them were anti-N-methyl-D-aspartate (NMDA) receptor AE, followed by antileucine-rich glioma-inactivated-1 (LGI1), contactin-associated protein-like-2 (CASPR2), and antiglutamic acid decarboxylase 65 (GAD65). Heterogeneity of the subtypes and retrospective nature were the significant limitations of the study. However, it still has significant value in the absence of a good prospective study. Good treatment response was obtained with rituximab in CASPR2 AE. No response was obtained in GAD65 antibody disease, which is considered to be T-cell mediated. Relapse rates were less with rituximab. Early treatment resulted in better outcomes. This study supports the use of the short-term, early rituximab in AE. However, better prospective case–control studies are needed to make decision regarding the dose and duration of therapy.

ARTICLE 4

Characterization of LRP4/Agrin Antibodies from a Patient with Myasthenia Gravis

Yu Z, Zhang M, Jing H, Chen P, Cao R, Pan J, et al. Characterization of LRP4/agrin antibodies from a patient with myasthenia gravis.
Neurology. 2021;97(10):e975-e987.

Abstract

Summary: The purpose of the study was to assess whether anti-LRP4/agrin antibodies are pathogenic in mice and to determine their mechanisms of pathogenesis. The anti-LRP4/agrin antibodies were extracted from a patient with myasthenia gravis (MG) and administered to mice.

The antibodies' effects on agrin-induced muscle-specific tyrosine kinase (MuSK) activation and acetylcholine receptor (AChR) clustering were evaluated, and their epitopes were discovered. The antibody-injected mice had MG symptoms, including weight loss and muscle weakness. Compound muscle action potentials (CMAPs) were decreased, twitch and tetanus force were reduced, the neuromuscular transmission was impaired, and the neuromuscular junction (NMJ) was fragmented and distorted in the mice. Agrin-induced MuSK activation and AChR clustering were blocked by patient immunoglobulin. The study revealed that anti-LRP4/agrin antibodies are pathogenic in MG patients.

COMMENT

Classically, myasthenia gravis is an antibody-mediated disease characterized by postsynaptic neuromuscular junction dysfunction. In nearly 90% of the cases, the disease is mediated by acetylcholine receptor antibodies. The majority of the seronegative cases are caused by antimuscle-specific tyrosine kinase (MuSK) antibodies. Later, LRP4 and anti-agrin antibodies were described in the causation. To prove the autoimmune pathogenesis, Witebsky's postulates need to be satisfied. One of the important components of the postulate is the reproduction of the autoimmune disease in experimental animal models by passive transfer. In this experiment, antibodies from the patient were transferred to animals to see if the disease manifestation occurred. In this study, the authors undisputedly demonstrated disease manifestation in mice after passive transfer of antibodies, thus establishing the pathogenic role of LRP4/agrin antibodies in myasthenia gravis.

ARTICLE 5

Autoimmune Encephalitis Resembling Dementia Syndromes

Bastiaansen AE, van Steenhoven RW, de Bruijn MA, Crijnen YS, van Sonderen A, van Coevorden-Hameete MH, et al. Autoimmune encephalitis resembling dementia syndromes.
Neurol Neuroimmunol Neuroinflamm. 2021;8(5):e1039.

Abstract

Summary: Autoimmune encephalitis (AE) can sometimes mimic neurodegenerative dementia syndromes, and the patients do not always show symptoms of encephalitis. This article analyses how often AE resembles dementia syndromes that are neurodegenerative and identifies red flags in middle-aged and older patients. Patients with antileucine-rich glioma-inactivated-1 (LGI1), anti-N-methyl-D-aspartate receptor (NMDAR), anti-gamma-aminobutyric acid B receptor (GABABR), or anticontactin-associated protein-like-2 (CASPR2) encephalitis were included in this observational cohort study. They also had to meet three additional criteria: be 45 years old, satisfy dementia criteria, and have no significant seizures during the first 4 weeks of the disease. There were 290 patients with AE, 175 of whom were 45 years or older. 67 patients (38%) met the criteria for dementia without significant seizures early in the disease's course. Anti-LGI1 was found in 42 cases (48%), anti-NMDAR was found in 13 cases (52%), anti-GABABR was found in 8 cases (22%), and anti-CASPR2 was found in four cases (15%). A neurodegenerative dementia syndrome was suspected in half of the patients ($n = 33$), while 48 patients (76%) had rapidly progressing cognitive decline. Subtle seizures were overlooked in 17 patients (27%; 16/17 anti-LGI1). There were 16 patients (25%) without any inflammatory changes identified by brain magnetic resonance imaging (MRI) or cerebrospinal fluid (CSF) pleocytosis. At least one CSF biomarker, which is frequently sought when dementia is suspected, was abnormal in 27 of 44 patients (61%), while 8 had positive 14-3-3 findings (19%). With immunotherapy, the majority of patients (84%) improved.

COMMENT

This is an important study from Netherland with a significant impact on day-to-day clinical practice. Dementia presentation of autoimmune encephalitis (AE) is very well described. Here the authors attempt to identify how many of the AE mimic degenerative dementia syndromes. 38% met the criteria for dementia after excluding those with encephalitis and seizures. Interestingly many of them were thought to be degenerative, and markers of degeneration like tau protein and 14-3-3 were positive in a good number of cases. A quarter of them had normal magnetic resonance imaging (MRI) and cerebrospinal fluid (CSF). There was an excellent response to immunotherapy. The important message here is to strongly consider and evaluate patients with dementia for autoimmunity, especially if it is rapidly progressive and if the seizures are subtle at the onset of the illness.

ARTICLE 6

Discontinuation of Immunosuppressive Therapy in Patients with Neuromyelitis Optica Spectrum Disorder with Aquaporin-4 Antibodies

Kım SH, Jang H, Park NY, Kim Y, Kim SY, Lee MY, et al. Discontinuation of immunosuppressive therapy in patients with neuromyelitis optica spectrum disorder with aquaporin-4 antibodies.
Neurol Neuroimmunol Neuroinflamm. 2021;8(2):e947.

Abstract

Summary: The authors try to assess the effects of stopping immunosuppressive therapy (IST) in individuals with neuromyelitis optica spectrum disease (NMOSD) after a sustained period of remission. The medical records of 17 patients with antiaquaporin-4 antibody-positive NMOSD who discontinued IST after a 3-year relapse-free period were reviewed. After a median relapse-free period of 62 months [interquartile range (IQR) 52–73], IST was withdrawn at a median age of 40 years (IQR 32–51). After the withdrawal of IST, 14 (82%) of the 17 patients relapsed at a median interval of 6 months (IQR 4–34). Three of them (18%) had severe attacks, and all three of these patients had a history of severe attacks before IST initiation. These three patients were treated with steroids and plasma exchange for acute treatment, but two of them showed poor recovery and significant disability with worsening 6 months after relapse. The study showed that discontinuing IST may raise the relapse risk in seropositive patients with NMOSD even 5 years after they were in remission. Given the potentially devastating consequences of a single NMOSD event, IST cessation should be approached with caution, especially in patients who had a severe attack prior to starting IST.

COMMENT

An important question that every neurologist and patient will ask is how long to treat a case of neuromyelitis optica spectrum disease (NMOSD). There is no evidence-based answer for this. Most of them believe that lifelong treatment is required as the consequences of a relapse can be disastrous, including vision loss or limb weakness. Treatment was stopped for various reasons after a 5-year disease-free interval; however, the majority of patients relapsed within 6 months. Two patients had serious relapses that did not reverse with steroids or plasma exchange. The majority of those who were seronegative at the time of discontinuation of IST became aquaporin-4-immunoglobulin G (AQP4-IgG) seropositive. This study strongly warns the clinician against discontinuation of immunotherapy in AQP4-positive NMOSD. The study's major drawbacks are its retrospective nature and limited sample size.

ARTICLE 7

Overlapping Central and Peripheral Nervous System Syndromes in Myelin Oligodendrocyte Glycoprotein Antibody-associated Disorders

Rinaldi S, Davies A, Fehmi J, Beadnall HN, Wang J, Hardy TA, et al. Overlapping central and peripheral nervous system syndromes in MOG antibody-associated disorders.
Neurol Neuroimmunol Neuroinflamm. 2020;8(1):e924.

Abstract

Summary: Antibodies against myelin oligodendrocyte glycoprotein (MOG) are linked to central nervous system (CNS) demyelination, including optic neuritis (ON) and transverse myelitis (TM). The study was conducted in an Australasian MOG antibody-associated diseases (MOGADs) cohort to determine if peripheral nervous system (PNS) involvement is linked with MOGAD. 271 adults with MOGAD (2013–2018) who were diagnosed using a live cell-based assay were identified, and comprehensive clinical and immunologic characterization was done on those with suspected PNS involvement. There were 19 patients without past TM who had MOGAD and PNS involvement. A CNS involvement was found in all patients, such as ON [bilateral ($n = 3$), unilateral ($n = 3$), and recurrent ($n = 7$)], cortical lesions ($n = 1$), meningoencephalitis ($n = 1$), and subsequent TM ($n = 4$). The clinical phenotyping and neurophysiology were consistent with acute inflammatory demyelinating polyneuropathy (1 case), myeloradiculitis (3 cases), multifocal motor neuropathy (1 case), brachial neuritis (2 cases), migrant sensory neuritis (3 cases), and paresthesia and/or radicular limb pain (10 cases). The initial magnetic resonance imaging (MRI) spine study in 3/19 showed nerve root enhancement consistent with myeloradiculitis and was normal in 16/19 cases. In 12/15 (80%) cases, immunotherapy resulted in partial or complete resolution of PNS symptoms. In 4/16 MOGAD PNS patients, serum antibodies targeting neurofascin 155, contactin-associated protein 2, or GM1 were found, compared to 0/30 controls ($p = 0.01$).

COMMENT

Myelin oligodendrocyte glycoprotein antibody-associated disease (MOGAD) is typically associated with central nervous system (CNS) demyelination optic neuritis, transverse myelitis, and acute disseminated encephalomyelitis (ADEM). Myeloradiculopathy, combined central and peripheral demyelination (CCPD), and inflammatory neuropathy are being described in this study by the Australian and New Zealand study group. As there has never been a report of MOG antigen expressed in the peripheral nervous system in humans, this finding must be interpreted in the broader context of autoimmunity. Autoimmune diseases may present with autoimmunity that is organ-specific or nonorgan-specific, and as a result, patients may harbor autoimmunity to multiple organs. This is supported by the multiple coexisting antibodies, such as neurofascin 155, GM1, and contactin-associated protein 2.

ARTICLE 8

Use and Safety of Immunotherapeutic Management of N-methyl-D-aspartate Receptor Antibody Encephalitis: A Meta-analysis

Nosadini M, Eyre M, Molteni E, Thomas T, Irani SR, Dalmau J, Dale RC, et al. Use and safety of immunotherapeutic management of N-methyl-d-aspartate receptor antibody encephalitis: A meta-analysis.
JAMA Neurol. 2021;78(11):1333-44.

Abstract

Summary: Immunotherapy has been demonstrated to enhance outcomes and decrease relapses in people with N-methyl-D-aspartate receptor antibody encephalitis (NMDARE). However, the superiority of specific treatments and combinations is unknown. The purpose of this study was to map the use and safety of immunotherapies in people with NMDARE, identify early predictors of poor functional outcome and relapse, assess changes in immunotherapy use and disease outcome over the 14 years since NMDARE was first reported, and determine the anti-NMDAR encephalitis 1-year functional status (NEOS) score. Patients with NMDARE who had positive NMDAR antibodies and available individual immunotherapy data were identified by a systematic search in PubMed from inception to January 1, 2019. Multivariable logistic regression models were used to enter individual patient data on immunotherapies, clinical features at presentation, disease progression, and final functional outcome [modified Rankin Scale (mRS) score]. Data from 1,550 patients were analyzed from 652 publications. 1,105 of 1,508 were females (73.3%), and 707 of the 1,526 (46.3%) were under the age of 18 at the time of disease onset. Adolescent age and first-line treatment with therapeutic apheresis, corticosteroids plus intravenous immunoglobulin (IVIG), or corticosteroids plus IVIG plus therapeutic apheresis were strongly associated with good functional status at the first episode. Age < 2 years or 65 years or older at onset, intensive care unit admission, excessive delta brush pattern on electroencephalography (EEG), lack of immunotherapy during the first 30 days of onset, and maintenance IVIG usage for 6 months or longer were all associated with poor functional outcome. Rituximab use or maintenance IVIG use for 6 months or longer was found to be strongly associated with nonrelapsing illness. Relapsing illness was highly associated with adolescent age at onset. Another interesting finding was the increased use of rituximab from 13.5 (52 of 384; 2007–2013) to 28.3% (311 of 1,100; 2013–2019) ($p < 0.001$), which was accompanied by a decrease in relapse rates over time [22% (12 of 55) in 2008 and earlier; 10.9% (35 of 322) in 2017; and later $p = 0.006$]. The modified NEOS score was linked to the likelihood of poor functional status after 1 year [20.1% (40 of 199) for a score of 0 to 1 point; 43.8% (77 of 176) for a score of 3 to 4 points; $p = 0.05$].

COMMENT

This meta-analysis, which includes 1,550 cases, is quite extensive. It has identified potential factors for poor outcomes, such as advanced age, treatment delay, intensive care unit (ICU) admission, and excessive delta brush—all of which are self-explanatory. There has been a trend of increased use of rituximab in the last few years. The study's retrospective nature as well as reporting bias is its weaknesses. Despite this, this study emphasizes the importance of early immunotherapy and, if necessary, second-line therapy in anti-N-methyl-D-aspartate receptor (NMDAR) autoimmune encephalitis (AE).

ARTICLE 9

Characterization of Extracranial Giant Cell Arteritis with Intracranial Involvement and its Rapidly Progressive Subtype

Beuker C, Wankner MC, Thomas C, Strecker JK, Schmidt-Pogoda A, Schwindt W, et al. Characterization of extracranial giant cell arteritis with intracranial involvement and its rapidly progressive subtype.
Ann Neurol. 2021;90(1):118-29.

Abstract

Summary: The goal of this study was to determine the characteristics of patients with extracranial giant cell arteritis (GCA) who also had intracranial involvement. 31 patients with systemic GCA with intracranial involvement were included in this multicenter retrospective analysis. Assessment of the clinical characteristics, the pattern of arterial involvement, and cytokine profiles were done. Controls were patients with GCA without intracranial involvement ($n = 17$) and with intracranial atherosclerosis ($n = 25$). The erythrocyte sedimentation rate (ESR) was observed to be high in 18 individuals (69.2%) with intracranial involvement and 16 patients (100%) without intracranial involvement ($p = 0.02$). Headache was reported by 15 patients (50.0%) with intracranial involvement and 13 individuals (76.5%) without intracranial involvement ($p = 0.03$). In 26 patients (83.9%), posterior circulation arteries were involved, anterior circulation arteries were affected in 17 patients (54.8%), and both territories were affected in 12 patients (38.7%). The V_4 segment of the vertebral artery after the posterior inferior cerebellar artery (PICA) origin was found to be involved in individuals with atherosclerosis, whereas the V_3 and V_4 segment before the PICA origin was shown to be affected in patients with GCA. 11 patients (37.9%) with GCA and intracranial involvement had a rapidly progressing disease course marked by short-term recurrent ischemic episodes. At follow-up, the median modified Rankin Scale (mRS) score was 4 [interquartile range (IQR) = 2.0–6.0], and four patients (36.4%) died. In patients with a rapidly progressive course, interleukin (IL)-6 and IL-17 expression on vessel walls were considerably higher.

COMMENT

Data showing intracranial artery involvement in giant cell arteritis (GCA) are sparse and are reported in approximately 4% of patients with a high potential of cerebrovascular complications. The German researchers employed biopsies and imaging to reach the diagnosis in this study. In patients with GCA with intracranial involvement, typical clinical manifestations such as headache and increased erythrocyte sedimentation rate (ESR) were frequently absent. V_3–V_4 stenosis of the vertebral artery before posterior inferior cerebellar artery (PICA) origin was the classical pattern observed. Progressive disease was noted in one-third of cases. As is inherent in rare disease studies, this study also had several limitations, including its retrospective nature and small sample size. The limitations of vascular intervention in GCA, the potential lack of efficacy of cyclophosphamide, and the necessity to evaluate interleukin (IL)-6 and IL-17A receptor blockers in the treatment are all concerns that need to be addressed in future prospective research.

ARTICLE 10

Clinical Features and Risk of Relapse in Children and Adults with Myelin Oligodendrocyte Glycoprotein Antibody-associated Disease

Cobo-Calvo A, Ruiz A, Rollot F, Arrambide G, Deschamps R, Maillart E, et al.; NOMADMUS, KidBioSEP, and OFSEP study groups. Clinical features and risk of relapse in children and adults with myelin oligodendrocyte glycoprotein antibody-associated disease.
Ann Neurol. 2021;89(1):30-41.

Abstract

Summary: The study's major goal was to compare clinical characteristics, disease progression, and myelin oligodendrocyte glycoprotein (MOG) antibody (Ab) dynamics in children and adults with MOG-Ab-associated disease (MOGAD). 98 children and 268 adults with MOGAD were included in this retrospective multicenter study between January, 2014 and September, 2019. In both children (40.8%) and adults (55.9%, $p = 0.013$), isolated optic neuritis was the most common clinical manifestation, while acute disseminated encephalomyelitis (ADEM) syndrome was more common in children (36.7% vs. 5.6%, $p < 0.001$). Children had better recovery when compared to adults. Adults had a higher risk of relapse than children in the multivariate analysis [hazard ratio 1.41; 95% confidence interval (CI) 1.12–1.78; $p = 0.003$]. In nonrelapsing children, 64.2% (95% CI 40.9–86.5) of MOG-Ab was negative at 2 years, while only 14.1% (95% CI 4.7–38.3) was negative in children who relapsed (log-rank $p < 0.001$). This difference was not observed in adults.

COMMENT

In the study of demyelinating diseases, a common question is whether or not patients will relapse after their first attack of myelin oligodendrocyte glycoprotein antibody-associated disease (MOGAD). This multicentric French study attempts to answer this issue partially. The researchers found that adults had severe disease and suffered more relapses than children. Antibody negativity occurred earlier in nonrelapsing children than in relapsing children. The difference in oligodendrocyte structural conformation and the reduced compactness of myelin sheaths could explain the more significant occurrence of acute disseminated encephalomyelitis (ADEM) in children. However, a better recovery could be attributed to the pediatric brain's greater reserve. The results are severely limited due to the study's retrospective character. However, the study clearly indicates that adult and pediatric cases require different therapeutic strategies.

Section 13: Rehabilitation

Section Editor: Nirmal Surya

Associate Editor: Hitav Someshwer

ARTICLE 1

Effect of Aquatic versus Land Motor Dual Task Training on Balance and Gait of Patients with Chronic Stroke: A Randomized Controlled Trial

Saleh MSM, Rehab NI, Aly SMA. Effect of aquatic versus land motor dual task training on balance and gait of patients with chronic stroke: A randomized controlled trial.
NeuroRehabilitation. 2019;44(4):485-92.

Abstract

Background: Stroke is one of the leading causes of morbidity and mortality. There are certain psychological consequences that stroke survivors face due to difficulty in performing activities of daily living (ADLs). Balance and gait abnormalities are common symptoms seen in stroke survivors leading to an increase in the risk of falls and also participation restrictions and activity limitations. Land-based exercises have their benefits and shortcomings as well, hence water-based exercises are a better and safer environment to perform exercises to improve balance in stroke survivors.

Objective: A randomized control trial was conducted to evaluate the effect of water-based dual task exercises on balance and gait abnormalities in chronic stroke survivors when compared to land-based dual task exercises.

Methodology: 67 patients were screened for inclusion and exclusion criteria, out of which 50 chronic stroke survivors of both sexes in the age group of 45–65 years, were finally recruited in the study. They were randomly assigned to either of the two groups, i.e., aquatic or land group. The participants received the same motor dual task exercise protocol for 45 minutes, three times a week for 6 weeks irrespective of the group they belonged to. The participants were assessed for balance and gait parameters using the Biodex balance system and Biodex gait trainer, respectively. They were assessed at the time of recruitment and at the end of 6 weeks of treatment.

Results: There was no significant difference between the baseline demographic values, balance parameters, and gait parameters among the participants of the two groups. Post treatment there was significant decrease in the overall stability index, anteroposterior stability index, and mediolateral stability index in both the groups when compared to baseline values. There is a significant decrease in the aquatic group when compared to the land-based group in the balance parameters. There was a significant increase in the walking speed, step length, and time of support in both the groups when compared with the baseline values. There was a significant increase in the aquatic group when compared to land-based group in the gait parameters.

Conclusion: We conclude that water-based dual task exercise training has a better effect on the gait and balance parameters of chronic stroke survivors when compared with land-based motor dual task training.

COMMENT

Stroke is one of the leading causes of morbidity and mortality. The physical and emotional impacts of poststroke are negative. In a randomized controlled trial, Saleh M and his group attempted to examine the effect of aquatic versus land motor dual task training on the balance and gait of patients with chronic stroke. 50 patients with chronic stroke of both sexes, aged 45–55 years, were randomly assigned to the aquatic or land group to determine the difference they chose. For 45 minutes, 3 days a week for 6 weeks, all groups underwent the same motor dual task instruction, either in water or on ground. The dynamic balance indices tested using the Biodex balance method as well as kinematic gait parameters were calculated using the Biodex gait trainer before and after the intervention. Baseline characteristics for both the groups on the basis of demographics, balance parameters, and gait parameters were same. Compared to the baseline value, both groups have shown significant difference overall stability index, anteroposterior stability index, and mediolateral stability index. There was a significant improvement in patients who received the motor dual task training in water compared with patients treated on the land in overall stability index ($p = 0.02$), anteroposterior stability index ($p = 0.03$), mediolateral stability index ($p = 0.002$), walking speed ($p = 0.01$), step length of affected limb ($p = 0.03$), step length of nonaffected limb ($p = 0.01$), and time of support on the affected limb ($p = 0.002$). On the basis of this authors concluded that aqua therapy dual task exercise training had a better effect on the gait and balance parameters of chronic stroke patients when compared with only land-based motor dual task training.

ARTICLE 2

Early Mobilization and Quality of Life after Stroke: Findings from AVERT

Cumming TB, Churilov L, Collier J, Donnan G, Ellery F, Dewey H, et al.; AVERT Trial Collaboration Group. Early mobilization and quality of life after stroke: Findings from AVERT.
Neurology. 2019;93(7):e717-e728.

Abstract

Background: Stroke is a complex neurological condition; it has an effect on the physical, social, psychological, and spiritual wellbeing of survivor. Stroke also has an effect on the perceived quality of life of stroke survivors. Physical rehabilitation helps in early return to daily activities and return to work.

Objective: The study was aimed at evaluating the effect of a very early rehabilitation following stroke on the quality of life of stroke patients.

Methodology: A multicenter, pragmatic, parallel, single-blinded randomized control trial was conducted. Patients older than 18 years with stable hemodynamic parameters were recruited in the study. They recruited 2,104 participants, were then randomly assigned to either the early intervention group or usual care group. In the early intervention group, the patients were mobilized within 24 hours and more frequent mobilizations were done. The participants were assessed at 3 and 12 months postintervention on the assessment of quality of life-four dimension (AQOL-4D) scale, which consists of 12 items which covers four domains. Those patients who expired before 12 months of the intervention were assigned a score of 0 on the outcome measure.

Results: Out of the 2,104 participants recruited only 2,017 participants followed up at 12 months postintervention which also included 257 participants who died in the 12 months. At 12 months the mean score of AQOL-4D was 0.46 ± 0.37 for the interventional group and 0.47 ± 0.36 for the control group. There was no significant difference between the quality of life scores. Similar results were seen at 3-month assessment as well. Similarly, there was no significant difference noted among the four domains of the scales among both the groups. There was inverse relationship between age and quality of life, there was a direct relation between educational qualification and quality of life.

Conclusion: A very early mobilization in poststroke survivors does not have any effect on the quality of life of patient's 12-months postintervention.

COMMENT

More individuals survive stroke with advances in healthcare, but many have to contend with the physical, psychological, social, and functional sequelae, resulting in higher personal and public costs. Cerebral stroke causes a major decline in the functioning of the patient and a deterioration in the quality of life of the patient. A common issue in all countries is long-term disability caused by stroke and its incidence rises markedly with advancing age. The quality of life assessment may also be the evaluator of stroke sequelae as a measure of poststroke recovery effectiveness. In an attempt to evaluate the impact of early mobilization on quality of life of stroke patients Cumming and group did a multicenter, pragmatic, parallel, single blinded randomized control trial. In the study, patients over the age of 18 with healthy hemodynamic parameters were recruited. 2,104 participants were then recruited and randomly allocated either to the early intervention group or the normal treatment group. The patients in the early intervention group were mobilized within 24 hours and more regular mobilizations were carried out in the early intervention community. Quality of life assessment was done at 3 and 12 months postintervention. The scale had 12 items from the four main domains of health. For those patients who expired before 12 months postintervention. A total of 257 patients out of the 2,104 patients enrolled has expired before the follow-up at 12 months. We followed up on a total of 2,017 patients. Their quality of life was similar between both groups. Hence the authors concluded that, very early mobilization of survivors after stroke has no effect on the quality of life of patients 12 months after intervention.

ARTICLE 3

Botulinum Toxin and Occupational Therapy for Writer's Cramp

Park JE, Shamim EA, Panyakaew P, Mathew P, Toro C, Sackett J, et al. Botulinum toxin and occupational therapy for writer's cramp.
Toxicon. 2019;169:12-7.

Abstract

Background: Writer's cramp is a form of upper limb task-specific dystonia condition which leads to reduction in writing and thereby affecting the quality of life of the patient. Botulinum neurotoxin (BoNT) helps in reducing dystonia and spasticity. There are various noninvasive therapies also for the rehabilitation of writer's cramp.

Objective: In this study, they aimed to compare the effect of combination therapy of BoNT and occupational therapy and single therapy of botulinum toxin in patients with writer's cramp.

Methodology: A randomized clinical trial was conducted on 12 patients which were randomly assigned to either BoNT plus occupational therapy or BoNT alone group. The outcome measures used in this study were a patient-rated subjective scale, writer's cramp rating scale (WCRS), writer's cramp impairment scale (WCIS), writer's cramp disability scale (WCDS), and kinetic parameters. The patient was assessed at baseline and the end of 20 weeks postinjection. Patients of both groups were injected BoNT by a trained neurologist under electromyography (EMG) guidance, the patients were injected at week 1 and week 12 by the same neurologist. Patients in the combination group received isometric splints which were worn for half an hour per day and some finger exercises.

Results: All 12 patients completed the 20 weeks of study duration; there was no significant difference in the patient-rated subjective scale between patients of both the groups. There was a significant decrease seen in the WCIS score in the combination group. There was a significant increase in the WCRS score in the BoNT group alone. No significant difference was seen in the WCDS, handgrip, and kinematic data scores.

Conclusion: There was no difference of patient rate subjective scale between both the groups. The combination of BoNT and occupational therapy group had a better outcome but this was limited by due to small sample size and the two groups being heterogenous. A further large scale study should be conducted to show there is in an improved efficacy of BoNT.

COMMENT

There are many types of task-specific dystonia which affect the upper extremity, the most common form is Writer's cramp (WC). Although the focal botulinum neurotoxin (BoNT) injection of the dystonic muscles may be beneficial, the drawback of BoNT is its transient effects

Repetitive writing is the major reason for its occurrence hence the name. Various forms of therapy have been developed as WC therapy, of which BoNT injections are considered to be the most effective at this time. Although the focal BoNT injection of the dystonic muscles may be beneficial, the drawback of BoNT is its transient effects. Park and Group evaluated the effect of combination therapy of BoNT and occupational therapy and single therapy of botulinum toxin in patients with writer's cramp. A randomized clinical trial was performed in 12 patients randomized to either BoNT plus occupational therapy or BoNT alone.

The patients were tested preintervention and at the end of 20 weeks after intervention on patient-rated subjective scale, the writer's cramp rating scale (WCRS), the writer's cramp impairment scale (WCIS), the writer's cramp disability scale (WCDS), and the kinetic parameters. Patients in both groups were injected with BoNT by a qualified neurologist under the supervision of the electromyography (EMG), and patients were injected at week 1 and week 12 by the same neurologist.

Patients in the combination category got isometric splints that were worn for half an hour a day and some finger exercises. All 12 patients completed 20 weeks of study duration; A substantial decrease was seen in the WCIS score in the combination category. In the BoNT category alone, there was a substantial improvement in the WCRS ranking. Authors noticed that there was no difference in the subjective scale of the patient rate between the two classes. The combination of the BoNT and the occupational therapy community had a better result, but this was limited due to small sample size and heterogeneous two groups. A further large-scale research should be performed to demonstrate that BoNT has increased efficacy.

ARTICLE 4

A Newly Designed Intensive Caregiver Education Program Reduces Cognitive Impairment, Anxiety, and Depression in Patients with Acute Ischemic Stroke

Zhang L, Zhang T, Sun Y. A newly designed intensive caregiver education program reduces cognitive impairment, anxiety, and depression in patients with acute ischemic stroke.
Braz J Med Biol Res. 2019;52(9):e8533.

Abstract

Background: Acute ischemic stroke leads to degeneration and dysfunction of the cortical and subcortical regions of the brain. It is a complex condition which could lead to cognitive impairments and also psychological comorbidities such as anxiety and depression. This may interfere with the recovery process and thus increase morbidity.

Objective: They aimed to understand the effectiveness of a newly designed intensive caregiver education program (ICEP) to reduce cognitive impairment, anxiety, and depression in acute ischemic stroke patients.

Methodology: A randomized control trial was conducted, where acute ischemic stroke patients and their caregivers were recruited. The patients upon recruitment were enrolled in either ICEP group or the control group using a block randomization method. In the ICEP group the caregivers received intervention from a trained nurse and a physical therapy. The sessions were divided into two parts, hospitalization phase and discharge phase. They received the first session 7 days after hospitalization of the patient followed by one session every week for 1 hour till discharge. Post discharge the caregivers were given intervention for 90 minutes every 2 weeks. The educational intervention consisted of six topics. In control group they were given normal education. All patients were given same conventional therapy in both groups. All participants were assessed on the following outcome measures, Mini Mental State Examination (MMSE), Montreal Cognitive Assessment (MoCA), Hospital Anxiety and Depression Scale (HADS), Zung Self-rating Anxiety Scale (SAS), and Zung Self-rating Depression Scale (SDS). The patients were assessed at baseline, at 3 months, at 6 months, and at 12 months.

Results: A total of 196 patients and caregivers were recruited for this study, there was no significant difference in the baseline scores across all the outcome measures. The MMSE score of the patients in both the groups had no significant difference at the baseline reading, 3 and 6 months readings but there was significant improvement in the 12-month reading in the ICEP group. The MoCA score had no significant difference at baseline and 3-month reading but had a significant improvement in the 6 and 12 months readings in the ICEP group. There was no significant change on the HADS scores at baseline, 3, 6, and 12 months readings. There was a significant reduction in the score of SAS scale in the 12-month reading in the ICEP group. There was significant reduction in SDS scores at 12-month reading only.

Conclusion: They concluded that caregiver education plays an important rehabilitation of acute ischemic stroke patients. The caregiver program helps in improving cognitive impairments and reduces depression and anxiety in the acute ischemic stroke patients.

COMMENT

Cognitive deficiency as a complication affecting more than one-third patients with strokes are increasingly deteriorating and followed by neuropsychological disorders, including anxiety and depression. In addition, anxiety and depression are also widespread in poststroke patients and associated with increased risk of functional dependency as well as decreased quality of life. Reduce cognitive decline, depression, and anxiety in acute ischemic stroke patients are important. A randomized controlled trial was performed in which acute ischemic stroke patients and their caregivers were recruited. Patients on recruitment were enrolled in either the intensive caregiver education program (ICEP) group or the control group using a block randomization process. In the ICEP group, the caregivers received the intervention of a qualified nurse and physical therapy. The sessions were divided into two parts, the phase of hospitalization and the phase of discharge. The first session was given 7 days after the hospitalization of the patient, followed by one session every week for 1 hour until discharge. After discharge, the caregivers were given an intervention for 90 minutes every 2 weeks. Educational intervention consisted of six subjects. Standard education was given in the control group. In both types, both patients received the same traditional therapy. Both participants were tested on the following outcome measures: Mini Mental State Test (MMSE), Montreal Cognitive Evaluation (MoCA), Hospital Anxiety and Depression Scale (HADS). A total of 196 patients and caregivers have been recruited for this analysis, with no substantial difference in baseline scores across all outcome measures. The MMSE score for patients in both groups had no substantial difference in baseline readings, 3 and 6 months, but there was a significant increase in ICEP 12-month reading. The MoCA score had no substantial difference in baseline and 3-month reading but had a significant increase in 6 and 12 months readings in the ICEP community. There was no noticeable improvement in baseline, 3, 6, and 12 months HADS ratings. In the 12-month reading in the ICEP community, there was a substantial reduction in the Self-rating Anxiety Scale (SAS) score. There was a substantial decrease in Self-rating Depression Scale (SDS) scores at 12-month reading only. They concluded that caregiver education plays an important role in the recovery of acute ischemic stroke patients. The caregiver program aims to enhance cognitive disability and decreases stress and anxiety in acute ischemic stroke patients.

ARTICLE 5

Combining Virtual Reality Motor Rehabilitation with Cognitive Strategy Use in Chronic Stroke

Boone AE, Wolf TJ, Engsberg JR. Combining virtual reality motor rehabilitation with cognitive strategy use in chronic stroke.
Am J Occup Ther. 2019;73(4):7304345020p1-7304345020p9.

Abstract

Background: Rehabilitation professionals use interventions in the chronic stage based on the impairments. Cognitive training helps in improving the patient's functional outcomes. The combination therapy of virtual reality and cognitive training has not been studied.

Objective: To evaluate acceptability, recruitment, and retention rate and determine which outcome measures best capture the effect of the intervention.

Methodology: A single group quasi-experimental study was conducted on 10 chronic stroke patients, Fugl-Meyer scale was used to assess the upper extremity motor performance. Performance quality rating scale and the Canadian occupational performance measure were used to measure the occupational performance on trained and untrained goals. The assessment was done preintervention, postintervention, and after 3 months. A 12-week intervention was conducted where Kinect-based virtual reality to encourage high numbers of upper extremity movement repetitions was a 2 weekly session and use of cognitive strategies with practice of client-centered goals was the focus of third weekly session.

Results: The intervention was perceived as acceptable. Recruitment rate was 15%, and retention rate was 100%. Large effects were found on outcomes of upper extremity motor performance, occupational performance, and participation at follow-up.

Conclusion and Relevance: Combination therapy is feasible for adults with chronic stroke. The maximal effects are seen in of upper extremity motor performance, occupational performance, and participation.

COMMENT

More than half of poststroke individuals appear to have trouble performing daily functional activities even after recovery. In particular, bathing and dressing are the most problematic areas of chronic stroke, with 68% and 59% of individuals having ongoing difficulty, respectively, at 1 year poststroke. People often self-report needing high levels of assistance with instrumental activities of daily life, including meal planning (77%), housekeeping (70%), and shopping (52%), at 1 year poststroke. Despite frequent demands for occupational testing and intervention, occupational therapy professionals expend the bulk of their time on rehabilitation to treat impairments. A single group quasi-experimental study was conducted in 10 chronic stroke patients, Fugl-Meyer scale was used to assess upper extremity motor performance. The occupational performance quality rating scale and the Canadian occupational performance measure were used to measure occupational performance on the basis of trained and untrained objectives. The assessment was carried out before, after, and after 3 months of action. A 12-week intervention was conducted in which Kinect-based virtual reality to encourage high numbers of upper extremity movement repetitions was a 2-week session and the use of cognitive strategies with client-centered goal practice was the focus of the third weekly session.

The intervention was considered acceptable. The recruitment rate was 15% and the retention rate was 100%. Effects have been identified on the results of upper extremity motor performance, occupational performance, and follow-up participation.

ARTICLE 6

Virtual Reality Rehabilitation versus Conventional Physical Therapy for Improving Balance and Gait in Parkinson's Disease Patients: A Randomized Controlled Trial

Feng H, Li C, Liu J, Wang L, Ma J, Li G, et al. Virtual reality rehabilitation versus conventional physical therapy for improving balance and gait in Parkinson's disease patients: A randomized controlled trial.
Med Sci Monit. 2019;25:4186-92.

Abstract

Background: Prevalence of Parkinson's disease (PD) is increasing in the world and rehabilitation helps in improving quality of life by improving balance and gait in them. Virtual reality (VR) is a new innovative method of rehabilitation developed over the last decade.

Objective: To investigate the effect of VR technology on balance and gait in patients with PD.

Methodology: A total of 28 Parkinson patients were included in this single-blinded randomized control trial where $n = 14$ were randomly assigned to intervention and the remaining $n = 14$ were the control group. Patients performed 45 minutes per session, 5 days a week, for 12 weeks in which experiment group received VR training and the other group received the regular physiotherapy. Berg Balance Scale (BBS), Timed Up and Go Test (TUGT), third part of Unified Parkinson's Disease Rating Scale (UPDRS3), and Functional Gait Assessment (FGA) were used as outcome measures.

Results: After treatment, BBS, TUGT, and FGA scores had improved significantly in both groups ($p < 0.05$). However, there was no significant difference in the UPDRS3 between the pre- and postrehabilitation data of the control group ($p > 0.05$). VR training resulted in significantly better performance compared with the conventional physical therapy group ($p < 0.05$).

Conclusion: The results of this study indicate that 12 weeks of VR rehabilitation resulted in a greater improvement in the balance and gait of individuals with PD when compared to conventional physical therapy.

COMMENT

Gait freezing is one of the common complications of Parkinson's disease (PD) patients, often in advanced stages. This complication limits the progression to the feet, raises the risk of falling and causes problems in patient care, in spite of the patient's tentative to walk.

Medicines aimed at freezing gait in PD currently do not have a completely successful response for the patient. Studies indicate that the motor functions of PD patients can be further enhanced by physical care. Virtual reality (VR), a visual, auditory, and somatosensory stimuli that can help enhance the gait for people suffering from PD, is one of the most successful therapies. This encourages people to engage with an artificial VR, while health workers can track and measure their progress. External stimuli are strong in improving gait for PD patients with more acceleration in combination with the use of visual details.

In this single-randomized control study, 28 patients with Parkinson have been included in a total of $n = 14$ and the remaining $n = 14$ were distributed randomly for intervention. Patients had 45 minutes a session, 5 days a week, during 12 weeks of VR-training in the experiment group and routine physiotherapy in the other group. The result measures were the third part of Unified Parkinson's Disease Rate Scale (UPDRS3), Berg Balance Scale (BBS), Timed Up and Go Tests (TUGT), and Functional Gait Assessment (FGA). The BBS, TUGT, and FGA ratings in both groups significantly improved after treatment ($p < 0.05$). However, in the UPDRS3 there was no substantial difference between the control group data before and after rehabilitation ($p > 0.05$). Compared with the traditional physical therapy community ($p < 0.05$), VR training yielded substantially better results. The results of this study indicate that 12 weeks of VR rehabilitation resulted in a greater improvement in the balance and gait of individuals with PD when compared to conventional physical therapy.

ARTICLE 7

Urinary Symptoms in Patients with Parkinson's Disease and Progressive Supranuclear Palsy: Urodynamic Findings and Management of Bladder Dysfunction

Gupta A, Krishnan UKR, Nageshkumar S, Pal PK, Khanna M, Taly AB. Urinary symptoms in patients with Parkinson's disease and progressive supranuclear palsy: Urodynamic findings and management of bladder dysfunction. *Ann Indian Acad Neurol. 2019;22(4):432-6.*

Abstract

Background: Parkinson's disease (PD) is a motor neurodegenerative disorder secondary to basal ganglia dysfunction. PD patients frequently present with lower urinary tract symptoms, often typical of overactive bladder and associated with the urodynamic finding of neurogenic detrusor overactivity.

Objective: To observe urinary symptoms in PD patients and progressive supranuclear palsy patients and based on the urodynamic study (UDS) findings manage the bladder dysfunction.

Methods: A sample size of 22 patients was taken with 15 patients with PD and 7 patients with progressive supranuclear paralysis (PSP) patients and only 1 patient was not on levodopa and carbidopa. All the patients had urinary dysfunction and were assessed using UDS.

Results: 60.4 ± 8.4 years was the mean age of the study participants. The mean duration was 14.8 months for their urinary symptoms and 31.9 months for their illness. 12 out of 22 patients had absence of voluntary anal contraction on per-rectal examination. UDS was suggestive of 12 patients with neurogenic detrusor overactivity with or without sphincter dyssynergy. Six patients had normal detrusor pressure, and four patients were found to have contractile detrusor. 10 patients had significant postvoid residual. 18 patients reported nocturia and 16 patients had urgency with or without urge incontinence. Three patients had retention and straining to void and three had mixed urinary complaints.

Conclusion: Urinary symptoms are common symptoms in patients of PD and PSP. The severity of symptoms and UDS results do not correlate. UDS is necessary for bladder training as patients have urinary complaints during the course of illness.

COMMENT

Patients with Parkinson's disease (PD) often present with symptoms of the lower urinary tract, often characteristic of overactive bladder, and associated with the neurogenic detrusor overactivity (NDO) urodynamic finding. Because neurogenic bladder dysfunction can lead to significant upper and lower urinary tract injury, early diagnosis and treatment is needed for this disorder. There is also a need to assess patients at the earliest on the basis of urinary symptoms. In different studies, the incidence of urinary symptoms is stated to vary from 29 to 73%, which correlates with the seriousness of the disease and has an adverse effect on the quality of life. Patients have lower urinary tract symptoms (LUTS) of both storage and voiding types—LUTS is more frequent with the former.

Progressive supranuclear paralysis (PSP) is a prevalent atypical neurodegenerative Parkinsonian condition, which is a sporadic disease with more common occurrence in the fifth to seventh decade of life, first identified by Steele, Richardson, and Olszewski in the early 1960s as a separate clinicopathological entity. A proportion of PSP patients are known to develop urinary complaints. Current studies found that urinary storage dysfunction does not vary from PD or multiple system atrophy (MSA) in patients with PSP, but voiding dysfunction is milder and more severe in patients with MSA than in patients with PD. Authors: A sample size of 22 patients was taken in 15 patients with PD and 7 patients with PSP patients and only 1 patient was not on levodopa and carbidopa. Both patients had urinary dysfunction and were tested using UDS. Authors conducted a cross-sectional study in the department of neurological rehabilitation of a quaternary hospital-based research institute. The mean age of the study participants was 60.4 ± 8.4 years. The mean length was 14.8 months for their urinary symptoms and 31.9 months for their disease.

12 of the 22 patients had no voluntary anal contraction on a per-rectal test. UDS was indicative of 12 patients with neurogenic detrusive overactivity with or without sphincter dyssynergia. Six patients had natural detrusor pressure and four patients had a contractile detrusor. 10 patients had a large residual postvoid. 18 patients had nocturnal symptoms and 16 patients had emergency incontinence or not. Three patients were held back and strained to void, and three had mixed urinary problems. Urinary symptoms are common symptoms in patients of PD and PSP. The severity of symptoms and urodynamic study results do not correlate. UDS is necessary for bladder training as patients have urinary complaints during the course of illness.

ARTICLE 8

The Effects of Vestibular Rehabilitation on Dizziness and Balance Problems in Patients after Traumatic Brain Injury: A Randomized Controlled Trial

Kleffelgaard I, Soberg HL, Tamber AL, Bruusgaard KA, Pripp AH, Sandhaug M, et al. The effects of vestibular rehabilitation on dizziness and balance problems in patients after traumatic brain injury: A randomized controlled trial. *Clin Rehabil. 2019;33(1):74-84.*

Abstract

Objective: To analyze the consequences of group-based vestibular rehabilitation in patients with traumatic brain injury.

Methodology: A single-blind randomized controlled trial was conducted at a university hospital (recruitment and baseline assessments) (experimental intervention); a complete of 65 patients (45 women) with mild-to-moderate traumatic brain injury (mean age 39.4 ± 13.0 years) were randomly assigned to intervention ($n = 33$) or control group ($n = 32$). Group-based vestibular rehabilitation was done for 8 weeks. Participants were tested at baseline (3.5 ± 2.1 months after injury) and at two postintervention follow-ups (2.7 ± 0.8 and 4.4 ± 1.0 months after baseline testing). *Primary outcome*: Dizziness Handicap Inventory. *Secondary outcome*: High-level Mobility Assessment Tool. *Other outcomes*: Vertigo Symptom Scale, Rivermead Postconcussion Symptoms Questionnaire, Hospital Anxiety and Depression Scale, and Balance Error classification system. Between-group differences were analyzed with a linear mixed-model analysis for repeated measurements.

Results: At baseline, no group differences were revealed (personal factors, clinical characteristics, and outcome measures). At the primary follow-up, statistically significant mean differences in favor of the intervention were found within the primary [−8.7, 95% confidence interval (CI) −16.6 to −0.9] and secondary outcomes (3.7 points, 95% CI 1.4–6.0). At the second follow-up, no significant between-group differences were found. No significant between-group differences within the other outcomes were found at the two follow-ups.

Conclusion: The intervention gave the impression to speedup recovery for patients with dizziness and balance problems after traumatic brain injury. However, the advantages had dissipated 2 months after the top of the intervention.

COMMENT

Vestibular rehabilitation is an accepted and frequently used treatment for dizziness and balance problems. Vestibular rehabilitation is a broad concept that includes compensation and balance training after a vestibular lesion and in other causes of vertigo dizziness and balance problems. Current vestibular rehabilitation includes a combination of exercises mainly addressing the patient's impairments and activity limitations. Kleffelgaard and team planned single-blind randomized controlled study to analyze the consequences of group-based vestibular rehabilitation in patients with traumatic brain injury. A total of 65 patients (45 women) with mild-to-moderate traumatic brain injury (mean age 39.4 ± 13.0 years) were randomly assigned to the intervention ($n = 33$) or control group ($n = 32$) at the university hospital (recruitment and baseline assessments) and the metropolitan university (experimental intervention). 8 weeks of group-based vestibular therapy. The patients were assessed at baseline (3.5 ± 2.1 months after injury) and two postintervention follow-ups (2.7 ± 0.8 and 4.4 ± 1.0 months after baseline testing). *Main output*: Dizziness Handicap Inventory. *Secondary Outcome*: High-level Mobility Evaluation Method. *Other results*: Vertigo Symptom Scale, Rivermead Postconcussion Symptoms Questionnaire, Hospital Anxiety and Depression Scale, and Balance Error Classification System. Intergroup variations were evaluated with a linear mixed-model analysis for repeated measurements. No group differences (personal factors, clinical characteristics, and outcome measures) were established at baseline. In the primary follow-up, statistically significant mean differences in favor of intervention were established between the primary [−8.7, 95% confidence interval (CI) −16.6 to −0.9] and secondary outcomes (3.7, 95% CI 1.4−6.0). No major differences between groups were reported during the second follow-up. No major differences between groups within the other outcomes were reported in the two follow-ups. The intervention gave the appearance of accelerating recovery in patients with dizziness and balance issues following traumatic brain injury. The advantages had, however, dissipated 2 months after the top of the intervention.

ARTICLE 9

Effects of High- and Low-frequency Repetitive Transcranial Magnetic Stimulation on Motor Recovery in Early Stroke Patients: Evidence from a Randomized Controlled Trial with Clinical, Neurophysiological and Functional Imaging Assessments

Du J, Yang F, Hu J, Hu J, Xu Q, Cong N, et al. Effects of high- and low-frequency repetitive transcranial magnetic stimulation on motor recovery in early stroke patients: Evidence from a randomized controlled trial with clinical, neurophysiological and functional imaging assessments.
Neuroimage Clin. 2019;21:101620.

Abstract

Background: Repetitive transcranial magnetic stimulation (rTMS) can modulate cortical excitability, and will be beneficial for motor recovery after stroke. However, the neuroplasticity effects of rTMS have not been thoroughly investigated within the early stage after stroke.

Objective: To comprehensively assess the results of high- and low-frequency (LF) rTMSs on motor recovery in early stroke patients, employing a randomized controlled trial supported clinical, neurophysiological and functional imaging assessments.

Methods: Sixty hospitalized, first-ever apoplexy patients (within 2 weeks after stroke) with motor deficits were randomly allocated to receive, additionally to straightforward therapy, five consecutive sessions of either: (1) high-frequency (HF) rTMS at 10 Hz over the ipsilesional primary motor region (M1); (2) LF rTMS at 1 Hz over the contralesional M1, and (3) sham rTMS. The first outcome measure was a motor impairment score (upper extremity Fugl-Meyer) evaluated at baseline, after rTMS intervention, and at 3-month follow-up. Cortical excitability and functional magnetic resonance imaging (fMRI) data were obtained within 24 hours before and after rTMS intervention. Analyses of variance were conducted to check the recovery effects among the three rTMS groups, assessed using clinical, neurophysiological, and fMRI tests.

Results: Motor improvement was considerably larger inside the two rTMS teams than inside the management cluster. The HF-rTMS cluster showed considerably inflated plant tissue excitability and motor-evoked fMRI activation in ipsilesional motor areas, whereas the LF-rTMS cluster had considerably reduced plant tissue excitability and motor-evoked fMRI activation in contralesional motor areas. Activity in ipsilesional area considerably related to with motor perform, when intervention still as at 3-month follow-up.

Conclusion: HF-rTMS and LF-rTMS will each improve motor perform by modulating motor cortical activation inside the early phase of stroke.

COMMENT

The interhemispheric inhibition (IHI) model is the theoretical model widely adopted for guiding the use of repetitive transcranial magnetic stimulation (rTMS) after stroke in motor recovery. According to the neuronal excitability of each cerebral hemisphere in the IHI model, the contralateral effect exerts an inhibitory effect, so that the brain between hemispheres, operation is usually balanced. In patients with strokes, however, stroke can disrupt the equilibrium by reducing the IHI of the affected hemisphere and moving the equilibrium to the unaffected hemisphere. Which contributes to the overactivity of as compared to the affected one, in the unaffected hemisphere. Therefore, promoting the excitability of the motor cortex of the ipsilesian (high rTMS frequency > 1 Hz) or suppression of contralesional motor cortex excitability (low rTMS frequency > 1 Hz) may be helpful for correcting and promoting the interhemispheric imbalance. To validate this hypothesis, the randomized controlled trial was done by Jung Du and group. The objective of the study was to comprehensively assess the results of high-frequency (HF) and low-frequency (LF) repetitive transcranial magnetic stimulations on motor recovery in early stroke patients. In addition to straightforward therapy, 60 hospitalized first-time apoplexy patients (within 2 weeks after stroke) with motor defects were randomly assigned to undergo five consecutive sessions of either: (1) HF-rTMS at 10 Hz over the ipsilesian primary motor region (M1), (2) LF-rTMS at 1 Hz over the contralesional region (M1), and (3) sham rTMS. A motor disability score (upper extremity Fugl-Meyer) measured at baseline, after rTMS intervention, and at follow-up for 3 months was the first outcome test. Within 24 hours before and after rTMS intervention, cortical excitability and functional magnetic resonance imaging (fMRI) data were obtained. Variance studies were carried out to check the recovery effects of the three classes of rTMS, evaluated using clinical, neurophysiological, and fMRI measures.

Within the two rTMS classes, motor enhancement was substantially greater than within the control group. In ipsilesional motor regions, the HF-rTMS group displayed significantly increased cortical excitability and motor-evoked fMRI activation, while in contralesional motor areas the LF-rTMS group had significantly decreased cortical excitability and motor-evoked fMRI activation. Activity in the ipsilesian cortical area was strongly associated with motor function, even at 3-month follow-up after intervention. By modulating motor cortical activity during the early phase of stroke, HF- and LF-rTMS can also enhance motor function.

ARTICLE 10

A Randomized Control Trial Comparing the Effects of Motor Relearning Programme and Mirror Therapy for Improving Upper Limb Motor Functions in Stroke Patients

Jan S, Arsh A, Darain H, Gul S. A randomized control trial comparing the effects of motor relearning programme and mirror therapy for improving upper limb motor functions in stroke patients.
J Pak Med Assoc. 2019;69(9):1242-5.

Abstract

Objective: To check the effectiveness of motor relearning program with mirror therapy in upper limb motor functions of stroke patients.

Methods: A randomized controlled trial was conducted in Rafsan Neuro Rehabilitation Center, Peshawar, Pakistan, from June to December 2017, which they recruited stroke patients with Mini Mental State Examination (MMSE) score of over 24. They were randomly allocated into treatment and control groups. The treatment group underwent a motor relearning program, while the control group received mirror therapy. Upper limb subscales of the motor assessment scale were used as data collection tool.

Results: 46 (69.7%) were males and 20 (30.3%) were females out of the total 66 patients recruited. The mean age of the study population was 55.44 ± 9.21 years. Left hemiplegia was found in 31 (47%) subjects, while 35 (53%) had right hemiplegia. There was a significant improvement in the upper arm functions, hand function, and advance hand activities in the treatment group ($p < 0.001$).

Conclusion: Motor relearning program and mirror therapy were found to be effective in improving upper limb motor functions of stroke patients, but the previous was found to be more practical than the latter.

COMMENT

Different studies have used different forms of intervention and different durations of therapy to assess the efficacy of these treatments in promoting upper limb function recovery. Proprioceptive neuromuscular facilitation (PNF), Brunnstorm, Bobath therapy, the motor relearning program (MRP), constrained-induced movement therapy (CIMT), and mirror therapy (MT) are the main therapeutic approaches for the rehabilitation of upper limb functions in stroke patients. In literature, success is rare. The study was designed to compare the efficacy of MRP with MT in upper limb motor functions of stroke patients to demonstrate the hypothesis that there would be a substantial difference in the impact of MRP and MT in improving upper limb motor functions of stroke patients.

From June to December 2017, the randomized control trial was performed at the Rafsan Neuro Rehabilitation Center, Peshawar, Pakistan, and consisted of stroke patients with a Mini Status Test score above 24. Participants were allocated randomly into groups of care and supervision. The treatment group underwent an MRP, while MT was received by the control group. As a data collection instrument, the upper limb subscales of the motor evaluation scale were used. For data processing, SPSS 20 was used. 46 (69.7%) of the 66 subjects were males and 20 (30.3%) were females. The mean age was 55.44 ± 9.21 years. In 31 (47%) participants, left hemiplegia was observed, while 35 (53%) had right hemiplegia. There were 33 (50%) topics in each of the two classes. There were important variations between the upper arm functions, hand function, and advanced hand movements of the two groups ($p < 0.05$ each) between pretreatment and posttreatment. Compared to the control group, all three variables changed substantially within the treatment group ($p < 0.001$). It was found that the MRP and MT were successful in enhancing stroke patients' upper limb motor functions, although the former one was found to be more realistic than the latter.

ARTICLE 11

The Use of Virtual Reality Rehabilitation for Individuals Post Stroke

Moreira GM, de Lima EMR, Machado IT, Cunha Loureiro APC, Manffra EF. The use of virtual reality rehabilitation for individuals post stroke.
J Rehab Therapy.2019;1(1):21-7.

Abstract

Background: Stroke causes somatosensory and motor deficits that compromise the static and equilibrium. The recovery of those skills is a vital goal within the rehabilitation process and physiotherapy treatments have employed video games (VGs) for therapeutic purposes.

Objective: To research the results of employing VG in static and equilibrium of people after stroke.

Method: A quasi-experimental study was conducted. The sample consisted of 28 individuals with hemiparesis, divided into experimental group (EG) and control group (CG), with 14 participants in each. The EG underwent conventional physiotherapy and commercial VGs training. The interventions were individualized, with duration of half-hour, twice per week, for 10 sessions. The CG received only conventional physiotherapy. The groups were evaluated before and immediately after completion of the study. Individuals were assessed with Berg Balance Scale, Mini-BESTest, Postural Assessment Scale for Stroke, Functional Reach Test, and 1-minute sit-to-stand Test.

Results: Both groups increased their scores on the scales. However, this increase was significant just for the EG within the Berg Balance Scale ($p = 0.001$), Mini-BESTest ($p = 0.001$), and Functional Reach Test ($p = 0.041$). Correlation analysis indicated that the rise in functional scales was associated with progress within the Tightrope game.

Conclusion: These results suggest that VG is a valuable tool for physiotherapy practice, bringing potential benefits to enhance static, and equilibrium in stroke individuals.

COMMENT

The recovery of equilibrium after a stroke is a significant target for physiotherapy, which has a variety of treatment modalities such as traditional physiotherapy, aquatic physiotherapy, electrostimulation therapy, proprioceptive neuromuscular facilitation, and the approach to Bobath. There is, however, an increasing need for more motivational therapies to facilitate neurofunctional rehabilitation and strengthen adherence to therapy. Digital technology may be an interesting resource to be connected to other therapeutic techniques in this way. Despite the possible benefits of video games as therapeutic tools, commercial ones were not initially designed for people with disabilities, as games with activities involving weight transfer between the paretic and nonparetic lower limbs could be an interesting alternative in the case of poststroke hemiparetic patient balance training. In this research, in standing posture, attempts were made to promote lateral weight shifting and multidirectional balance. The purpose of this study was to check the effects of a commercial video game (VG) on improving balance between persons with chronic stroke in relation to improving balance with the use of various functional scales. A quasi-experimental research has been carried out. The study consisted of 28 hemiparesis patients, divided into experimental group (EG) and control group (CG), each with 14 participants. The EG obtained traditional instruction in physiotherapy and commercial VGs. The treatments for 10 sessions were individualized, with a length of half an hour, twice a week. Only traditional physiotherapy was obtained by the CG. Before and immediately after completion of the analysis, the groups were measured. With the Berg Balance Scale, Mini-BESTest, Postural Evaluation Scale for Stroke, Functional Reach Test, and 1-minute sit-to-stand Test, individuals were tested. Both classes on the scales raised their ratings. However, it was only for the EG inside the Berg Balance Scale ($p = 0.001$), Mini-BESTest ($p = 0.001$), and Functional Reach Test ($p = 0.041$) that this increase was important. Correlation research showed that improvement within the Tightrope game was correlated with the increase in functional scales. These results suggest that VG is a valuable tool for physiotherapy practice, bringing potential benefits to enhance static, and equilibrium in stroke individuals.

ARTICLE 12

A Stimulus for Eating. The Use of Neuromuscular Transcutaneous Electrical Stimulation in Patients Affected by Severe Dysphagia after Subacute Stroke: A Pilot Randomized Controlled Trial

Simonelli M, Ruoppolo G, Iosa M, Morone G, Fusco A, Grasso MG, et al. A stimulus for eating. The use of neuromuscular transcutaneous electrical stimulation in patients affected by severe dysphagia after subacute stroke: A pilot randomized controlled trial.
NeuroRehabilitation. 2019;44(1):103-10.

Abstract

Background: Oropharyngeal dysphagia could be a common problem in subacute stroke patients resulting in bronchopneumonia and malnutrition. Noninvasive neuromuscular electrical stimulation (NMES) let alone traditional therapy can be best treatment option for patients with poststroke dysphagia, however, results are still inconclusive and more studies are requested.

Objective: The aim of the study was to analyze the effect of laryngopharyngeal NMES on dysphagia caused by stroke.

Methods: We recruited 33 patients suffering from stroke and dysphagia in the subacute period. They were divided into NMES plus traditional dysphagia training ($n = 17$) and traditional dysphagia training alone in a time matched condition ($n = 16$). All participants were given treatment 5 days/week for 8 weeks. Assessment was done pre and post 8 weeks. There was single blinding done. Primary outcomes were considered the status of swallowing function in step with the Functional Oral Intake Scale (FOIS), the instrumental Fiberoptic Endoscopic Examination of Swallowing examination, the Penetration Aspiration Scale, and therefore, the pooling score and the presence of oropharyngeal secretion. Secondary outcomes were the kind of diet taken by mouth, the requirement for postural compensations, and also the duration of the dysphagia training.

Results: A functional improvement was observed in both groups but treatment group showed a better improvement for primary outcome with the exception of the pooling score ($p = 0.015$, $p = 0.203$, $p = 0.003$, and $p = 0.048$, respectively) and for secondary outcome $p < 0.005$. The results confirm that laryngopharyngeal NMES in poststroke patients with dysphonia improve outcome of the training.

Conclusion: Laryngopharyngeal NMES could also be considered as an extra and effective treatment option for dysphagia after stroke.

COMMENT

Oropharyngeal dysphagia can be a common problem in patients with subacute stroke, leading to bronchopneumonia and malnutrition. Noninvasive neuromuscular electrical stimulation (NMES) let alone conventional therapy may be best treatment choice for patients with poststroke dysphagia, but findings are still inconclusive and further research are needed. To evaluate the effect of electrical laryngopharyngeal neuromuscular stimulation on stroke-caused dysphagia, the study was planned. During this study, 33 patients suffering from subacute stroke and dysphagia took part. The themes were divided into NMES plus conventional training in dysphagia ($n = 17$) and traditional training in dysphagia alone in an overly time-matched situation ($n = 16$). Both groups were handled for 8 weeks, 5 days a week. Before and after the procedure, all the patients were examined. The study was conceived as a single-randomized controlled blind trial. The status of swallowing activity in accordance with the Functional Oral Intake Scale (FOIS), the instrumental Fiberoptic Endoscopic Swallowing Test, the Penetration Aspiration Scale and therefore the pooling score, and therefore, the occurrence of oropharyngeal secretion were considered primary results. The form of diet taken by mouth, the need for postural compensation, and also the length of dysphagia training were secondary outcomes. A functional change was found in both groups, but with the exception of the pooling score ($p = 0.015$, $p = 0.203$, $p = 0.003$, and $p = 0.048$, respectively) and the secondary outcome $p < 0.005$, the treatment group showed a significant improvement in primary outcome. The findings indicate that laryngopharyngeal NMES enhances the outcome of training in poststroke patients with dysphonia. It may also be considered that laryngopharyngeal NMES is an alternative and successful treatment choice for poststroke dysphagia.

ARTICLE 13

The Effects of Aerobic Exercise on Sleep Quality Measures and Sleep-related Biomarkers in Individuals with Multiple Sclerosis: A Pilot Randomized Controlled Trial

Al-Sharman A, Khalil H, El-Salem K, Aldughmi M, Aburub A. The effects of aerobic exercise on sleep quality measures and sleep-related biomarkers in individuals with multiple sclerosis: A pilot randomised controlled trial.
NeuroRehabilitation. 2019;45(1):107-15.

Abstract

Background: Sleep disturbances square measure extremely prevailing in folks with multiple sclerosis (MS), and square measure associated with pain, fatigue, depression, and reduced quality of life (QoL). Significantly, sleep has been thought of an essential brain state for motor learning and memory consolidation. Therefore, interventions that specialize in sleep management in folks with MS square measure required.

Objectives: To explore the results of a 6 weeks moderate-intensity cardiopulmonary exercise intervention on sleep characteristics and sleep-related biomarkers specifically monoamine neurotransmitter, melatonin, and corticosteroid in folks with MS using a pilot randomized controlled trial.

Methods: Participants were haphazardly allotted to either a moderate-intensity aerobic exercise program (MAE, $n = 20$) or a home exercise program (HEP, $n = 20$). Participants were assessed at baseline and follow-up. Subjective and objective measures were accustomed to assess sleep quality. The metropolis Pittsburgh Sleep Quality Index (PSQI) and sleep disorder Insomnia Severity Index (ISI) were accustomed subjectively to assess sleep whereas actigraphy was accustomed objectively assess sleep. Blood samples were collected for measure of corticosteroid, hormone, and monoamine neurotransmitter from MS participants in each teams at 8:00 AM ± 1 hour.

Results: 17 participants among the MAE and 13 among the informed cluster completed the study. Compared to the informed cluster, folks with MS who participated during a very moderate-intensity exercising knowledgeable vital enhancements ($p < 0.05$) on the PSQI, ISI, different and several other other objective sleep parameters measured exploitation actigraphy. Solely the monoamine neurotransmitter levels exaggerated considerably over the 6-week amount among the MAE cluster compared to the informed cluster. The modification score in monoamine neurotransmitter (from baseline to follow up assessment) was considerably correlated with the modification score in PSQI ($r = -0.97$, $p < 001$) and conjointly the modification score in ISI ($r = -0.56$, $p = 0.015$) solely among the MAE cluster however not the informed cluster.

Conclusion: Exercise might even be a nonpharmacological, cheap, and safe methodology to boost sleep quality in folks with MS. The event among the monoamine neurotransmitter level due to aerobic exercise might make a case for one in each of the physiological mechanisms driving these enhancements.

COMMENT

In individuals with multiple sclerosis (MS), sleep disturbances are highly prevalent and are associated with pain, exhaustion, depression, and decreased quality of life (QoL). Importantly, sleep for motor processing and memory consolidation has been considered a vital brain condition. Therefore, strategies are required that target sleep control in individuals with MS. A pilot randomized controlled trial was designed to investigate the effects of a 6-week moderate-intensity aerobic exercise (MAE) intervention on sleep characteristics and sleep-related biomarkers, specifically serotonin, melatonin, and cortisol, in people with MS.

A moderate-intensity aerobic exercise program (MAE, $n = 20$) or a home exercise program (HEP, $n = 20$) is randomly assigned to the participants. Baseline and follow-up tests were carried out on the participants. To test sleep efficiency, subjective and objective indicators were used. In order to subjectively measure sleep, the Pittsburgh Sleep Quality Index (PSQI) and the Insomnia Severity

Index (ISI) were used. Actigraphy was used to evaluate sleep critically. Blood samples were obtained at 8:00 AM ± 1 hour for cortisol, melatonin, and serotonin tests from MS participants in both classes.

The study was completed by 17 participants in the MAE and 13 in the HEP group. Important changes ($p < 0.05$) in PSQI, ISI, and several objective sleep parameters measured using actigraphy were observed in people with MS who engaged in MAE relative to the HEP population. Compared with the HEP group, serotonin alone increased dramatically over the 6-week period in the MAE group. The serotonin change score (from baseline to follow-up) was significantly associated with the PSQI change score ($r = -0.97, p < 001$) and the ISI change score ($r = -0.56, p = 0.015$) in the MAE group only, but not the HEP group. Exercise may be a healthy, affordable, nonpharmacological tool for improving the quality of sleep in people with MS. The increase in the amount of serotonin due to aerobic exercise may clarify one of the physiological mechanisms driving these improvements.

ARTICLE 14

Task-based Mirror Therapy Enhances the Upper Limb Motor Function in Subacute Stroke Patients: A Randomized Control Trial

Madhoun HY, Tan B, Feng Y, Zhou Y, Zhou C, Yu L. Task-based mirror therapy enhances the upper limb motor function in subacute stroke patients: A randomized control trial.
Eur J Phys Rehabil Med. 2020;56(3):265-71.

Abstract

Background: The advance of the upper limb disability, which is principally caused by stroke, continues to be one in all the rehabilitation treatment challenges. However, the effectiveness of task-based mirror therapy (TBMT) on subacute stroke with moderate and severe upper limb impairment has not been deeply explored.

Objective: To research the consequences of TBMT, compared to physiotherapy, in moderate and severe upper limb impairment by analyzing the motor function and activities of daily living in subacute stroke patients.

Methodology: A randomized controlled trial was conducted, 30 patients with moderate and severe subacute stroke recruited from the second affiliated hospital of Chongqing Medical University are randomly divided into two groups; the TBMT group ($n = 15$) and therefore, the control group ($n = 15$). The primary group received TBMT while the control group only underwent physiotherapy without mirror utilization. Taking into consideration that both groups received conventional therapy. The intervention time was equal for both groups consisting of 25 min/day for 25 days. Fugl-Meyer Assessment (FMA), Brunnstrom Assessment (BRS), modified

Barthel Index (MBI), and Modified Ashworth Scale (MAS) were wont to assess the outcomes for this study.

Results: After 25 sessions of treatment, the patients in both groups have shown improvement within the activities of daily living, motor recovery, and motor function. No significant differences between the two groups were observed on BRS and MBI. However, interestingly, the results of the TBMT group were significantly better than the control group in FMA ($p < 0.05$) and certain aspects of MAS (elbow flexion, wrist flexion, wrist extension, and fingers extension with $p < 0.05$).

Conclusion: This study shows that the mix of conventional rehabilitation treatment and TBMT is an efficient thanks to improve the functional recovery within the upper limb stroke patients.

COMMENT

Mirror therapy (MT) has been used in patients with various disorders, such as phantom limb pain, complex regional pain syndrome, brain paralysis, and stroke patients with acute, subacute, and chronic stroke at different severity stages. It can only be used in conjunction with other modalities, such as electrical stimulation. The primary principle of MT is to provide visual input from the reflection on the mirror of the unaffected limb, which contributes to the development of a visual illusion. The stimulation of the somatosensory cortex, prefrontal cortex, supplementary motor region, cingulate cortex, and superior temporal gyrus is thought to be possible with MT. In addition, MT activates the mirror neuron located in the premotor cortex, inferior frontal gyrus, and inferior parietal lobe, which may boost the motor control of the upper limb in patients with stroke. However, the effectiveness of task-based mirror therapy (TBMT) on subacute stroke with moderate and severe upper limb impairment has not been deeply explored. The study was designed to study the impact of TBMT compared to physiotherapy on moderate and extreme upper limb disability by evaluating motor function and daily living behaviors in patients with subacute stroke. 30 patients with moderate and severe subacute stroke recruited from the second affiliated hospital of Chongqing Medical University were randomly divided into two groups, the TBMT group ($n = 15$) and the control group ($n = 15$). 30 patients with moderate and severe subacute stroke were recruited from the second affiliated hospital of Chongqing Medical University. While the control group only underwent physiotherapy without mirror use the primary group received TBMT. Taking into consideration that both groups received conventional therapy. For both classes, the intervention time was the same, consisting of 25 minutes a day for 25 days. The findings of this analysis were not assessed by the Fugl-Meyer Assessment (FMA), the Brunnstrom Assessment (BRS), the modified Barthel Index (MBI), and the modified Ashworth Scale (MAS). After 25 therapy sessions, patients have demonstrated progress in daily life activities, motor rehabilitation, and motor control in both categories. No major variations in the BRS and MBI between the two groups were found. Interestingly, however, the findings of the TBMT group were slightly stronger than those of the FMA control group ($p < 0.05$) and certain aspects of MAS (elbow bending, wrist bending, wrist extension, and $p < 0.05$ finger extension). This research indicates that the combination of traditional rehabilitation therapy and TBMT is successful in improving the functional recovery of patients with upper limb stroke.

ARTICLE 15

Combined Cognitive-motor Rehabilitation in Virtual Reality Improves Motor Outcomes in Chronic Stroke: A Pilot Study

Faria AL, Cameirão MS, Couras JF, Aguiar JRO, Costa GM, Badia SBI. Combined cognitive-motor rehabilitation in virtual reality improves motor outcomes in chronic stroke – A pilot study.
Front Psychol. 2018;9:854.

Abstract

Background: Stroke is one in all the foremost common causes of acquired disability, leaving numerous adults with cognitive and motor impairments, and affecting patients' capability to measure independently. Virtual reality (VR)-based methods for stroke rehabilitation have mainly focused on motor rehabilitation but there is increasing interest toward the mixing of cognitive training for providing more practical solutions.

Objective: To investigate the feasibility for stroke recovery of a virtual cognitive-motor task, the Reh@Task, which mixes adapted arm reaching, and a focus and memory training.

Methodology: 24 participants within the chronic stage of stroke, with cognitive and motor deficits, were allocated to at least one of two groups (VR, control). Both groups were enrolled in conventional physiatrics, which mostly involves motor training. Additionally, the VR group underwent training with the Reh@Task and therefore the control group performed time-matched conventional physical therapy. Motor and cognitive competences were assessed at baseline, end of treatment (1 month) and at a 1 month follow-up through the Montreal Cognitive Assessment, Single Letter Cancelation, Digit Cancelation, Bells Test, Fugl-Meyer Assessment Test, Chedoke Arm and Hand Activity Inventory, modified Ashworth Scale, and Barthel Index.

Results: Both groups improved in motor function over time, but the Reh@Task group displayed significantly higher between-group outcomes within the arm subpart of the Fugl-Meyer Assessment Test. Improvements in cognitive function were significant and similar in both groups.

Conclusion: These results are supportive of the viability of VR tools that combine motor and cognitive training, like the Reh@Task.

COMMENT

Stroke is one in all the foremost common causes of acquired disability, leaving numerous adults with cognitive and motor impairments, and affecting patients' capability to measure independently. Virtual reality (VR)-based stroke rehabilitation approaches have focused largely on motor rehabilitation, but there is a growing trend in combining cognitive training to provide more realistic solutions. This study is planned to explore the feasibility of a simulated cognitive-motor task for stroke rehabilitation, the Reh@Task, which incorporates adapted arm reach and concentration and memory training.

At least one of the two classes (VR, control) was assigned to 24 participants in the chronic stage of stroke, with cognitive and motor deficits. In traditional physiatrics, which often includes motor exercise, both groups were enrolled. In addition, the VR group underwent training for the Reh@Task and thus undertook traditional physical therapy in a time-matched control group. The Montreal Cognitive Evaluation, Single Letter Cancelation, Digit Cancelation, Bells Test, Fugl-Meyer Assessment Test, Chedoke Arm and Hand Movement Inventory, modified Ashworth Scale, and Barthel Index measured motor and cognitive competencies at baseline, end of therapy (1 month) and 1 month follow-up. Both groups improved motor function over time, but within the arm subpart of the Fugl-Meyer Evaluation Test, the Reh@Task group showed significantly higher between-group performance. In both classes, changes in cognitive performance were substantial and identical. These findings support the viability of VR instruments that, like the Reh@Task, combine motor and cognitive training.

ARTICLE 16

Effects of Fluoxetine on Functional Outcomes after Acute Stroke (FOCUS): A Pragmatic, Double-blind, Randomized, Controlled Trial

FOCUS Trial Collaboration. Effects of fluoxetine on functional outcomes after acute stroke (FOCUS): A pragmatic, double-blind, randomised, controlled trial.
Lancet. 2019;393(10168):265-74.

Abstract

Background: Results of tiny trials indicate that selective-serotonin reuptake inhibitor would possibly improve purposeful outcomes when stroke. The most target trial aimed to provide a certain estimate of these effects.

Methodology: FOCUS (Fluoxetine Or Control Under Supervision) was a sensible, multicenter, parallel cluster, double-blind, randomized, placebo-controlled trial done at 103 hospitals at intervals in the United Kingdom. Patients were eligible if they were aged 18 years or older, had a clinical stroke identification, were listed and haphazardly assigned between 2 and 15 days when onset, and had focal medicine deficits. Patients were haphazardly allotted selective-serotonin reuptake inhibitor 20 mg or matching placebo orally once daily for 6 months via a web-based system by use of a minimization algorithmic rule. The primary outcome was purposeful standing, measured with the modified Rankin Scale (mRS), at 6 months. Patients, carers, healthcare workers, and conjointly the trial team were covert to treatment allocation. Purposeful standing was assessed at 6 and 12 months. Patients were analyzed to keep with their treatment allocation. This trial is registered with the International Standard Randomised Controlled Trial Number (ISRCTN) written record, range ISRCTN83290762.

Results: Between September 10, 2012 and March 31, 2017, 3,127 patients were recruited. 1,564 patients were allotted selective-serotonin reuptake inhibitor and 1,563 allotted placebo. mRS knowledge at 6 months were accessible for 1,553 (99.3%) patients in every treatment cluster. The distribution across mRS classes at 6 months was similar at intervals the selective-serotonin reuptake inhibitor and placebo teams {common odds magnitude relation adjusted for minimization variable 0.951 [95% confidence interval (CI) 0.839–1.079]; $p = 0.439$}. Patients allotted selective-serotonin reuptake inhibitor were less possible than those allotted placebo to develop new depression by 6 months [210 (13.43%) patients vs. 269 (17.21%), distinction 3.78% (95% CI 1.26–6.30); $p = 0.0033$], however, they had additional bone fractures [45 (2.88%) vs. 23 (1.47%), distinction 1.41% (95% CI 0.38–2.43); $p = 0.0070$]. There are no important variations within the alternative event at 6 or 12 months.

Conclusion: Selective-serotonin reuptake inhibitor 20 mg given daily for 6 months when acute stroke does not appear to spice up purposeful outcomes. Though the treatment reduced the incidence of depression, it increased the frequency of bone fractures. These results do not support the routine the results of the FOCUS trial show that fluoxetine 20 mg given daily for 6 months after an acute stroke did not influence patients' functional outcomes but did decrease the occurrence of depression and increase the occurrence of bone fractures.

COMMENT

Fluoxetine was suggested in the FLAME analysis when given to patients with a recent ischemic disorder. A motor deficit, a stroke, and a median National Institute of Health Stroke Scale (NIHSS) 13, enhanced motor recovery function as calculated by the motor score of Fugl-Meyer at about for 3 months. In a post hoc analysis released, the proportion of patients in everyday life who were independent [modified Rankin Scale (mRS) 0–2] were in the fluoxetine group, considerably higher than in the placebo group, (26% vs. 9%, $p = 0.015$) party. Nonetheless, an ordinary study of the mRS data did not indicate a substantial difference between groups.

The FOCUS (Fluoxetine Or Control Under Supervision) trial was designed to assess whether, relative to placebo, patients with a clinical stroke diagnosis would have better functional results with a 6-month course of fluoxetine. Identifying any other advantages or harms and determining whether any benefits existed from the end of the treatment period to 12 months after stroke were significant secondary objectives. In 103 hospitals in the UK, FOCUS was a practical, multicenter, parallel group, double-blind, randomized placebo-controlled experiment. Patients were eligible if they were 18 years of age or older, had a history of clinical stroke, were registered and randomly assigned and had focal neurological defects between 2 and 15 days after onset. Patients were randomly assigned fluoxetine 20 mg or placebo-matched orally once daily for 6 months using a minimization algorithm using a web-based system. The first result was functional status, assessed at 6 months using the mRS. For treatment allocation, patients, caregivers, healthcare workers, and even the trial team were masked. 6 and 12 months after randomization, functional status was evaluated. In line with their care allowance, patients were examined. This trial has been registered with the International Standard Randomised Controlled Trial Number (ISRCTN) registry under the number ISRCTN832907622. 3,127 patients were recruited between September 10, 2012 and March 31, 2017. Fluoxetine was assigned to 1,564 patients and placebo was allocated to 1,563. For 1,553 (99.3%) patients in each treatment category, mRS data at 6 months was available. Within the fluoxetine and placebo classes, the distribution across mRS categories at 6 months was identical {common odds ratio adjusted for minimization variables 0.951 [95% confidence interval (CI) 0.839–1.079]; $p = 0.439$}. Fluoxetine allocated patients were less likely to experience new depression by 6 months than placebo allocated patients [210 (13.43%) vs. 269 (17.21%), 3.78% difference (95% CI 1.26–6.30); $p = 0.0033$], but they had more bone fractures [45 (2.88%) vs. 23 (1.47%), 1.41% difference (95% CI 0.38–2.43); $p = 0.0070$]. At 6 or 12 months, there were no major variations in the other cases. Fluoxetine 20 mg, administered daily for 6 months following an acute stroke, does not seem to improve functional performance. Although the treatment reduced the occurrence of depression, it increased the frequency of bone fractures. These findings do not support the regular use of fluoxetine, either to avoid post-stroke depression or to facilitate functional recovery.

Section 14: Neurogenetics

Section Editor: Sunil Narayan

Associate Editor: KP Vinayan

NOVEL THERAPIES

ARTICLE 1

Onasemnogene Abeparvovec Gene Therapy for Symptomatic Infantile-onset Spinal Muscular Atrophy in Patients with Two Copies of SMN2 (STR1VE): An Open-label, Single-arm, Multicentre, Phase 3 Trial

Day JW, Finkel RS, Chiriboga CA, Connolly AM, Crawford TO, Darras BT, et al. Onasemnogene abeparvovec gene therapy for symptomatic infantile-onset spinal muscular atrophy in patients with two copies of SMN2 (STR1VE): An open-label, single-arm, multicentre, phase 3 trial.
Lancet Neurol. 2021;20(4):284-93.

Abstract

Background: A motor neuron condition called spinal muscular atrophy type 1 causes death or the requirement for ongoing ventilation by the age of 2 years. Our goal was to assess the safety and effectiveness of onasemnogene abeparvovec (formerly known as AVXS-101), a gene therapy that delivers the survival motor neuron (*SMN*) gene, in symptomatic patients with infantile-onset spinal muscular atrophy who were identified through clinical evaluation.

Methods: STR1VE was a phase 3 open-label, single-arm, single-dose trial conducted at 12 hospitals and universities across the United States. Patients with spinal muscular atrophy who have biallelic SMN1 mutations (deletion or point mutations) and one or two copies of SMN2 were eligible. For 30–60 minutes, patients were given an intravenous infusion of onasemnogene abeparvovec (1.1×10^{14} vector genomes per kg). Patients were assessed once per week beginning on day 7 postinfusion for 4 weeks and then once per month until the end of the study during the outpatient follow-up (age 18 months or early termination). At the 18-month trial visit, independent sitting for 30 seconds or more (Bayley-III item 26) and survival (lack of death or permanent ventilation at age 14 months) were coprimary efficacy outcomes. Through the analysis of adverse events, concurrent medication use, physical examinations, vital sign assessments, cardiac assessments, and laboratory evaluations, safety was determined. From the Pediatric Neuromuscular Clinical Research (PNCR) dataset, primary effectiveness endpoints for the intention-to-treat population were compared with untreated children aged 6 months or younger ($n = 23$) with spinal muscular atrophy type 1 (biallelic deletion of SMN1 and two copies of SMN2).

Findings: A total of 22 individuals with spinal muscular atrophy type 1 who were eligible between October 24, 2017 and November 12, 2019, were given onasemnogene abeparvovec. At the 18-month study visit, 13 [59%; 97.5% confidence interval (CI) 36–100] of 22 patients were able to sit independently for at least 30 seconds (compared to 0 of 23 patients in the PNCR cohort who were not receiving treatment; $p < 0.0001$). Compared to the untreated PNCR cohort [6 (26%), 8–44; $p < 0.0001$, 20 patients (91%, 79–100)] survived without the need for permanent ventilation at age 14 months. Onasemnogene abeparvovec had at least one side effect in every patient (most common was pyrexia). Bronchitis, pneumonia, respiratory distress, and respiratory syncytial virus bronchiolitis were the most frequently reported major adverse effects. Three significant side effects were connected to the therapy or may have been connected (two patients had elevated hepatic aminotransferases, and one had hydrocephalus).

Interpretation: Results from this multicenter trial demonstrate the safety and effectiveness of commercial grade onasemnogene abeparvovec, building on those from the phase 1 START research. When compared to findings from the PNCR natural history cohort, onasemnogene abeparvovec demonstrated statistical superiority and clinically significant responses. Onasemnogene abeparvovec may be used to treat symptomatic children with genetic or clinical traits suggestive of infantile-onset spinal muscular atrophy type 1 because of the favorable benefit–risk profile demonstrated in this trial.

COMMENT

Spinal muscular atrophy type 1 is a motor neuron disorder resulting in death or the need for permanent ventilation by age 2 years. Onasemnogene abeparvovec is a single intravenous infusion of a recombinant adeno-associated virus serotype 9 vector-based gene therapy designed to deliver a full-length functional copy of the human survival motor neuron (*SMN*) gene via a self-complementary adeno-associated virus serotype 9 vector that crosses the blood–brain barrier. Results from the STRIVE study (built on the background of the phase 1 START study), a phase 3 multicenter trial study, showed safety, superiority, and clinically meaningful responses onasemnogene abeparvovec, in symptomatic patients with infantile-onset spinal muscular atrophy when compared with a natural history cohort of type 1 spinal muscular atrophy.

ARTICLE 2

Safety and Efficacy of Omaveloxolone in Friedreich Ataxia (MOXIe Study)

Lynch DR, Chin MP, Delatycki MB, Subramony SH, Corti M, Hoyle JC, et al. Safety and efficacy of omaveloxolone in Friedreich ataxia (MOXIe Study).
Ann Neurol. 2021;89(2):212-25.

Abstract

Objective: There is no known cure for the inherited neurodegenerative condition Friedreich ataxia (FA), which progresses over time. In FA model, omaveloxolone, a Nrf2 activator, enhances mitochondrial activity, returns the redox equilibrium, and lowers inflammation. In patients with FA, we looked into the efficacy and safety of omaveloxolone.

Methods: At 11 institutions in the US, Europe, and Australia, we carried out a global, double-blind, randomized, placebo-controlled, parallel-group, registrational phase 2 trial (NCT02255435, EudraCT2015-002762-23). Patients who met the criteria—those 16–40 years old with genetic confirmation of FA and baseline modified Friedrich's ataxia rating scale (mFARS) scores between 20 and 80 were randomized 1:1 to receive a placebo or 150 mg of omaveloxolone daily. The mFARS score change from baseline in those receiving omaveloxolone versus those receiving a placebo at 48 weeks was the primary outcome.

Result: The whole analysis set included 40 patients who received omaveloxolone and 42 patients who received a placebo. Out of the 135 individuals who underwent screening, 103 were randomly assigned to receive either the drug ($n = 51$) or a placebo ($n = 52$). Omaveloxolone (-1.55 ± 0.69) and placebo (0.85 ± 0.64) individuals' changes from baseline in mFARS scores revealed a difference between treatment groups of -2.40 ± 0.96 ($p = 0.014$). Omaveloxolone caused brief, transitory elevations in aminotransferase levels but no changes in total bilirubin or other symptoms of liver damage. Patients taking omaveloxolone also experienced greater headaches, nausea, and weariness.

Interpretation: Omaveloxolone dramatically enhanced neurological performance in the MOXIe substitute experiment with 'Trial' as compared to placebo, and it was typically well-tolerated and safe. It stands for a possible treatment for FA.

COMMENT

Friedreich ataxia (FA) is a progressive genetic neurodegenerative disorder with no approved treatment. Omaveloxolone, is an Nrf2 activator which improves mitochondrial function, restores redox balance, and reduces inflammation in models of FA. FA is caused by a biallelic trinucleotide (GAA) repeat expansion in the first intron of the *FXN* gene, which impairs transcription and significantly reduces the amount of functional frataxin protein. The pathological consequences of frataxin deficiency include disruption of iron–sulfur cluster biosynthesis, cellular iron dysregulation, mitochondrial dysfunction, and increased sensitivity to oxidative stress in vitro, leading to the clinical features of FA. The MOXIE part 2 trial, an international, double-blind, randomized, placebo-controlled trial of Omaveloxolone conducted in US, Europe, and Australia with 40 FA and 42 control subjects, showed that the primary outcome mFARS (modified Friedrich's ataxia rating scale) improved in each component (bulbar, upper limb coordination, lower limb coordination, and upright stability) relative to placebo, with the greatest effects documented on the upright stability. The main outcome measure was mFARS after 48 weeks. The severe adverse events (SAEs) were mainly limited to rise in liver enzymes. This is one of the most promising first-ever successful trials in inherited ataxia and is therefore of great significance.

ARTICLE 3

Hematopoietic Stem- and Progenitor-cell Gene Therapy for Hurler Syndrome

Gentner B, Tucci F, Galimberti S, Fumagalli F, De Pellegrin M, Silvani P, et al.; MPSI Study Group. Hematopoietic stem- and progenitor-cell gene therapy for Hurler syndrome.
N Engl J Med. 2021;385(21):1929-40.

Abstract

Background: The recommended treatment for Hurler syndrome is allogeneic hematopoietic stem-cell transplantation [mucopolysaccharidosis type I, Hurler variant (MPSIH)]. The downside of this therapy is that it has side effects and is only partially curative.

Methods: We have eight MPSIH children who are participating in an ongoing study. The kids had developmental quotient or intelligence quotient scores above 70 and were enrolled despite not having a suitable allogeneic donor (i.e., none had moderate or severe cognitive impairment). Following myeloablative conditioning, the kids were given autologous hematopoietic stem and progenitor cells (HSPCs) that had been ex vivo transduced with a lentiviral vector encoding α-L-iduronidase (IDUA). The main end goals were security and correction of blood IDUA activity up to supraphysiologic levels. Development of the skeleton and the nervous system were evaluated as secondary and exploratory end points, together with the clearance of lysosomal storage material. The study is expected to last 5 years.

Result: We now present preliminary findings. At the time of *HSPC* gene therapy, the children's mean [± standard deviation (SD)] age was 1.9 ± 0.5 years. The treatment exhibited a safety profile that was comparable to autologous hematopoietic stem-cell transplantation at a median follow-up of 2.10 years. Within a month, all of the patients displayed supraphysiologic blood IDUA activity, which they had all maintained up until the most recent follow-up. They also all demonstrated prompt and persistent engraftment of gene-corrected cells. In four of the five patients who could be assessed, urinary glycosaminoglycan (GAG) excretion reduced sharply and returned to normal levels after a year. After gene therapy, previously undetectable levels of IDUA activity in the cerebrospinal fluid (CSF) were detectable and were linked to local GAGs clearance. Patients displayed stable cognitive function, stable motor abilities consistent with ongoing motor development, better or stable findings on brain and spine magnetic resonance imaging, decreased joint stiffness, and normal growth according with World Health Organization growth charts.

Conclusion: When *HSPC* gene therapy was administered to MPSIH patients, the peripheral tissues and the central nervous system underwent considerable metabolic correction.

COMMENT

The delivery of hematopoietic stem- and progenitor-cell-based (*HSPC*) gene therapy in patients with mucopolysaccharidosis (MPS)-type 1, Hurler's disease is expected to induce extensive metabolic correction in peripheral tissues and the central nervous system. Investigators from planned a 5-year follow-up study on eight children with Hurler's disease of mean age of 2 years, with autologous HSPCs transduced ex vivo with an α-L-iduronidase (IDUA)-encoding lentiviral vector. On an interim analysis after 2 years, they found that the safety profile was excellent and the children had achieved stable cognitive performance, motor skills, continued motor development, improved or stable magnetic resonance imaging of the brain and spine as well as reduced joint stiffness, and normal growth. They had prompt and sustained engraftment of gene-corrected cells and had supraphysiologic blood IDUA activity within a month, which was maintained. This is yet another remarkable success story in the therapy of inborn errors of metabolism. 5-year follow-up results are awaited. This trial was funded by an Italian biomedical charity group.

ARTICLE 4

Treatment of Infantile-onset Spinal Muscular Atrophy with Nusinersen: Final Report of a Phase 2, Open-label, Multicentre, Dose-escalation Study

Finkel RS, Chiriboga CA, Vajsar J, Day JW, Montes J, De Vivo DC, et al. Treatment of infantile-onset spinal muscular atrophy with nusinersen: Final report of a phase 2, open-label, multicentre, dose-escalation study.
Lancet Child Adolesc Health. 2021;5(7):491-500.

Abstract

Background: At the interim analysis of a phase-2 clinical study, participants with infantile-onset spinal muscular atrophy (SMA) demonstrated nusinersen to have a favorable benefit–risk profile. We now provide the study's final analysis, which evaluates the 3-year effectiveness and safety of nusinersen.

Methods: In three university hospital sites in the United States and one in Canada, this phase-2 open-label, multicenter, dose-escalation trial was conducted. Infants with infantile-onset SMA with two or three copies of the *SMN2* gene between the ages of 3 weeks and 6 months were eligible for inclusion. Participants who met the criteria were given several intrathecal loading doses of nusinersen corresponding to 6 mg (for cohort 1) or 12 mg (for cohort 2), followed by maintenance doses of nusinersen equivalent to 12 mg. The Hammersmith Infant Neurological Examination section 2 (HINE-2) was used to measure reaching motor milestones at the last study visit in all participants who successfully completed the loading dose period and day 92 assessment. The protocol was amended on January 25, 2016, changing the primary efficacy endpoint from safety and tolerability to reaching motor milestones. On February 10, 2016, the statistical analysis plan was changed to include further studies of the participant subgroup with two SMN2 copies. All individuals who received at least one dosage of study therapy were evaluated for adverse events.

Findings: 20 symptomatic infantile-onset SMA participants [12 boys and 8 girls; median age at diagnosis 78 days (range 0–154)] were enrolled between May 3, 2013 and July 9, 2014. The median length of time spent studying was 36.2 months [interquartile range (IQR) 20.6–41.3]. Twelve (63%) of the 19 evaluable individuals met the primary goal of an incremental improvement in HINE-2 developmental motor milestones. The HINE-2 motor milestone total score steadily climbed in the 13 participants with two SMN2 copies treated with 12 mg nusinersen from a baseline mean of 1.46 [standard deviation (SD) 0.52] to 11.86 (6.18) at day 1,135, showing a clinically significant rise of 10.43 (6.05). At the end of the study (August 21, 2017), 15 (75%) of the 20 participants were still alive. In 16 (80%) of the 20 participants, 101 serious adverse events were reported; all five deaths (one in cohort 1 and four in cohort 2) were most likely related to the progression of SMA disease.

Interpretation: Our results are in line with those of other nusinersen studies, and they demonstrate better survival and achievement of motor milestones over the course of 3 years in patients with infantile-onset SMA. They also demonstrate a favorable safety profile.

COMMENT

In a phase-2 open-label, multicentric dose-escalation study of 20 infants of 3–6 months of age, with spinal muscular atrophy (SMA), with two or three copies of *SMN1* gene, were treated with intrathecal nusinersen 8 and 12 mg at the end of 3 years of follow-up, the motor outcome measured by Hammersmith Infant Neurological Examination section 2 (HINE-2) scores. At 3-year follow-up point, primary endpoint of an incremental improvement in HINE-2 developmental motor milestones was reached by 12 of 19 evaluable participants. In the 13 participants with two SMN2 copies treated with 12 mg nusinersen, the HINE-2 motor milestone total score increased steadily from a baseline mean of 1.5–11.9 at day 1,135, representing a clinically significant change. 75% of 20 participants were alive. Five deaths that occurred were likely to be related to SMA disease progression. The study was funded by the industry.

ARTICLE 5

A Major Successful Early Step towards Effective Vaccination for Arresting Progression of IDH1 Grade III Glioma – Phase I Human Trial

Platten M, Bunse L, Wick A, Bunse T, Le Cornet L, Harting I, et al. A vaccine targeting mutant IDH1 in newly diagnosed glioma.
Nature. 2021;592(7854):463-8.

Abstract

Mutated isocitrate dehydrogenase 1 (IDH1) is defined as molecularly different subtype of diffuse glioma (1–3). In gliomas, the most common IDH1 mutation has an effect on codon 132; it also encodes IDH1(R132H) that has shared clonal neoepitopes, which presents on major histocompatibility complex (MHC) class II (4,5). Particular therapeutic T-helper cell responses are induced by an IDH1(R132H)-specific peptide vaccine (IDH1-vac). These responses are found to be effective against IDH1(R132H)(+) tumors among syngeneic MHC-humanized mice (4,6–8). This multicenter, single-arm, open-label, first-in-humans phase I trial included 33 patients who had newly diagnosed World Health Organization grade 3 and 4 IDH1(R132H)(+) astrocytomas [Neuro-Oncology Working Group of the German Cancer Society trial 16 (NOA16), ClinicalTrials.gov identifier NCT02454634]. The primary safety endpoint of this trial was achieved with adverse events related to vaccine restricted to grade 1. The majority of patients (93.3%) had vaccine-induced immune responses across multiple MHC alleles. 3-year progression-free rate was 0.63 and death-free rates were 0.84. Among patients having immune responses, there was 2-year progression-free rate of 0.82. In two patients without an immune response, there was tumor progression within 2 years of first diagnosis. An association was found between mutation-specificity score [including duration and level of vaccine-induced IDH1(R132H)-specific T-cell responses] and intratumoral presentation of the IDH1(R132H) neoantigen in pretreatment tumor tissue. Increased frequency of pseudoprogression was found, indicating intratumoral inflammatory reactions. There was an association between pseudoprogression and enhanced vaccine-induced peripheral T-cell responses. Among patient with pseudoprogression, combined single-cell RNA and T-cell receptor sequencing demonstrated that tumor-infiltrating CD40LG(+) and CXCL13(+) T helper cell clusters were dominated by a single IDH1(R132H)-reactive T-cell receptor.

COMMENT

In this NIH clinical trials registered phase 1 trial, an important breakthrough in the treatment of grade III and IV malignant gliomas was found using clonal neoepitope-specific peptide vaccine with an immune response dependent 3-year progression-free rate of 0.63 and death-free rate of 0.84 and side effects restricted to grade 1 tumor. A early but major step towards the development of an effective vaccine for arresting the progression of a type of grade III glioma.

ARTICLE 6

Safety and Sustained 6 Years Effects of Treatment for Adult SMA Therapy – Phase I Trial

Mendell JR, Al-Zaidy SA, Lehman KJ, McColly M, Lowes LP, Alfano LN, et al. Five-year extension results of the phase 1 START trial of onasemnogene abeparvovec in spinal muscular atrophy.
JAMA Neurol. 2021;78(7):834-41.

Abstract

Importance: This ongoing study assesses long-term safety and durability of response in infants with spinal muscular atrophy (SMA) type 1 after dosing with onasemnogene abeparvovec gene replacement therapy.

Objective: The primary objective of this ongoing study is to assess safety. The secondary objective is to determine whether developmental milestones achieved in the START phase 1 clinical trial were maintained and new milestones gained.

Design, Setting, and Participants: This study is an ongoing, observational, follow-up study for continuous safety monitoring for 15 years in patients from the START phase I study (conducted May 5, 2014, through December 15, 2017) at Nationwide Children's Hospital in Columbus, Ohio. Participants were symptomatic infants with SMA type 1 and 2 copies of SMN2 previously treated with an intravenous dose of onasemnogene abeparvovec (low dose, $6.7 \times 1,013$ vg/kg; or therapeutic dose, $1.1 \times 1,014$ vg/kg) in START. Thirteen of 15 original START patients are included in this analysis; 2 patients' families declined follow-up participation. Data were analyzed from September 21, 2017 to June 11, 2020.

Exposures: Median time since dosing of 5.2 (range, 4.6–6.2) years; 5.9 (range, 5.8–6.2) years in the low-dose cohort and 4.8 (range, 4.6–5.6) years in the therapeutic-dose cohort.

Main Outcomes and Measures: The primary outcome measure was the incidence of serious adverse events (SAEs).

Results: At data cutoff on June 11, 2020, 13 patients treated in START were enrolled in this study [median age, 38.9 (range, 25.4–48.0) months; 7 females; low-dose cohort, $n = 3$; and therapeutic-dose cohort, $n = 10$]. Serious adverse events occurred in 8 patients (62%), none of which resulted in study discontinuation or death. The most frequently reported SAEs were acute respiratory failure [$n = 4$ (31%)], pneumonia [$n = 4$ (31%)], dehydration [$n = 3$ (23%)], respiratory distress [$n = 2$ (15%)], and bronchiolitis [$n = 2$ (15%)]. All 10 patients in the therapeutic-dose cohort remained alive and without the need for permanent ventilation. Prior to baseline, 4 patients (40%) in the therapeutic-dose cohort required noninvasive ventilatory support, and 6 patients (60%) did not require regular ventilatory support, which did not change in long-term follow-up. All 10 patients treated with the therapeutic dose maintained previously acquired motor milestones. Two patients attained the new milestone of "standing with assistance" without the use of nusinersen.

Conclusions and Relevance: The findings of this ongoing clinical follow-up of patients with SMA type 1 treated with onasemnogene abeparvovec supports the long-term favorable safety profile up to 6 years of age and provides evidence for sustained clinical durability of the therapeutic dose.

COMMENT

In the longest available follow-up study monitoring the safety and durability of response to therapy for a period of 15 years on onasemnogene abeparvovec gene replacement therapy in terms of long-term safety as well as durability of response among the 13 symptomatic spinal muscular atrophy (SMA) type 1 patients who took part in START phase 1 clinical trial. Only eight patients had serious adverse events, mainly related to respiratory difficulties, but no discontinuation or death were reported. All but three maintained previous milestones and two achieved a new milestone of standing with assistance. This is a remarkable milestone in clinical care and in therapeutic bioscience.

ARTICLE 7

Long-term (1 Year) Safety and Efficacy of High-dose Pyridoxine in IGD Deficiency Epilepsy

Tanigawa J, Nabatame S, Tominaga K, Nishimura Y, Maegaki Y, Kinosita T, et al. High-dose pyridoxine treatment for inherited glycosylphosphatidylinositol deficiency.
Brain Dev. 2021;43(6):680-7.

Abstract

Objective: The aim of this study was to evaluate the efficacy as well as safety of high-dose pyridoxine treatment among patients with seizures. This study also aimed to assess its effects on development among individuals having inherited glycosylphosphatidylinositol deficiencies (IGDs).

Material and Methods: The design of the present study was prospective open-label multicenter pilot study, where study population included individuals who were diagnosed with IGDs through genetic tests and flow cytometry. The treatment given to patients included oral pyridoxine at the dose of 20–30 mg/kg/day for duration of 1 year, along with previous treatment.

Result: The mean age of the enrolled patients ($n = 9$) was 66.3 ± 44.3 months. There was significant reduction in levels of CD16, which is a glycosylphosphatidylinositol-anchored protein, present on blood granulocytes. Among the underlying genetic etiology of IGDs included gene mutations like *PIGO* to be present in two patients, *PIGL* in two patients, and unknown in five patients. Seizures were present in six patients, and developmental delay in all patients. The mean developmental age was 11.1 ± 8.1 months. In patients with seizures, there was marked reduction in frequency of seizures (>50%) in three patients and drastic decrease (>90%) in one patient. Exacerbation of seizures was not seen in study period. There was modest improvement in development in eight out of nine patients ($p = 0.14$). None of the patients had adverse events, with exceptions being mild transient diarrhea in one patient.

Conclusion: High-dose pyridoxine daily treatment for duration of 1 year was found to be effective in treating seizures among >50% of the patients having IGDs, which resulted in modest improvement in development in most of the patients. Treatment was found to be quite safe. The results of this study suggest high-dose pyridoxine treatment to be effective in treatment of seizures among those with IGDs. However, more studies should be conducted for confirming the findings.

COMMENT

High-dose pyridoxine daily treatment for duration of 1 year was found to be effective in treating seizures among >50% of the patients having inherited glycosylphosphatidylinositol deficiencies (IGDs), which resulted in modest improvement in development in most of the patients. Treatment was found to be quite safe. The results of this study suggest high-dose pyridoxine treatment to be effective in treatment of seizures among those with IGDs. However, more studies should be conducted for confirming the findings.

ARTICLE 8

Oral Prednisolone up to 1 mg/kg Orally Improved the Functional Status of Children with Congenital Fukuyama Myopathy (as for DMD)

Murakami T, Sato T, Adachi M, Ishiguro K, Shichiji M, Tachimori H, et al. Efficacy of steroid therapy for Fukuyama congenital muscular dystrophy.
Sci Rep. 2021;11(1):24229.

Abstract

Despite the fact that only symptomatic treatment exists for Fukuyama congenital muscular dystrophy (FCMD), multiple reports recommended that steroid therapy may be effective. But, there is lack of independent intervention studies. The aim of the present study was to assess the efficacy of steroid therapy in restoration of motor functions among those with FCMD. The study population included FCMD patients (3–10 years) with reduction in motor functions, and required steroid therapy. Patients who gave their consent received 0.5 mg/kg prednisolone every other day, which was increased to 1.0 mg/kg when there was inadequate response. The Gross Motor Function Measure (GMFM) was used for assessing and comparing the motor functions of all patients. For statistical analysis, the Wilcoxon signed-rank test, with significance level being $p \leq 0.05$. The mean age of FCMD patients at initiation of steroid therapy was 8.10 years [standard deviation (SD) 2.14 years]. The mean GMFM difference between before and after the steroid therapy was found to be +1.23 (SD, 1.10); there was significant improvement in GMFM ($p = 0.015$). The findings of this study suggested that steroid therapy may help patients with advanced-stage FCMD maintain and improve their motor functions.

COMMENT

Prednisolone and deflazacort have established effects on the treatment of XR muscular dystrophies such as Duchenne and Becker muscular dystrophy. Fukuyama congenital muscular dystrophy, is due to a mutation of gene named Fukutin inducing abnormalities in the sugar chain of α-dystroglycan (α-DG) reducing its binding to laminin within the basal membrane, resulting in the weakening of myocyte membranes and necrosis/denaturation of muscle cells. Prednisolone was also found to be effective. In a pilot study from the Tokyo National Center of Neurology on nine children including boys and girls with Fukuyama congenital muscular dystrophy, the second common muscular dystrophy in Japan. The dosage of steroids was 0.5–1 mg/kg, the average duration of follow-up 9 months and the outcome parameters assessed was gross motor function measure (GMFM).

ARTICLE 9

In Parkinson's Disease, Yearlong Administration of Sargramostim 3 µg/kg, Stopped UPDRS Progression, Decreased Numbers and Severity of Adverse Events and Restored Peripheral Immune Function Correlating with Increased Numbers and Function of Treg: Phase 1b Study

Olson KE, Namminga KL, Lu Y, Schwab AD, Thurston MJ, Abdelmoaty MM, et al. Safety, tolerability, and immune-biomarker profiling for year-long sargramostim treatment of Parkinson's disease.
EBioMedicine. 2021;67:103380.

Abstract

Background: There is pathogenic role of neuroinflammation in Parkinson's disease (PD). Immunotherapies that restore brain homeostasis can help to slow neurodegeneration by changing T-cell phenotypes. Sargramostim has received a lot of attention in form of immune transformer in laboratory bench to bedside clinical trials. However, its therapeutic application has been hampered by dose-dependent adverse events (AEs). Thus, this study used a lower drug dose regimen for 1 year for evaluating safety and discovering novel disease-linked biomarkers during 5 days/week sargramostim treatments.

Methods: For evaluating safety as well as tolerability of 3 µg/kg/day sargramostim, five patients with PD were included in a phase 1b, unblinded, open-label study. The investigations included complete blood counts and chemistry profiles. Physical examination was done, and information related to AEs, Movement Disorder Society-sponsored revision of the Unified Parkinson's Disease Rating Scale (MDS-UPDRS) scores, immune profiling, DNA methylation, T-cell phenotypes/function, and gene and protein patterns was collected.

Result: On administering Sargramostim (3 µg/kg/day), there was significant reduction in number as well as severity of AEs/subject/month in comparison to 6 µg/kg/day treatment. The reductions in MDS-UPDRS part III score was found. There was an increase in peripheral blood immunoregulatory phenotypes as well as function. An increase in hypomethylation of upstream FOXP3 DNA elements was seen.

Conclusion: Treatment with sargramostim at dose of 3 µg/kg/day for long term is well-tolerated as well as effective in restoration of immune homeostasis. AEs were less in numbers as well as severity. The restored peripheral immune function coordinated with increase in number and function of Treg. number worsening of MDS-UPDRS part III scores was seen. Large sample size studies should be conducted for evaluating the conclusive drug efficacy.

COMMENT

Sargramostim, a yeast-derived granulocyte-macrophage colony-stimulating factor (GM-CSF), is a molecularly cloned, pleiotropic cytokine which supports proliferation, differentiation, maturation, and survival of cells. In Alzheimer's disease, Sargramostim treatment had altered innate immune system markers, with no drug-related serious adverse events or worsening of amyloid-related imaging abnormalities and improvement in cognitive parameters. In this phase 1b study in Parkinson's disease, yearlong administration of Sargramostim stopped Unified Parkinson's Disease Rating Scale (UPDRS) progression, decreased numbers and severity of adverse events, and restored peripheral immune function markers.

ARTICLE 10

Long 5.5-year Follow-up of Adeno-associated Vector-mediated Intracerebral Gene Therapy Encoding Human α-N-acetylglucosaminidase (rAAV2/5-hNAGLU) plus Immunotherapy in Sanfilippo B was Safe and Showed Sustained Enzyme Production

Deiva K, Ausseil J, de Bournonville S, Zérah M, Husson B, Gougeon ML, et al. Intracerebral Gene Therapy in Four Children with Sanfilippo B Syndrome: 5.5-Year Follow-Up Results.
Hum Gene Ther. 2021;32(19-20):1251-9.

Abstract

This study aimed to report the safety, which was the primary endpoint of the study, along with efficacy (which was secondary endpoint) of a new intracerebral gene therapy at follow-up of 5.5 years among children having Sanfilippo B. This was an uncontrolled, phase 1/2 clinical trial that included in four patients of age 20, 26, 30, and 53 months, respectively. The treatment given to the patients comprised of 16 intracerebral and cerebellar deposits of a recombinant adeno-associated viral vector encoding human α-N-acetylglucosaminidase (rAAV2/5-hNAGLU) plus immunosuppression. An intermediate 30-month report had previously been published. There were 30 adverse events caused by treatment between 30 and 66 months following surgery, which included three categorized as severe with no serious drug reactions. NAGLU activity was consistently detected in the lumbar cerebrospinal fluid (18% of unaffected control level) at 5.5 years. There was presence of circulating T-cells reacting against NAGLU peptides, which indicated absence of acquired tolerance. Progressive brain atrophy and neurocognitive evolution were present in patients 2, 3, and 4 that was similar to those of untreated Sanfilippo A/B children.

As compared to three other patients and untreated patients, patient 1 (who was enrolled at 20 months of age) had milder disease with normal findings on brain imaging and significantly better cognitive outcomes, however, it was not similar to normal children. The study achieved primary endpoint of the study after 5.5 years was achieved, along with good safety profile of the proposed treatment. There was sustained production of enzyme in the brain and lack of immunological tolerance. Among three oldest patients, confirmation of cognitive benefit was not done. The presence of mild disease in the youngest patient promotes more investigations of adeno-associated vector-mediated intracerebral gene therapy in Sanfilippo B.

COMMENT

5.5 years long follow-up of Sanfilippo disease treatment with adeno-associated vector-mediated intracerebral gene therapy which encoded human α-N-acetylglucosaminidase, along with immunotherapy showed that the regimen was safe and led to sustained enzyme production in children with this mucopolysaccharidosis (MPS). In one young child enrolled at 20 months of age, the disease was milder with normal brain imaging and significantly better cognitive outcomes, rising hopes of effectiveness of the gene therapy.

ARTICLE 11

European Pompe Consortium: In Classic Infantile Pompe Disease, High ERT Dosage of 40 mg/kg/week (Alglucosidase α had Significantly Improved Survival when Compared with Patients Treated with the Standard Recommended ERT Dosage of 20 mg/kg Every Other Week. Recommend Dosage Reconsideration

Ditters IAM, Huidekoper HH, Kruijshaar ME, Rizopoulos D, Hahn A, Mongini TE, et al; European Pompe Consortium project group on classic infantile Pompe disease. Effect of alglucosidase alfa dosage on survival and walking ability in patients with classic infantile Pompe disease: A multicentre observational cohort study from the European Pompe Consortium.
Lancet Child Adolesc Health. 2022;6(1):28-37.

Abstract

Introduction: Enzyme replacement therapy (ERT) with alglucosidase alpha is reported to result in improvement of outcomes among patients having classic infantile Pompe disease, who if not treated will die before the age of 1 year. Due to varying responses to the standard recommended dosage, optional dosing strategies have been developed. The aim of this study was to evaluate the impact of real-world ERT regimens in terms of survival as well as walking ability of such patients.

Methods: This was an observational cohort study, in which data was collected as part of a collaborative study within the European Pompe Consortium among patients having classic infantile Pompe disease (diagnosed between October 26, 1998 and March 8, 2019) from Germany, Netherlands, France, and Italy. Those who were eligible for the study had classic infantile Pompe disease with onset of disease and proven diagnosis prior to 1 year of age, and hypertrophic cardiomyopathy. The definition of proven diagnosis of classic infantile Pompe disease included confirmed deficiency of α-glucosidase in lymphocytes or leukocytes, muscle or fibroblasts, or two pathogenic acid α-glucosidase (GAA) variants in trans, or presence of both of these conditions. Data related to demographic characteristics, ERT dosage, GAA variants, age at death, as well as walking ability was also collected. Kaplan–Meier curves, Cox regression, and log-rank tests were used for analyzing effects of ERT dosage on survival as well as walking ability.

Result: Total 124 patients who had classic infantile Pompe disease were included. Out of these, 116 received treatment with ERT; the median age at treatment initiation was 3.3 months [interquartile range (IQR) 1.8–5.0, range 0.03–11.8]). The mean duration of follow-up was 60.1 months (SD 57.3) ($n = 115$). Follow-up of 116 patients was possible, out of which 36 (31%) died. The patients received 39 different ERT dosing regimens. Total 64 patients remained on the same dosage; at final follow-up, 16 (52%) of 31 patients who received the standard dosage (20 mg/kg every other week), 12 (80%) of 15 patients who received an intermediate dosage (20 mg/kg/week or 40 mg/kg every other week), and 16 (89%) of 18 patients who received the high dosage (40 mg/kg/week) were alive. High-dosage group had significant improvement in survival than standard dosage group [hazard ratio (HR) 0.17 (95% CI 0.04–0.76); $p = 0.02$]. The intermediate dosage group and the standard dosage group had similar survival [HR 0.44 (0.13–1.51); $p = 0.19$]. Among 86 patients who attained 18 months of age, 44 (51%) were able to walk. There was no significant difference in ability to walk in standard dosage regimen ($n = 19$), intermediate dosage regimens ($n = 9$), and high-dosage regimens ($n = 15$) [10 (53%) vs. 6 (67%) vs. 14 (93%)].

Conclusion: A significant improvement was seen in survival of patients with classic infantile Pompe disease who received treatment with the high ERT dosage (40 mg/kg/week) in comparison to those who received the standard recommended ERT dosage (20 mg/kg every other week). On the basis of findings of this study, it is suggested to reconsider existing registered dosage.

COMMENT

In a cohort observational study in collaboration with the European Pompe Consortium illustrated that in classic infantile Pompe disease, enzyme replacement therapy (ERT) with dosage of 40 mg/kg/week of alglucosidase α had significantly better effects on survival and walking ability of children with a mean recruitment age of 3 years, when compared with the standard recommended ERT dosage of 20 mg/kg every other week, on a mean follow-up of 5 years. Considering the high fatality of infantile Pompe's, these results are very encouraging.

ARTICLE 12

In NF1, No Evidence of Neurotoxicity on 1 Year of Treatment with an MEKi and a Potential Clinical Signal of Cognitive Improvement, Supporting Future Research of Mitogen Activated Protein Kinase Inhibitor (MEKi) as a Cognitive Intervention

Walsh KS, Wolters PL, Widemann BC, Del Castillo A, Sady MD, Inker T, et al. Impact of MEK Inhibitor Therapy on Neurocognitive Functioning in NF1.
Neurol Genet. 2021;7(5):e616.

Abstract

Introduction and Objectives: Cognitive impairments caused by neurofibromatosis type 1 (NF1) are associated with significant long-term morbidity. A significant unmet requirement is the lack of targeted biologic treatments. The study examined at how cognition changes in NF1 patients during the first 48 weeks of mitogen-activated protein kinase inhibitor (MEKi) treatment.

Methods: The study considered 59 patients who had NF1 (5–27 years) on an MEKi clinical trial receiving treatment for plexiform neurofibroma. In all patients, pretreatment and follow-up cognitive evaluations were done over 48 weeks of treatment. The primary outcomes considered in the study included performance tasks (Cogstate) as well as observer-reported functioning (BRIEF). The study used group-level (paired T-tests) and individual-level analyses (reliable change index, RCI).

Result: It was found that there were significant improvements on BRIEF in comparison to baseline [24-week behavioral regulation index: $t(58) = 3.03$, $p = 0.004$, $d = 0.24$; 48-week Meta-cognition Index: $t(39) = 2.70$, $p = 0.01$, $d = 0.27$]. RCI demonstrated more number of patients to have clinically significant improvement at 48 weeks as compared to that expected by chance [$\chi2 = 11.95$, $p = 0.001$, odds ratio (OR) = 6.3]. On group-level analyses, there was stable performance on Cogstate ($p > 0.05$). Significantly more improvement was seen in working memory (24-week $\chi2 = 8.36$, $p = 0.004$, OR = 4.6, and 48-week $\chi2 = 9.34$, $p = 0.004$, OR = 5.3) on RCI statistics; however, no such improvement was seen in visual learning/memory. As compared to nonimpaired patients, those with baseline impairments on BRIEF had significantly more improvement (at 24 weeks: 46% vs. 8%; $\chi2 = 9.54$, $p = 0.008$, OR 9.22; at 48 weeks 63% vs. 16%; $\chi2 = 7.50$, $p = 0.02$, OR 9.0).

Conclusion: The findings of this study showed no case of neurotoxicity after treatment with an MEKi for period of 48 weeks, and gives potential clinical signal that supports more research in future indicating MEKi as a cognitive intervention.

COMMENT

One year of treatment with a mitogen-activated protein kinase inhibitor (MEKi) was found to improve the cognitive state in neurofibromatosis type 1 (NF1) in 59 patients and this effect is thought to be mediated through the targeted biologic treatment. The cognitive assessment was primarily using a performance task (Cogstate). This is one of the first-ever breakthrough treatment for this otherwise frustratingly progressive and disabling and disabling familial neurological disorder.

SYMPTOMATIC THERAPY

ARTICLE 1

Prevention of Epilepsy in Infants with Tuberous Sclerosis Complex in the EPISTOP Trial

Kotulska K, Kwiatkowski DJ, Curatolo P, Weschke B, Riney K, Jansen F, et al.; EPISTOP Investigators. Prevention of epilepsy in infants with tuberous sclerosis complex in the EPISTOP trial.
Ann Neurol. 2021;89(2):304-14.

Abstract

Objective: Epilepsy develops in approximately 70–90% of children with tuberous sclerosis complex (TSC). It is a drug-resistant form. In recent years, scientists have proposed preventive antiepileptic treatment to alter the natural history of epilepsy. EPISTOP, a clinical trial, was designed to compare preventive and conventional antiepileptic methods of treatment in infants with TSC.

Methods: This is a multicenter study, involving 94 infants with TSC and without any prior seizure history. These infants were followed with monthly video electroencephalography (EEG). The infants received vigabatrin either as a conventional antiepileptic treatment, started either after the first electrographic or clinical seizure, or preventively when an epileptiform EEG activity before seizures were detected. Participants were randomly allocated to treatment group in a 1:1 ratio in a randomized controlled trial (RCT) at six study sites. However, allocation to the treatment was fixed at four sites. This was referred as an open-label trial (OLT). Participants were then followed until 2 years of age. The time to first clinical seizure was noted as the primary endpoint of the study.

Result: Epileptiform EEG abnormalities were identified before seizures in 54 participants. Of these, 27 participants were included in the RCT and 27 participants were included in the OLT. The time to the first clinical seizure was significantly longer with preventive than the conventional treatment {RCT: 364 days [95% confidence interval (CI) 223–535] vs. 124 days [95% CI 33–149]; OLT: 426 days [95% CI 258–628] vs. 106 days [95% CI 11–149]}. Our pooled analysis demonstrated that preventive treatment decreased the risk of clinical seizures [odds ratio (OR) 0.21; $p = 0.032$], drug-resistant epilepsy (OR 0.23; $p = 0.022$), and infantile spasms (OR 0; $p < 0.001$) at 24 months. In addition, no adverse events because of the preventive treatment were noted.

Interpretation: Preventive treatment with vigabatrin was reported to be a safer approach. This modified the natural history of seizures in infants with TSC, thereby decreasing the risk and severity of epilepsy.

COMMENT

Ninety four infants with tuberous sclerosis without seizure history were followed with monthly video electroencephalography (EEG), and received vigabatrin as conventional antiepileptic treatment, after first electrographic or clinical seizure, in a randomized controlled trial (RCT). At four of the sites, treatment was on open-label trial (OLT). Subjects were followed until 2 years of age. At 24 months, preventive treatment significantly reduced the risk of clinical seizures, drug-resistant epilepsy, and infantile spasms.

ARTICLE 2

Pharmacogenetic Predictors of Cannabidiol Response and Tolerability in Treatment-resistant Epilepsy

Davis BH, Beasley TM, Amaral M, Szaflarski JP, Gaston T, Grayson LP, et al.; UAB CBD Study Group (includes all the investigators involved in the UAB EAP CBD program). Pharmacogenetic predictors of cannabidiol response and tolerability in treatment-resistant epilepsy.
Clin Pharmacol Ther. 2021;110(5):1368-80.

Abstract

Cannabidiol (CBD) is known to provide variable improvement in controlling seizures in patients who are reported to have treatment-resistant epilepsy (TRE). The study enrolled patients from the University of Alabama at Birmingham CBD Expanded Access Program (EAP) in this genomic study and were genotyped using the Affymetrix drug metabolizing enzymes and transporters plus array. Associations between variants and CBD response (≥50% seizure reduction) and tolerability (diarrhea, sedation, and abnormal liver function) were examined under dominant and recessive models. Expression quantitative trait loci (eQTL) influencing potential CBD targets were evaluated in the UK Brain Expression Consortium data set (Braineac), and genetic coexpression was examined. Of 169 EAP patients, 112 (54.5% pediatric and 50% female) were included in the genetic analyses. Patients with AOX1 rs6729738 CC [aldehyde oxidase; odds ratio (OR) 6.69; 95% confidence interval (CI) 2.19–20.41; $p = 0.001$] or ABP1 rs12539 (diamine oxidase; OR 3.96; 95% CI 1.62–9.73; $p = 0.002$) were more likely to respond. In contrast, patients with SLC15A1 rs1339067 TT had lower odds of response (OR 0.06; 95% CI 0.01–0.56; $p = 0.001$). ABCC5 rs3749442 was reported to be associated with lower likelihood of response and abnormal liver function tests and higher likelihood of sedation. The eQTL revealed that rs1339067 decreased GPR18 expression (endocannabinoid receptor) in white matter ($p = 5.6 \times 10^{-30}$), and rs3749442 decreased hippocampal HTR3E expression (serotonin 5-HT$_{3E}$; $p = 8.5 \times 10^{-50}$). In addition, 75% of the genes that were associated with a lower likelihood of response coexpressed. Pharmacogenetic variation is associated with CBD response and influences expression of CBD targets in TRE. Involved pathways, including cholesterol metabolism and glutathione conjugation, show potential interactions between CBD and common medications (e.g., statins and acetaminophen) that might require a close monitoring. These results signify the role of pharmacogenes in basic biologic processes and likely genetic underpinnings of resistance to treatment.

COMMENT

In patients with treatment-resistant epilepsy (TRE), cannabidiol produces variable improvement in seizure control. TRE patients in the University of Alabama at Birmingham on Cannabinoids, were assessed for the genotypes of aldehyde oxidase, diamine oxidase with favorable response to Cannabinoids, or SLC15A1 and ABCC5 variations had unfavorable response.

PHARMACOGENOMICS

ARTICLE 1

Association between COMT Methylation and Response to Treatment in Children with ADHD

Fageera W, Chaumette B, Fortier MÈ, Grizenko N, Labbe A, Sengupta SM, et al. Association between COMT methylation and response to treatment in children with ADHD.
J Psychiatr Res. 2021;135:86-93.

Abstract

Background: Catechol-O-methyltransferase (COMT) is considered a promising candidate gene in pharmacogenetic studies in attention deficit hyperactivity disorder (ADHD). However, the findings from previous studies have been not consistent. These inconsistencies could be in part related to the epigenetic mechanisms (including DNA methylation). This study investigated the role of genetic variants of the *COMT* gene on the methylation levels of CpG sites in the same gene and examined the effects of methylation on methylphenidate (MPH) and placebo (PBO) response in children with ADHD.

Methods: A total of 230 children with ADHD (6–12 years) were included in a randomized, double-blind, PBO-controlled crossover trial with MPH. Associations between genotypes in the

COMT gene and DNA methylation in the same genetic loci were analyzed by univariate analysis. Association between the DNA methylation of 11 CpG sites and PBO/MPH responses were then examined by performing Spearman's correlation analysis in 212 children. Interaction between these factors while accounting for sex was tested by performing multiple linear regression analyses.

Result: Associations were studied between specific genetic variants and methylation level of cg20709110. Homozygous genotypes of GG (rs6269), CC (rs4633), GG (rs4818), Val/Val (rs4680), and the haplotype (ACCVal/GCGVal) were significantly associated with higher level of methylation. This CpG demonstrated a significant correlation with PBO response ($r = -0.15$, $p = 0.045$) based on the teachers' evaluation, and a close-to significance correlation with response to MPH on the basis of the evaluation by parents ($r = -0.134$, $p = 0.051$). Regression analysis exhibited that in the model including rs4818, sex, and DNA methylation of cg20709110 contributed significantly to response to treatment.

Conclusion: These preliminary findings could provide evidence for the impacts of genetic variations on methylation level and involvement of the epigenetic variation of *COMT* loci in modulating the treatment response in ADHD.

Trial Registration: Clinicaltrials.gov, number NCT00483106.

Keywords: Attention-deficit/hyperactivity disorder (ADHD), COMT, Conners', Methylation, Pharmacoepigenetics, Treatment response

COMMENT

In 230 children with attention-deficit/hyperactivity disorder (ADHD), the effects of methylation on response to therapy with methylphenidate or placebo was studied and it was found that the genetic variations on methylation level and the involvement of the epigenetic variation of catechol-O-methyltransferase (*COMT*) loci in modulating the response to treatment in ADHD.

ARTICLE 2

Integrative Network-based Analysis Reveals Gene Networks and Novel Drug Repositioning Candidates for Alzheimer's Disease

Gerring ZF, Gamazon ER, White A, Derks EM. Integrative Network-Based Analysis Reveals Gene Networks and Novel Drug Repositioning Candidates for Alzheimer Disease.
Neurol Genet. 2021;7(5): e622.

Abstract

Background and Objectives: This study aimed at integrating data of genome-wide association study with information of tissue-specific gene expression for identifying biological pathways, coexpression networks, and drug repositioning candidates for Alzheimer's disease (AD).

Methods: This study involved integration of genome-wide association summary statistics for AD with tissue-specific gene coexpression networks from samples of brain tissue in the Genotype-Tissue Expression study. The gene coexpression networks enriched with genetic signals for AD were identified and the related networks were characterized by us of biological pathway analysis. The study used disease-implicated modules as molecular substrate for a computational drug repositioning analysis, including (1) imputed genetically regulated gene expression within AD implicated modules; (2) integration of the imputed gene expression levels with drug-gene signatures from the connectivity map for recognizing compounds causing normalization of dysregulated gene expression causing AD; and (3) prioritization of drug compounds as well as mechanisms of action on the basis of their ability to normalize dysregulated expression signatures.

Result: The genetic factors related to AD are found to be enriched in brain gene coexpression networks included in the immune response. Computational drug repositioning analyses of expression alterations in the disease-related networks derived established drugs of AD (such as memantine) and biologically meaningful drug categories (such as glutamate receptor antagonists).

Conclusion: The findings of this study help in improvement of the biological interpretation of genetic data for AD and give information of possible antidementia drug repositioning candidates whose efficacy need to be studied in functional validation studies.

COMMENT

Integrative network-based analysis of gene networks of drug and neurotransmitter molecules helped develop novel drugs and repositioned drugs as candidates for Alzheimer's disease (AD), including memantine, and N-methyl-D-aspartate (NMDA) agonists.

GENETIC MARKERS

ARTICLE 1

KCNT1-related Epilepsies and Epileptic Encephalopathies: Phenotypic and Mutational Spectrum

Bonardi CM, Heyne HO, Fiannacca M, Fitzgerald MP, Gardella E, Gunning B, et al. KCNT1-related epilepsies and epileptic encephalopathies: Phenotypic and mutational spectrum.
Brain. 2021;144(12):3635-50.

Abstract

Variants in KCNT1, which encodes a sodium-gated potassium channel (subfamily T member 1), have been associated with a range of epilepsies and neurodevelopmental disorders. These vary from familial autosomal dominant or sporadic sleep-related hypermotor epilepsy to epilepsy of infancy with migrating focal seizures (EIMFS) and include developmental and epileptic encephalopathies. This study provides a broad overview of the phenotypic and genotypic spectrum of KCNT1 mutation-related epileptic disorders. A total of 248 individuals (66 previously unpublished and 182 published cases) were included in this cohort that has been the largest cohort reported so far. The analysis gave four phenotypic groups: (1) EIMFS (152 individuals, 33 previously unpublished); (2) developmental and epileptic encephalopathies other than EIMFS (non-EIMFS developmental and epileptic encephalopathies) (37 individuals, 17 unpublished); (3) autosomal dominant or sporadic sleep-related hypermotor epilepsy (53 patients, 14 unpublished); and (4) other phenotypes (6 individuals, 2 unpublished). In this cohort comprising 66 new cases, the most common phenotypic features that were observed were as follows: (1) in EIMFS, heterogeneity of seizure types, including epileptic spasms, epilepsy improvement over time, no epilepsy-related deaths; (2) in non-EIMFS developmental and epileptic encephalopathies, possible onset with West syndrome, occurrence of atypical absences, possible evolution to developmental and epileptic encephalopathies with sleep-related hypermotor epilepsy features; one case of sudden unexplained death in epilepsy; (3) in autosomal dominant or sporadic sleep-related hypermotor epilepsy, we found a high prevalence of resistance to drugs. Although frequency of seizures improved with age in some individuals, appearance of cognitive regression after onset of seizures in all patients, none of them reported severe psychiatric disorders, though behavioral/psychiatric comorbidities were reported in approximately 50% of the patients, sudden unexplained death in epilepsy in one individual; and (4) other phenotypes in individuals with mutation of KCNT1 included temporal lobe epilepsy, and epilepsy with tonic–clonic seizures and cognitive regression. Genotypic analysis of the entire cohort of 248 individuals revealed only missense mutations and one inframe deletion in KCNT1. Although the KCNT1 mutations in affected individuals were observed to be distributed among the various domains of the KCNT1 protein, genotype–phenotype considerations found most of the autosomal dominant or sporadic sleep-related hypermotor epilepsy-associated mutations to be clustered around the RCK2 domain in the C terminus, distal to the NADP domain. Mutations associated with EIMFS/non-EIMFS developmental and epileptic encephalopathies did not reveal a particular pattern of distribution in the KCNT1 protein. Recurrent KCNT1 mutations were found to be associated with both severe and less severe phenotypes. Our study further elaborates and broadens the phenotypic and genotypic spectrums of KCNT1-related epileptic conditions and focusses on the crucial role of this gene in the pathogenesis of early onset developmental and epileptic encephalopathies and focal epilepsies, such as autosomal dominant or sporadic sleep-related hypermotor epilepsy.

Keywords: KCNT1, Developmental and epileptic encephalopathies, Epilepsy of infancy with migrating focal seizures, Epileptic encephalopathies, Sleep-related hypermotor epilepsy

COMMENT

In a comprehensive review of the largest cohort of epileptic disorders related to variants in *KCNT1* gene, encoding the sodium-gated potassium channel, among 248 individuals, four phenotypic groups emerged. They were (1) EIMFS (epilepsy of infancy with migrating focal seizures), (2) developmental and epileptic encephalopathies other than EIMFS (non-EIMFS developmental and epileptic encephalopathies), (3) autosomal dominant or sporadic sleep-related hypermotor epilepsy, and (4) other phenotypes which included temporal lobe epilepsy, and epilepsy with tonic–clonic seizures and cognitive regression. Genotypic analysis of the whole cohort of 248 individuals showed only missense mutations and one inframe deletion in KCNT1. Many of the mutations were clustered around the RCK2 domain in the C terminus, distal to the NADP domain. EIMFS/non-EIMFS developmental and epileptic encephalopathies did not show a particular pattern of distribution in the KCNT1 protein. This study further defines and broadens the phenotypic and genotypic spectrums of KCNT1-related epileptic conditions and emphasizes the increasingly important role of this gene in the pathogenesis of early onset developmental and epileptic encephalopathies as well as of autosomal dominant or sporadic sleep-related hypermotor epilepsy.

ARTICLE 2

APOE Genotype Contributes to the Heterogeneity in Rate of Clinical Progression in AD

Qian J, Betensky RA, Hyman BT, Serrano-Pozo A. Association of APOE genotype with heterogeneity of cognitive decline rate in Alzheimer disease.
Neurology. 2021;96(19):e2414-e2428.

Abstract

Objective: The aim of this study was testing the hypothesis that in clinical progression of Alzheimer's disease (AD), one of the significant drivers of heterogeneity is the APOE genotype; this can have significant effects design and interpretation of clinical trials.

Material and Methods: In the present study, new reverse-time longitudinal models were applied for evaluating the trajectories of clinical dementia rating-sum of boxes (CDR-SOB) as well as Mini-Mental State Examination (MMSE) scores, which were two common outcome measures in AD clinical trials. The study population included 1,102 patients with AD, which were autopsy proven (moderate/frequent neuritic plaques and Braak tangle stage III or greater), from the National Alzheimer's Coordinating Center Neuropathology database that resembled individuals having mild-to-moderate AD in therapeutic clinical trials.

Section 14: Neurogenetics

Result: Compared to than APOE ε3/ε3 carriers, there was nearly 1.5 times faster CDR-SOB increase in APOE ε4 carriers (2.12 points/year vs. 1.44 points/year). APOE ε4 carriers had about 1.3 times faster increase in comparison to APOE ε2 carriers (1.65 points/year). However, there was no significant difference between APOE ε2 and APOE ε3/ε3.

APOE ε4 carriers exhibited nearly 1.1 times faster MMSE reduction compared to APOE ε3/ε3 carriers (−3.45 vs. −3.03 points/year) and about 1.4 times faster reduction in comparison with APOE ε2 carriers (−2.43 points/year), while APOE ε2 carriers exhibited about 1.2 times slower decrease compared to APOE ε3/ε3 carriers (−2.43 vs. −3.03 points/year). After controlling for the impact of AD neuropathologic changes on the rate of cognitive decline and for the presence as well as severity of comorbid pathologies, there was no change in findings.

Conclusion: There is opposite effect of APOE ε2 and ε4 alleles (slowing and accelerating, respectively) on the rate of cognitive decline when compared to the APOE ε3/ε3 reference genotype, which are significant clinically and mainly independent of the differential APOE allele effects on AD as well as comorbid pathologies. Therefore, APOE genotype has a significant contribution to the heterogeneity in rate of AD clinical progression.

COMMENT

The association of *APOE* gene alleles ε2 and ε4 with cerebrovascular disease, Cognition and Alzheimer's disease (AD) has been realized for some time now, but their role in progression of dementia in AD had been unclear. This study, from over a thousand mild to moderate AD patients, from various trials, in a US national neuropathology database, showed the association between the *APOE* gene alleles and cognitive outcome scales indicating important predictive role of the APOE allele status for CVD, AD, and cognitive status.

ARTICLE 3

Adult GBA Variants, Parkinsonism is Linked to a more Aggressive Motor Disease Course over 7 Years from Diagnosis in Patients. Recruiting only GBA Carriers can Reduce Trial Size by up to 65% Compared to a Trial Recruiting all Patients with PD

Maple-Grødem J, Dalen I, Tysnes OB, Macleod AD, Forsgren L, Counsell CE, et al. Association of GBA genotype with motor and functional decline in patients with newly diagnosed Parkinson disease.
Neurology. 2021;96(7):e1036-44.

Abstract

Objective: The aim of this study was to find the importance of glucocerebrosidase gene (*GBA*) carrier—status on motor impairment among patients having incident Parkinson disease (PD).

Methods: The study included data from three studies including 528 European patients diagnosed with PD. For evaluation of GBA variants, 440 patients with genomic DNA were studied from baseline. Motor and functional impairment was assessed every year through Unified Parkinson's Disease Rating Scale (UPDRS) motor and activities of daily living (ADL) sections. Mixed random and fixed effects models were used for assessing differential effects of classes of GBA variants on disease progression.

Result: The study enrolled patients who had idiopathic disease ($n = 387$) (mean age at baseline 70.3 ± 9.5 years; 60.2% were males) and GBA carriers ($n = 53$) (mean age at baseline 66.8 ± 10.1 years; 64.2% were males). At diagnosis, there was clinically indistinguishable motor profile of the groups. In GBA carriers, there was faster annual increase in UPDRS scores measuring ADL [1.5 point/year, 95% confidence interval (CI) 1.1–2.0] as well as motor symptoms (2.2 points/year, 95% CI 1.3–3.1) in comparison with noncarriers (ADL, 1.0 point/year, 95% CI 0.9-1.1; $p = 0.003$; motor, 1.3 point/year, 95% CI 1.1–1.6; $p = 0.007$). Simulations of clinical trial designs demonstrated that recruitment of only GBA carriers can result in reduction of trial size by nearly 65% in comparison to trial that recruited patients with PD only.

Conclusion: Glucocerebrosidase gene variants are associated with a more aggressive motor disease course in PD patients 7 years after diagnosis. An improved knowledge of PD progression in genetic subpopulations may result in improvement of management of disease and has direct impact on improving the clinical trials design.

COMMENT

In a longitudinal study of clinically indistinguishable and matched 387 idiopathic Parkinson's disease (PD) and 53 glucocerebrosidase gene (*GBA*) carriers, the GBA variants parkinsonism was found to have a more aggressive motor disease course over 7 years from diagnosis. Recruiting only GBA carriers can reduce trial size by up to 65% when simulations of clinical trials were carried out. Better knowledge on the natural history and progression in genetic subpopulations of parkinsonism may result in improvement of management of disease.

ARTICLE 4

1,250 plus Finnish Ageing Clinical Trial on Multidomain Interventions Facilitated LTL Maintenance among Subgroups of Older People and LTL (Telomere Length) Maintenance was Associated with more Pronounced Cognitive Intervention Benefits

Sindi S, Solomon A, Kåreholt I, Hovatta I, Antikainen R, Hänninen T, et al; FINGER Study Group. Telomere Length Change in a Multidomain Lifestyle Intervention to Prevent Cognitive Decline: A Randomized Clinical Trial.
J Gerontol A Biol Sci Med Sci. 2021;76(3):491-8.

Abstract

Introduction: Shorter leukocyte telomere length (LTL) is reported to show association with aging as well as dementia. There is lack of randomized controlled trials (RCTs) that evaluated effect of changes of lifestyle on LTL, and association with cognition as well as genetic susceptibility in patients with dementia.

Methods: Finnish Geriatric Intervention Study to Prevent Cognitive Impairment and Disability was an RCT that was conducted for duration of 2 years; the study enrolled 1,260 individuals (60–77 years) who were at risk for dementia from the general population. The randomization of patients (1:1) was done to either multidomain lifestyle intervention group or control group. Cognitive change (neuropsychological test battery Z-score) was considered as the primary outcome. The quantitative real-time polymerase chain reaction was used for measuring relative LTL (trial registration: NCT01041989).

Result: In this exploratory LTL substudy, 756 individuals were included [intervention group ($n = 377$), control group ($n = 379$)]. LTL measurements were taken at baseline as well as 24 months. In the intervention and control groups, the mean annual LTL change (SD) was −0.016 (0.19) and −0.023 (0.17), respectively. There was nonsignificant between-group difference [unstandardized β-coefficient 0.007, 95% confidence interval (CI) 0.015–0.030]. On interaction analyses, there were better LTL maintenance in apolipoprotein E (APOE)-ε4 carriers versus noncarriers [0.054 (95% CI 0.007–0.102)]; younger versus older patients [0.005 (95% CI −0.010 to −0.001)]; and those with more versus less healthy lifestyle changes [0.047 (95% CI 0.005–0.089)]. There were more pronounced cognitive intervention benefits in patients with better LTL maintenance for executive functioning (0.227, 95% CI 0.057–0.396) as well as long-term memory (0.257, 95% CI 0.024–0.489), and similar trend was observed for neuropsychological test battery total score [0.127, 95% CI −0.011 to 0.264].

Conclusion: To the best of our knowledge, this was the first large RCT demonstrating that multidomain lifestyle intervention improved maintenance of LTL in subgroups of old age individuals who at risk for dementia, comprising APOE-ε4 carriers. An association was found between LTL maintenance and more pronounced cognitive intervention advantages.

COMMENT

Finnish Geriatric Intervention study is looking at the effects of multidomain lifestyle modifications on cognitive changes over 2 years in a cohort of 1,260 aging persons. Using qPCR, they estimated LTL (leukocyte telomere length) among subgroups of older people. Better LTL maintenance was associated with apolipoprotein E (APOE)-ε4, younger people, better lifestyle maintenance and with better cognition (more pronounced intervention benefits).

ARTICLE 5

Most known CSF Biomarkers of Parkinsonism Predict Cognitive Decline in PD during Follow-up but only α-syn help Dissociate it from Healthy Controls

Bartl M, Dakna M, Galasko D, Hutten SJ, Foroud T, Quan M, et al; Parkinson's Progression Markers Initiative. Biomarkers of neurodegeneration and glial activation validated in Alzheimer's disease assessed in longitudinal cerebrospinal fluid samples of Parkinson's disease.
PLoS One. 2021;16(10):e0257372.

Abstract

Introduction and Objective: In Parkinson's disease (PD), many pathophysiological processes are included, which could provide information about vivo biomarkers. This study aimed at evaluation of a well-known biomarker panel, which is validated in Alzheimer's disease, among cohort of PD patients.

Methods: The study included Parkinson's progression markers initiative (PPMI) [PD ($n = 252$), healthy controls (HC, $n = 115$)]. The analysis of longitudinal cerebrospinal fluid (CSF) samples was done at six time points (baseline, and at 6, 12, 24, 36, and 48 months follow-up) through Elecsys® electrochemiluminescence immunoassays for quantifying soluble TREM2 receptor (sTREM2), S100, interleukin-6 (IL-6), neurofilament light chain (NfL), glial fibrillary acidic protein (GFAP), chitinase-3-like protein 1 (YKL40), and total α-synuclein (αSyn).

Result: There was significantly lower mean αSyn in PD compared to HC [103 vs. 127 pg/mL, $p < 0.01$; area under the curve (AUC) 0.64], whereas other biomarkers were similar (AUC NfL: 0.49, sTREM2: 0.54, YKL40: 0.57, GFAP: 0.55, IL-6: 0.53, S100: 0.54, $p > 0.05$), with none demonstrating significant difference longitudinally. There were significantly greater levels of all these markers between PD patients in whom cognitive decline developed during follow-up; however, no such difference was seen in α-syn and IL-6.

Conclusion: With the exception of Syn, the other biomarkers did not distinguish between PD and HC, and none demonstrated longitudinal differences; however, majority of markers predicted cognitive decline in PD during follow-up.

COMMENT

A cerebrospinal fluid (CSF) biomarker panel, validated for Alzheimer's disease consisting of soluble TREM receptors, S100, interleukin-6, and neurofilament light chain (NfL), glial fibrillary acidic protein (GFAP), chitinase-3-like protein 1 (YKL40), and alpha synuclein showed significant difference from healthy controls only in low synuclein levels. Other CSF biomarkers showed correlation with cognitive decline in Parkinson's disease (PD) during follow-up but only α-syn helps distinguished it from healthy controls. However, several other studies correlating the disease severity with these biomarkers had concluded that disease severity may not correlate with the biomarker levels thereby reducing their predictive value. Given the current access to the biomarker panels, more research is needed to derive at more robust biomarker panels for diagnosis, prognosis, and specific disease modifying therapeutics of specific neurodegenerative diseases.

ARTICLE 6

CMT: UK CMT 6-year and US Follow-up Cohorts and Two Mouse Models—NfL Light Chain not a Helpful Biomarker to Assess Response to Therapy in Clinical Trials

Rossor AM, Kapoor M, Wellington H, Spaulding E, Sleigh JN, Burgess RW, et al. A longitudinal and cross-sectional study of plasma neurofilament light chain concentration in Charcot–Marie–Tooth disease.
J Peripher Nerv Syst. 2022;27(1):50-57.

Abstract

The advancement in genetic technology as well as development of small molecule drug provided the path for clinical trials among patients with Charcot–Marie–Tooth disease (CMT). But, existing United States Food and Drug Administration (FDA)-approved clinical trial outcome measures were found to be insensitive in detecting meaningful clinical response. As a result, sensitive outcome measures or clinically relevant biomarkers must be identified. This study aimed at assessing whether plasma neurofilament light chain (NfL) may play role of disease biomarker among patients with CMT. SIMOA technology was used for evaluating plasma NfL in cross-sectional study of United States cohort of CMT patients and longitudinally over 6 years in United Kingdom CMT cohort. Moreover, measurement of plasma NfL was done longitudinally in two mouse models of CMT2D. In comparison to controls, plasma levels of NfL were found to be raised in American patients having CMT1X, CMT1B, and CMT2A but not CMT2E. In a cohort including patients from UK, in an interval of 6 years, plasma NfL level was not significantly changed in hereditary sensory neuropathy type 1 (HSN1) or CMT1A, however, small but significant decrease in those with CMT1X was seen. In comparison with GARS (C201R) mice, wild type mice had significant increase in plasma NfL. The plasma NfL was comparable in GARS (P278KY) and wild type mice. Among individuals having CMT1A, the small difference in cross-sectional NfL levels as compared to healthy controls and no change over time indicates that plasma NfL may not have adequate sensitivity for detecting clinically meaningful treatment response among adult patients.

COMMENT

It is important to pay attention to trials with negative outcomes. There is a lot of literature on the usefulness of serum and cerebrospinal fluid neurofilament light (CSF NfL) as a biomarker. Charcot-Marie-Tooth disease (CMT) 6-year follow-up studies in UK and US as well as those on two mouse models suggested that NfL light chain may not be a helpful biomarker to assess response to therapy in clinical trials.

ARTICLE 7

Increased Copy Number of APP is Sufficient to Cause AD and CAA, with likely Earlier Onset in Case of Triplication Compared with Duplication

Grangeon L, Cassinari K, Rousseau S, Croisile B, Formaglio M, Moreaud O, et al. Early-onset cerebral amyloid angiopathy and Alzheimer disease related to an APP locus triplication.
Neurol Genet. 2021;7(5):e609.

Abstract

Background and Objective: This study aimed at reporting a triplication of the amyloid-β precursor protein (APP) locus in addition to relative messenger RNA (mRNA) expression in a family with autosomal dominant early-onset cerebral amyloid angiopathy (CAA) as well as Alzheimer's disease (AD).

Methods: The identification of four copies of the *APP* gene was done through fluorescent in situ hybridization (FISH), quantitative multiplex polymerase chain reaction (PCR) of short fluorescent fragments, and array comparative genomic hybridization. The evaluation of levels of APP mRNA was done through reverse-transcription–digital droplet PCR in the proband's whole blood. Comparison was done with controls ($n = 10$) and APP duplication carriers ($n = 9$).

Result: Initiating at age of 39 years, there is development of severe episodic memory deficits in proband with cerebrospinal fluid (CSF) biomarker profile typical of AD and multiple lobar microbleeds in the posterior regions on brain magnetic resonance imaging (MRI). There was history of seizures as well as recurrent cerebral hemorrhage (since 37 years of age) in his father. On cerebral biopsy, there was presence of abundant perivascular amyloid deposits, which resulted in CAA diagnosis. In the proband, there were four copies of a 506-kb region present on chromosome 21q21.3 and comprising the whole APP gene without any other gene. On FISH analysis, genotype of the proband was found to be three copies/one copy corresponding to an APP locus triplication that was consistent with existence of two APP copies in the healthy mother and with the paternal medical history. On analyzing the APP mRNA level, twofold increase in the proband and 1.8-fold increase in APP duplication carriers were found in comparison to controls.

Discussion: Increase in copy number of APP is adequate for causing AD as well as CAA, and there is possibly earlier onset in those with triplication in comparison to duplication.

COMMENT

Increased copy number of amyloid precursor protein identified through fluorescent in situ hybridization (FISH) and quantitative multiplex polymerase chain reaction (PCR) was found to be correlated with amyloid-β precursor protein (APP) messenger RNA (mRNA) levels and was associated with cerebral amyloid angiopathy (CAA) and Alzheimer's disease (AD), with likely earlier onset in case of triplication compared with duplication strongly establishing a 'cause-effect' association of APP with CAA and AD.

ARTICLE 8

PME is One of the Best Genetically Defined Epilepsy Syndrome with Diagnostic Yield >80%. Using NGS Technology, Pathogenic Variants were Detected in both Established PME Genes and in Genes not Previously Associated with PME but Other Developmental Encephalopathies

Canafoglia L, Franceschetti S, Gambardella A, Striano P, Giallonardo AT, Tinuper P, et al. Progressive Myoclonus Epilepsies: Diagnostic Yield With Next-Generation Sequencing in Previously Unsolved Cases.
Neurol Genet. 2021;7(6):e641.

Abstract

Objective: The present study aimed to evaluate the present diagnostic accuracy of genetic testing for the progressive myoclonus epilepsies (PMEs) of an Italian series (conducted in 2014) where Unverricht–Lundborg as well as Lafora diseases were accountable for nearly 50% of the study population.

Methods: Out of 47/165 unrelated patients who had PME of indeterminate genetic origin, new molecular assessment was done in 38 patients. All patients underwent many next-generation sequencing (NGS) techniques comprising gene panel analysis in seven patients and/or whole-exome sequencing (WES) (WES singleton in 29 patients, WES trio in seven patients, and WES sibling in four patients). Homozygosity mapping and then targeted NGS were done in one family. On clinical basis, the categorization of patients was done in four phenotypic categories: "Unverricht–Lundborg disease-like PME," "late-onset PME," "PME plus developmental delay," and "PME plus dementia."

Result: The positive diagnosis was done in 16 (42%) out of 38 unrelated patients, which increased the overall number of solved families in the total series from 72 to 82%. There was presence of pathogenic variants among CERS1 (1 family), NEU1 (2 families), and among 13 nonfamilial patients in KCNC1 (3), SACS, DHDDS (3), CACNA2D2, NAXE, AFG3L2, STUB1, CLN6, and CHD2. Among different phenotypic categories, there was similar diagnostic rate; same gene could be present among different phenotypic categories.

Conclusion: The implementation of NGS technology to unsolved PME patients has demonstrated collection of very rarely found genetic causes. Pathogenic variants were found in established *PME* genes as well as genes that had not previously been linked to PME but were linked to progressive ataxia or developmental encephalopathies. PME is among best genetically defined epilepsy syndromes, with a diagnostic yield of more than 80%.

COMMENT

Progressive myoclonus epilepsy (PME) is one of the best genetically defined epilepsy syndromes with diagnostic yield >80%. Using next-generation sequencing (NGS) technology, pathogenic variants were detected in both established PME genes and in genes not previously associated with *PME* but with other developmental encephalopathies. These genes include *CERS1, EU1, KCNC1, SACS, DHDDS, CACNA2D2, NAXE, AFG3L2, STUB1, CLN6,* and *CHD2.* The candidate gene mutations were pathogenic leading to syndromic neuropathologies, but not always necessarily resulting in stereotyped phenotypes, determined additionally by other regulator genes and epigenetic influences.

NATURAL HISTORY AND CLINICAL TOOLS

ARTICLE 1

First Long-term (2-year) Systematic Study in Progression of FSHD – Slow Progress but Considerable Unpleasant Soft Symptoms

Dijkstra JN, Goselink RJM, van Alfen N, de Groot IJM, Pelsma M, van der Stoep N, et al. Natural history of facioscapulohumeral dystrophy in children: A 2-year follow-up.
Neurology. 2021;97(21):e2103-e2113.

Abstract

Introduction and Objective: There is limited data regarding the natural history of facioscapulohumeral dystrophy (FSHD) among children, which is important improvement of patient care and readiness of clinical trial. The aim of this study was to explain the disease course of FSHD among pediatric patients.

Material and Methods: This was nationwide, single-center, prospective cohort study, in which FSHD was assessed among children for evaluating muscle functioning, imaging, as well as quality of life during follow-up of 2 years.

Results: The study population comprised of 20 children (2–17 years) who had genetically confirmed FSHD. The symptoms were slowly progressive. There was an increase in mean FSHD clinical score from 2.1 to 2.8 ($p = 0.003$). There was high variation in progression rate. Among 20 children with symptoms, 16 had facial weakness at baseline, whereas 19 children had facial weakness after 2 years. There was no significant change in muscle strength between baseline and follow-up. Trapezius as well as deltoid were the most common and severely affected muscles. There was improvement in functional exercise capacity, which was measured through 6-minute walk test. Systemic features were less common as well as nonprogressive. Complications related to weakness like lumbar hyperlordosis and dysarthria were frequent; there was an increase in their prevalence during follow-up. The common complaints were pain and fatigue, with increased prevalence during follow-up. Echogenicity was found to be progressively increased on muscle ultrasonography.

Discussion: The course of FSHD in children is slowly progressive but variable during follow-up of 2 years. For detecting progression, the most promising outcome measures included FSHD clinical score and muscle ultrasound (USG). In spite of progression of disease, functional capacity may improve with growth of children. The common symptoms were fatigue, pain, and reduced quality of life, which should be addressed in the management of children with FSHD. The findings of this study may be useful for counseling patients and as baseline measures in treatment trials among children with FSHD.

COMMENT

In a 2-year follow-up of facioscapulohumeral dystrophy (FSHD) over 2 years in school children of Netherlands, the authors documented an improvement on functional capacity as the child grows up along with symptoms of pain, fatigue, and a decreased quality of life which serve as important baseline information in better understanding of the disease, for counseling patients as well as for assessing responses to intervention in treatment trials in childhood FSHD.

ARTICLE 2

Ongoing Study Designed to Understand Natural History of Specific Congenital Muscular Dystrophy as an Essential Step for Reaching Trials Readiness

Bouman K, Groothuis JT, Doorduin J, van Alfen N, Cate FEAUT, van den Heuvel FMA, et al. Natural history, outcome measures and trial readiness in LAMA2-related muscular dystrophy and SELENON-related myopathy in children and adults: Protocol of the LAST STRONG study.
BMC Neurol. 2021;21(1):313.

Abstract

Background: The characteristics of SELENON (SEPN1)-related myopathy (SELENON-RM), which is rarely found congenital myopathy, include respiratory insufficiency, slowly progressive proximal muscle weakness, and early onset spine rigidity. There is similar clinical phenotype of muscular dystrophy caused due to mutations in the *LAMA2* gene (LAMA2-associated muscular dystrophy, LAMA2-MD), with either a severe, early onset because of complete Laminin subunit α2 deficiency [merosin-deficient congenital muscular dystrophy type 1A (MDC1A)] or a mild, childhood or adult onset because of partial Laminin subunit α2 deficiency. There is no curative treatment available for these muscle diseases; however, preclinical studies are being conducted.

Presently, data related to natural history data is lacking, and adequate clinical as well as functional outcome measures are required for reaching trial readiness.

Material and Methods: LAST STRONG was natural history study including Dutch patients of all ages who were diagnosed with LAMA2-MD or SELENON-RM, which initiated on August, 2020. In duration of 4 years, patients visited four times. The investigations included functional measurements, hand-held dynamometry (age 5 years or more), standardized neurological examination, questionnaires (patient report and/or parent proxy, age 2 years or more), pulmonary function tests (maximal inspiratory and expiratory pressure, spirometry, sniff nasal inspiratory pressure, age 5 years or more), ultrasonography of muscle comprising diaphragm, and accelerometry for 8 days (age 2 years or more). Cardiac evaluation was done at visit 1 and 3 [which included echocardiography, electrocardiogram (age 2 years or more), dual-energy X-ray absorptiometry (DEXA) scan (age 2 years or more), spine X-ray (age 2 years or more), and full-body magnetic resonance imaging (MRI) (age 10 years or more)]. All of these investigations were adapted to the age and functional abilities of patients. The assessment of correlation among key parameters within and between subsequent visits was done.

Conclusion: This study described the natural history of patients who were diagnosed with SELENON-RM or LAMA2-MD, which helped in selecting important clinical as well as functional outcome measures to reach readiness of clinical trials. In addition, the detailed explanation (deep phenotyping) of the clinical features will improve the clinical management and develop well-characterized baseline cohort for prospective follow-up. This natural history study is a necessary step to reach trial readiness in SELENON-RM and LAMA2-MD.

COMMENT

Newer players on the therapeutic armamentarium against neurogenetic disorders are being introduced on a regular basis. Many of these disorders are rare and the phenotypes are variable and hence the clinical courses as well. The development of these drugs involve sophisticated and costly methods. Before starting clinical trials using newer drugs/synthetic molecules, whose natural histories are poorly understood, it is important to have an insight on the natural histories of these conditions. This is exactly the step what researchers from Netherlands undertook in 2020. They started a study on the natural history of patients diagnosed with SELENON-RM or LAMA2-MD myopathy in the Dutch-speaking patients of all ages. This is to prepare for clinical trials on SELENON-NM myopathy, for which new molecules are on exciting clinical trials. Sonlicromanol, a new clinical stage chemical entity with a dual activity as antioxidant and redox modulator, developed for mitochondrial oxidative phosphorylation disturbances, is one of those drugs, beneficial for patients with SELENON-RM.

ARTICLE 3

Bayesian Models Adequately Predict the Natural Evolution of Congenital (Centronuclear) Myopathy and Facilitate a Sufficiently Powerful Trial Design

Fouarge E, Monseur A, Boulanger B, Annoussamy M, Seferian AM, De Lucia S, et al.; NatHis-MTM Study Group. Hierarchical Bayesian modelling of disease progression to inform clinical trial design in centronuclear myopathy. *Orphanet J Rare Dis. 2021;16(1):3.*

Abstract

Introduction: Centronuclear myopathies are among the severe and rarely found congenital diseases. One of the main challenges in clinical trial design is caused by clinical variability as well as genetic heterogeneity of such myopathies. Optional approaches to large placebo-controlled trials, such as using surrogate markers or historical controls, have disadvantages that are addressed by Bayesian statistics. In this study, a Bayesian model is presented in which natural history study data of each patient was used for predicting progression when treatment is not available. The aim of this prospective multicenter natural history study was assessment of data of 4-year follow-up of 59 patients having mutations in the *DNM2* or *MTM1* genes.

Methods: The approach of this study laid focus on assessing forced expiratory volume in 1 second (FEV1) among children of 6–18 years of age. A patient was considered as a responder when there was an improvement following treatment and the predictive probability of such improvement when intervention was not available was below 0.01. An FEV1 response was defined to be clinically relevant when it increased by >8%.

Result: The rate of response was considered to be the primary endpoint of a clinical trial using this model. The power of the study is on the basis of posterior probability that the rate of response observed is higher as compared to the rate of response seen in the absence of treatment predicted on the basis of prior natural history of each patient. For properly controlling type 1 error, the threshold probability by which the difference in response rates was more than zero was adapted to 91%, which ensured an overall rate of type 1 error to be 5% for the trial.

Conclusion: The study was able to reliably simulate the evolution of symptoms for individual patients over time using Bayesian statistical analysis of natural history data, and then compare these simulated trajectories to actual observed post-treatment outcomes. The proposed model accurately predicted the natural evolution of patients over the course of the study, allowing for a sufficiently powerful trial design that can account for the rarity of disease. More research and dialogue with regulatory authorities are required before Bayesian statistics can be used in orphan disease research.

COMMENT

Optional approaches to large placebo-controlled trials, such as using surrogate markers or historical controls, have the disadvantages that are addressed by Bayesian statistics. Bayesian analysis of natural history allows reliable simulation of the evolution of symptoms over time and to compare the simulated disease course to observe post-treatment outcomes Bayesian models adequately predicted the natural evolution of congenital (centronuclear) myopathy which will facilitate a sufficiently powerful trial design which can address the rarity of the disease. But there will be a need for further research and engagement with the regulatory authorities to allow for more applications of Bayesian statistics in orphan disease research.

ARTICLE 4

Identification of Stage-dependent Progression Rates Provide Reliable Outcome Measures to Monitor Disease Progression, in all Trial Designs in Friedreich's Ataxia

Reetz K, Dogan I, Hilgers RD, Giunti P, Parkinson MH, Mariotti C, et al EFACTS study group. Progression characteristics of the European Friedreich's Ataxia Consortium for Translational Studies (EFACTS): A 4-year cohort study.
Lancet Neurol. 2021;20(5):362-72.

Abstract

Introduction and Objective: The natural history of Friedreich's ataxia was evaluated by the European Friedreich's Ataxia Consortium for Translational Studies (EFACTS). The aim of this study was to evaluate characteristics of progression and to find patient groups with differential progression rates on the basis of longitudinal 4-year data for informing future clinical trials in Friedreich's ataxia.

Methods: European Friedreich's Ataxia Consortium for Translational Studies is a prospective, observational cohort study that is on the basis of an ongoing and open-ended registry. The study population included participants having genetically confirmed Friedreich's ataxia, who were examined every year at 11 clinical centers in seven European countries (Austria, Belgium, France, Germany, Italy, Spain, and the UK). The present study included data from baseline to follow-up of 4 years. The primary endpoints considered in the study were the Scale for the Assessment and Rating of Ataxia (SARA) and the activities of daily living (ADL). For evaluating annual disease progression, linear mixed-effect models were used for the entire cohort as well as subgroups defined by age of onset and ambulatory abilities. The study performed power calculations for potential trial designs. The present study is registered with ClinicalTrials.gov, NCT02069509.

Result: During September 15, 2010 to November 20, 2018, evaluation of total 914 individuals was done; out of which, 602 participants were enrolled. Among these, data was provided by 552 (92%) patients with minimum one follow-up visit. Among the overall patients, the annual progression rate for SARA was 0.82 points (standard error 0.05); it was found to be greater among ambulatory patients [1.12 (0.07)] as compared to nonambulatory patients [0.50 (0.07)]. Among the overall patients, there was worsening of ADL by 0.93 (SE 0.05) points/year, and progression rates were comparable among ambulatory patients [0.94 (0.07)] and nonambulatory patients [0.91 (0.08)]. Slightly higher worsening was seen in SARA and ADL among those with typical onset (symptom onset at ≤24 years) as compared to patients with late onset (symptom onset ≥25 years), with difference in progression slopes being insignificant.

For a parallel-group trial conducted for duration of 2 years, 230 (115 per group) patients would be needed for detecting 50% decrease in SARA progression at 80% power: 118 (59/group) when only ambulatory participants are enrolled. Considering ADL to be the primary outcome, 190 (95/group) Friedreich's ataxia patients would be required, and lesser number of patients would be needed when only participants with early-onset are enrolled.

Conclusion: The findings of this study in terms of stage-dependent progression rates carry significant implications for researchers as well as, because they give accurate outcome measures for monitoring progression of disease, and allows calculation of tailored sample size for guiding future clinical trial designs among patients with Friedreich's ataxia.

COMMENT

The natural history of Friedreich's ataxia was evaluated by the European Friedreich's Ataxia Consortium for Translational Studies (EFACTS). They evaluated characteristics of progression and patient groups with differential progression rates on a 4-year data to help future clinical trials in Friedreich's ataxia. The findings of this study in terms of stage-dependent progression rates carried significant implications for researchers because they give accurate outcome measures for monitoring progression of disease, and allowed calculation of tailored sample size for guiding future clinical trial designs.

ARTICLE 5

In GNE Myopathy 3-year Natural History Study, Insight into the Appropriate Tools to Detect Clinically Meaningful Changes for Future Interventional Trials

Lochmüller H, Behin A, Tournev I, Tarnopolsky M, Horváth R, Pogoryelova O, et al. Results from a 3-year Non-interventional, Observational Disease Monitoring Program in Adults with GNE Myopathy.
J Neuromuscul Dis. 2021;8(2):225-34.

Abstract

Introduction: GNE myopathy is rarely found autosomal recessive, muscle disease resulted due to mutations in GNE. The characteristics of this disease include rimmed vacuoles on muscle biopsy as well as progressive distal to proximal muscle weakness.

Objective: The aim of this study was to evaluate the clinical presentation as well as progression of GNE myopathy.

Methods: The "GNE Myopathy Disease Monitoring Program", which was an international, prospective, observational study, included individuals having GNE myopathy. The evaluation of muscle strength was done through hand-held dynamometry (HHD). The upper extremity (UE) composite scores show upper and lower extremity (LE) muscle groups and LE composite scores demonstrate LE muscle groups. For evaluation of impaired mobility, function of UE, and self-care, the GNE myopathy-Functional Activity Scale (GNEM-FAS) was utilized.

Result: Total 101 participants were included. Out of these, trial was completed by 87 subjects till the time study was closed by the sponsor. 36 months were completed by 60 patients. There was significant reduction in mean (SD) HHD UE composite score from baseline [34.3 kg (32.0)] to month 36 [29.4 kg (32.6)] kg [LS mean change (95% CI) −3.8 kg (−5.9, −1.7); $p = 0.0005$]. There was significant reduction in mean (SD) HHD LE composite score from baseline [32.0 kg (34.1)] to month 36 [25.5 kg (31.2)] [LS mean change (95% CI) −4.9 (−7.7, −2.2); $p = 0.0005$]. More severe GNEM-FAS scores were found at baseline among individuals who walked <200 meters compared to ≥200 meters in 6 minutes. Reduction in GNEM-FAS total, UE, mobility as well as self-care scores was found in both groups from baseline to month 36.

Conclusion: The findings of this study show that muscle strength declines progressively in GNE myopathy and give insight into the suitable tools for detecting clinically changes in GNE myopathy interventional trials to be conducted in future.

COMMENT

The GNE myopathy is caused by mutations in the gene encoding the enzyme, glucosamine (UDP-N-acetyl)-2-epimerase/N-acetylmannosamine kinase characterized by rimmed vacuoles on muscle biopsy and progressive distal to proximal muscle weakness. GNE Myopathy Disease Monitoring Program conducted an international, prospective, and observational study of individuals having GNE myopathy. 3-year natural history study on 101 patients gave insight into the appropriate tools to detect clinically meaningful changes for future interventional trials. GNE myopathy-Functional Activity Scale (GNEM-FAS) was found valid and useful for outcome assessment.

ARTICLE 6

30-year Follow-up Study in 350 Patients of NF Type 2 to Guide Clinical Trial Design

Forde C, King AT, Rutherford SA, Hammerbeck-Ward C, Lloyd SK, Freeman SR, et al. Disease course of neurofibromatosis type 2: A 30-year follow-up study of 353 patients seen at a single institution.
Neuro Oncol. 2021;23(7):1113-24.

Abstract

Background: Limited data exist on the disease course of neurofibromatosis type 2 (NF2) to guide clinical trial design.

Methods: A prospective database of patients meeting NF2 diagnostic criteria, reviewed between 1990 and 2020, was evaluated. Follow-up to first vestibular schwannoma (VS) intervention and death was assessed by univariate analysis and stratified by age at onset, era referred, and inheritance type. Interventions for NF2-related tumors were assessed. Cox regression was performed to determine the relationship between individual factors from time of diagnosis to NF2-related death.

Results: Three hundred and fifty-three patients were evaluated. During 4643.1 follow-up years from diagnosis to censoring, 60 patients (17.0%) died. The annual mean number of patients undergoing VS surgery or radiotherapy declined, from 4.66 and 1.65, respectively, per 100 NF2 patients in 1990–1999 to 2.11 and 1.01 in 2010–2020, as the number receiving bevacizumab increased (2.51 per 100 NF2 patients in 2010–2020). Five patients stopped bevacizumab to remove growing meningioma or spinal schwannoma. 153/353 (43.3%) had at least one neurosurgical intervention/radiation treatment within 5 years of diagnosis. Patients asymptomatic at diagnosis had longer time to intervention and better survival compared to those presenting with symptoms. Those symptomatically presenting <16 and >40 years had poorer overall survival than those presenting at 26–39 years ($p = 0.03$ and $p = 0.02$, respectively) but those presenting between 16 and 39 had shorter time to VS intervention. Individuals with de novo constitutional variants had worse survival than those with de novo mosaic or inherited disease ($p = 0.004$).

Conclusion: Understanding disease course improves prognostication, allowing for better-informed decisions about care.

Keywords: Manchester criteria; ependymoma; meningioma; neurofibromatosis type 2; vestibular schwannoma.

COMMENT

30-year follow-up study in 350+ patients of neurofibromatosis type 2 (NF2) showed that there was a reduction in annual mean number of patients who underwent surgery or radiotherapy, for vestibular schwannoma, because there was an increase in number of patients who received bevacizumab (2.51% NF2 patients in 2010–2020).

ARTICLE 7

RESCUE and REVERSE LHON Studies: LHON Progresses Rapidly in the First Months Following Onset during the Subacute Phase, Followed by Relative Stabilization during the Dynamic Phase

Moster ML, Sergott RC, Newman NJ, Yu-Wai-Man P, Carelli V, Bryan MS, et al; LHON study group. Cross-Sectional Analysis of Baseline Visual Parameters in Subjects Recruited Into the RESCUE and REVERSE ND4-LHON Gene Therapy Studies. *J Neuroophthalmol. 2021;41(3):298-308.*

Abstract

Objective: The present report was cross-sectional analysis of the baseline parameters of patients who had Leber hereditary optic neuropathy (LHON) and included in the gene therapy trials RESCUE as well as REVERSE, for evaluating the evolution of visual parameters in the first year of following loss of vision.

Methods: Two phase III clinical trials, RESCUE and REVERSE, were designed for evaluating the efficacy of *rAAV2/2-ND4* gene therapy among subjects with ND4-LHON. The vision loss in participants in RESCUE was for ≤6 months, and in REVERSE between 6 and 12 months, at the time of enrollment. Before treatment, assessment of functional visual parameters [Humphrey visual field (HVF) and best-corrected visual acuity (BCVA)], and contrast sensitivity (CS)] and structural parameters (by spectral-domain optical coherence tomography) was done. The baseline values obtained in all eyes at two different visits were included in the cross-sectional analysis of functional as well as anatomic parameters (screening and inclusion).

Result: The study enrolled 76 subjects: RESCUE ($n = 39$) and REVERSE ($n = 37$). In comparison with REVERSE subjects, there was significantly worse mean BCVA among RESCUE subjects (1.29 and 1.61 LogMAR respectively, $p = 0.0029$). Compared to RESCUE subjects, REVERSE subjects had significantly more impairment in mean CS and HVF ($p < 0.005$). The monthly reduction in ganglion cell layer macular volume, BCVA, and retinal nerve fiber layer thickness was found to be much more pronounced in the first 6 months following onset (+0.24 LogMAR, −0.06 mm^3, and −6.00 μm, respectively) as compared to that between 6 and 12 months following onset (+0.02 LogMAR, −0.01 mm^3, and −0.43 μm, respectively).

Conclusion: A rapid progression occurs in LHON in the first months after onset during the subacute phase, which is followed by relative stabilization while in the dynamic phase.

COMMENT

The RESCUE and REVERSE are clinical trials on Leber hereditary optic neuropathy (LHON) using *rAAV2/2-ND4* gene therapy. Analysis of the baseline parameters showed that LHON progressed rapidly in the first months following onset during the subacute phase, followed by a relative stabilization during the dynamic phase. These important trials on ND4-LHON are still in progress and results are eagerly awaited on potential efficacy to control this devastatingly blinding disease.

ARTICLE 8

Different Rates of Progression of Disease in Subgroups of Patients with Different Deletions Amenable to Exon Skipping Therapy in Duchenne Muscular Dystrophy

Coratti G, Pane M, Brogna C, Ricotti V, Messina S, D'Amico A, et al; on behalf of the International DMD Group and the iMDEX Consortium. North Star Ambulatory Assessment changes in ambulant Duchenne boys amenable to skip exons 44, 45, 51, and 53: A 3 year follow up.
PLoS One. 2021;16(6):e0253882.

Abstract

Introduction: This study aimed at reporting longitudinal changes occurring in 36 months through the North Star Ambulatory Assessment (NSAA) among ambulatory patients affected by Duchenne muscular dystrophy amenable to skip exons 44, 45, 51, or 53.

Material and Methods: Total 101 patients were enrolled; out of these, deletions amenable to skip exon 44, 25 exon 45, 19 exon 51, and 28 exon 53 were present in 34 patients, who were not enrolled in any continuing clinical trials. Five patients were counted to skip exon 51 and 53 as there was single deletion of exon 52.

Result: There was significant difference between subgroups (skip 44, 45, 51, and 53) at 12 ($p = 0.043$), 24 ($p = 0.005$), and 36 months ($p \leq 0.001$). There were lower baseline values and more negative changes in mutations amenable to skip exons 53 and 51 as compared to the other subgroups. Whereas higher scores at baseline and follow-up were present in those amenable to skip exon 44.

Conclusion: The findings of this study results in confirmation of different progression of disease among subgroups of patients having deletions amenable to skip different exons. The information provided by study is important because the NSAA is currently being used in long-term clinical trials in these subgroups of mutations.

COMMENT

Using North Star Ambulatory Assessment (NSAA) as the outcome measure, different base severity and rates of progression of Duchenne muscular dystrophy (DMD) was demonstrated between subgroups of patients with different deletions amenable to exon skipping therapy in DMD with exon 51 and 53 deletions showing worse level of severity and progress, compared to 44 and 45 deletions. Given the specificity of antisense oligonucleotides effective for the different exon deletions, this study provided important clinical clues for targeted mutation studies and therapeutic decision making.

ARTICLE 9

Delphi-method Consensus-derived Canadian Outcome Measurement Toolkit Claimed to Improve Monitoring and Assessment of Adult SMA Patients

Slayter J, Hodgkinson V, Lounsberry J, Brais B, Chapman K, Genge A. A Canadian adult spinal muscular atrophy outcome measures toolkit: Results of a National Consensus using a Modified Delphi Method.
J Neuromuscul Dis. 2021;8(4):579-88.

Abstract

Introduction: Spinal muscular atrophy (SMA) is rarely found disease, known to affect 1 in 11,000 live births. Novel disease-modifying therapies which need high-quality data for informing decisions about therapy initiation as well as continuation have recently been developed in SMA treatments. There are no nationally agreed upon outcome measures (OMs) used in SMA among adults in Canada. Standardization of OM is required for obtaining high-quality data which is similar across neuromuscular clinics.

Objective: The present study aimed at developing recommended toolkit as well as timing of outcome measures for evaluation of SMA in adulthood.

Methods: With panel of expert clinicians who treated adult patients with SMA in Canada, modified Delphi method comprising of two virtual voting rounds followed by virtual conference was used.

Result: A toolkit (derived from consensus) comprising eight outcome measures was created in three domains of function, in addition to extra three optional measures. Optimal evaluation frequency was 12 months in case of majority of patients irrespective of therapeutic availability, whereas patients who were in 1st year of receiving disease-modifying therapy were suggested to be evaluated frequently.

Conclusion: Implementing the consensus-derived outcome measures toolkit may help in improvement of monitoring as well as evaluation of adult patients with SMA, and improve the quality of real-world evidence. As novel evidence is accessible, it is suggested that the toolkit must be updated on a regular basis.

COMMENT

Delphi-method Consensus-derived Canadian Outcome Measurement 8-outcome measures toolkit claimed to improve monitoring and assessment of adult spinal muscular atrophy (SMA) patients. Periodicity of follow-up recommended was frequent in the first year and thereafter, yearly.

ARTICLE 10

AI-based Model from Data of Two Largest Cohort Imaging Studies in HD TRACK-HD PREDICT-HD and Structural MRI Changes Together Predict Huntington Disease Progress

Wijeratne PA, Garbarino S, Gregory S, Johnson EB, Scahill RI, Paulsen JS, et al. Revealing the timeline of structural MRI changes in premanifest to manifest Huntington disease.
Neurol Genet. 2021;7(5):e617.

Abstract

Introduction: For finding progression of disease in neurodegenerative diseases, one of the powerful markers is longitudinal measurement of brain atrophy by using structural magnetic resonance imaging (sMRI).

Objective: In this study, we use a disease progression model was used in present study for learning individual-level disease times and therefore, demonstrate novel timeline of sMRI changes among patients with Huntington disease (HD).

Methods: For training and testing the model, data was taken from the two largest cohort imaging studies in HD: TRACK-HD (n = 284:104 premanifest, 80 manifest, and 100 controls) and PREDICT-HD (n = 159, 128 premanifest and 36 controls). The study involved longitudinally registering T1-weighted sMRI scans from three consecutive time points for decreasing intraindividual variability as well as calculating regional brain volumes through an automated segmentation tool with rigorous manual quality control.

Result: To the best of our knowledge, this is the first study that demonstrated the relative magnitude as well as timescale of subcortical and cortical atrophy changes among those with HD. It was found that there were largest (nearly 20% average change in magnitude) and earliest (about 2 years prior to average abnormality) alterations in the subcortex (pallidum, putamen, and caudate), and then subsequently cascade of changes occur in other subcortical and cortical regions during duration of about 11 years. It was also found that sMRI, on combining with the present study disease progression model, gives improvement in predicting onset compared to the present best method (root mean square error = 4.5 years and maximum error = 7.9 years versus root mean square error = 6.6 years and maximum error = 18.2 years).

Conclusion: The results of this study support using disease progression modeling for demonstrating novel information from sMRI that can possibly advise imaging marker selection for clinical trials.

COMMENT

Artificial intelligence (AI)-based model together from data of two largest cohort imaging studies from Huntington disease (HD) TRACK-HD and PREDICT-HD found that structural magnetic resonance imaging (MRI) changes predict HD progress.

GENETIC SCREENING

ARTICLE 1

WISCOSIN Newborn Screening for SMA: 1/10000 Prevalence; both Timely SMN2 Information and SMN1 and SMN2 Confirmation as Parts of the Algorithm Facilitated Timely Clinical Follow-up, Family Counseling, and Treatment Planning

Baker MW, Mochal ST, Dawe SJ, Wiberley-Bradford AE, Cogley MF, Zeitler BR, et al. Newborn screening for spinal muscular atrophy: The Wisconsin first year experience.
Neuromuscul Disord. 2022;32(2):135-41.

Abstract

Recently, addition of spinal muscular atrophy was done to the Wisconsin newborn screening panel. In this study, methods of screening, algorithm, as well as outcomes were reported. For recognition of newborns with homozygous survival motor neuron gene 1 (*SMN1*) exon 7 deletion, multiplex real-time PCR assay was utilized. The specimens of those newborns were subjected to droplet digital polymerase chain reaction (PCR) assay to evaluate SMN2 copy number. Collection of an independent dried blood spot specimen was done and evaluation was done for confirming the results of initial screening for SMN1 and SMN2. The screening of 60,984 newborns was done for spinal muscular atrophy during October 15, 2019 to October 14, 2020. Positive screening results were present in six newborns, which confirmed spinal muscular atrophy, rendering birth prevalence of Wisconsin spinal muscular atrophy to be 1 in 10,164. Among these six infants, two copies of SMN2 were present in two patients, three copies of SMN2 in two patients, and four copies of SMN2 in two patients. Zolgensma therapy was given to five newborns, and Spinraza therapy to one newborn. The positive predictive value of present study screening methods was 100%. The comprehensive approach of this study enabled timely clinical follow-up, family counseling, and planning of treatment by offering timely SMN2 information as well as SMN1 and SMN2 confirmation as part of the algorithm for newborn screening for spinal muscular atrophy.

COMMENT

Spinal muscular atrophy (SMA) was added to Newborn Screening in Wisconsin recently and this revealed a prevalence of 1/10,000 in the Wisconsin cohort registry. Survival motor neuron gene 1 (*SMA 1*) screening was done looking for SMN1 homozygosity and *SMA2* by looking for 2, 3, or 4 copies of SMN2. SMN1 and SMN2 confirmation as parts of the algorithm. SMN1 diagnosis used multiplex real-time polymerase chain reaction (M-PCR) for *SMN* gene exon seven deletions and for the SMN2 copy numbers, digital polymerase chain reaction (PCR) assays. The positive predictive value was 100%. Treatments like nusinersen and onasemnogene abeparvovec were given as treatment was given to all six newborns detected to have SMA.

PREVALENCE STUDIES

ARTICLE 1

The IPaNeMA Study: Using Clinical, CPK and GAA Fluorometric Method, Late-onset Pompe Prevalence in Academic, Tertiary Neuromuscular Practices in the United States and Canada is Estimated to be 1%, with an Equal Prevalence Rate of Pseudodeficiency Alleles

Wencel M, Shaibani A, Goyal NA, Dimachkie MM, Trivedi J, Johnson NE, et al. Investigating Late-Onset Pompe Prevalence in Neuromuscular Medicine Academic Practices.
Neurol Genet. 2021;7(6):e623.

Abstract

Background and Objectives: We investigated the prevalence of late-onset Pompe disease (LOPD) in patients presenting to 13 academic, tertiary neuromuscular practices in the United States and Canada.

Methods: All successive patients presenting with proximal muscle weakness or isolated hyperCKemia and/or neck muscle weakness to these 13 centers were invited to participate in the study. Whole blood was tested for acid alpha-glucosidase (GAA) assay through the fluorometric method, and all cases with enzyme levels of ≤10 pmoL/punch/h were reflexed to molecular testing for mutations in the *GAA* gene. Clinical and demographic information was abstracted from their clinical visit and, along with study data, entered into a purpose-built REDCap database, and analyzed at the University of California, Irvine.

Result: Acid alpha-glucosidase enzyme assay results were available on 906 of the 921 participants who consented for the study. LOPD was confirmed in nine participants (1% prevalence). Another nine (1%) were determined to have pseudodeficiency of GAA, whereas 19 (1.9%) were found to be heterozygous for a pathogenic *GAA* mutation (carriers). Of the definite LOPD participants, eight (89%) were Caucasian and were heterozygous for the common leaky (IVS1) splice site mutation in the *GAA* gene (c32-13T>G), with a second mutation that was previously confirmed to be pathogenic.

Discussion: The prevalence of LOPD in undiagnosed patients meeting the criteria of proximal muscle weakness, high creatine kinase, and/or neck weakness in academic, tertiary neuromuscular practice in the United States and Canada is estimated to be 1%, with an equal prevalence rate of pseudodeficiency alleles.

COMMENT

The IPaNeMA study: Based on clinical methods, CPK assay, and estimation of GAA by fluorometric methods, late-onset Pompe prevalence in an academic, and tertiary neuromuscular practice in the United States and Canada was estimated to be 1%, with an equal prevalence rate of pseudodeficiency alleles.

ARTICLE 2

CADASIL Defining Cysteine Altering Stroke Associated NOTCH3 Variants Common in Korean Population, Around 10/1000 Compared to Rare 2–5/1, 00,000 Prevalence in West

Kang CH, Kim YM, Kim YJ, Hong SJ, Kim DY, Woo HG, Kim YR et al. Pathogenic *NOTCH3* variants are frequent among the Korean general population.
Neurol Genet. 2021;7 (6):e639.

Abstract

Objective: The aim of present study was to find the prevalence of pathogenic *NOTCH3* variants in Korean patients.

Methods: The present study was a cross-sectional study, which involved assessment of pathogenic NOTCH3 variants among two Korean public genome databases: The Korean Reference Genome Database (KRGDB) and the Korean Genome Project (Korea1K). The study also involved screening of three most common pathogenic NOTCH3 variants (p.Arg544Cys, p.Arg75Pro, and p.Arg578Cys) in 1,000 individuals on Jeju Island, which reported highest number of patients in Korea who had cerebral autosomal dominant arteriopathy with subcortical infarcts and leukoencephalopathy (CADASIL).

Result: In the Korea1K database, 0.44% of sequences had three pathogenic variants—p. Arg182Cys, p.Arg75Pro, and p.Arg544Cys; 0.12% of sequences in the KRGDB had pathogenic NOTCH3 variant (p.Arg544Cys). Among 1,000 natives of Jeju Island, there were two cysteine-altering NOTCH3 variants (p.Arg544Cys variant in nine and p.Arg578Cys in one individual) among 1% of the participants (95% confidence interval 0.48–1.83%). There was significantly association between presence of cysteine-altering NOTCH3 variants and history of stroke ($p < 0.001$).

Discussion: NOTCH3 pathogenic variants are common in the general Korean population. Increased frequency of pathogenic variants can endanger health of the brain of tens of thousands to hundreds of thousands of old age Korean adults.

Cerebral autosomal dominant arteriopathy with subcortical infarcts and leukoencephalopathy was known as a rare genetic disorder with an estimated prevalence of 2–5/100,000. However, recent genomic database research clearly indicates an estimated global mutation prevalence of 3.4/1,000, much higher than that estimated previously. In particular, the East or South Asian regions showed the highest frequency of cysteine-altering NOTCH3 mutations with a prevalence of 9.0–11.7/1,000 individuals. This study aimed to determine the frequency of pathogenic NOTCH3 variants among Koreans.

COMMENT

Jeju Island, in Korea reported the highest number of patients in Korea. Cerebral autosomal dominant arteriopathy with subcortical infarcts and leukoencephalopathy (CADASIL) defining cysteine altering stroke associated NOTCH3 variants common in Korean population, Around 10/1,000 compared to rare 2–5/100,000 prevalence in West. On screening of three most common pathogenic NOTCH3 variants (p.Arg544Cys, p.Arg75Pro, and p.Arg578Cys) in 1,000 individuals, there was significantly association between presence of cysteine-altering NOTCH3 variants and history of stroke ($p < 0.001$).

Technical Abbreviations

SE	:	(Standard error) Deleted
CPK	:	Creatinine phosphokinase
rAAV	:	Recombinant adeno-associated virus
ND4	:	NADH dehydrogenase protein subunit 4
TREM	:	Triggering receptor expressed on myeloid cells
S100	:	Protein group with solubility in a 100%-saturated solution with ammonium sulphate at neutral pH
GARS	:	Glycyl-tRNA synthetase (A: Adenine; T: Thymine; G: Guanine; C: Cytosine; U: Uracil)
KCNC1	:	Potassium voltage-gated channel subfamily C member 1
SACS	:	Sacsin
DHDDS	:	Dehydrodolichyl diphosphate (dedol-PP) synthase
CACNA2D2	:	Voltage-dependent calcium channel subunit alpha2delta-2
NAXE	:	NAD(P)HX epimerase
AFG3L2	:	AFG3-like protein 2
STUB1	:	STIP1 homology and U-box containing protein 1
CLN6	:	Ceroid-lipofuscinosis neuronal protein 6
CHD2	:	Chromodomain-helicase-DNA-binding protein 2
CerS1	:	Ceramide synthase 1 (p.Arg544Cys, p.Arg75Pro, and p.Arg578Cys)

Section 15: Demyelination

Section Editor: Netravathi M

ARTICLE 1

Disease-modifying Therapies in Relapsing-remitting Multiple Sclerosis: A Systematic Review and Network Meta-analysis

Liu Z, Liao Q, Wen H, Zhang Y. Disease modifying therapies in relapsing-remitting multiple sclerosis: A systematic review and network meta-analysis.
Autoimmun Rev. 2021;20(6):102826.

Abstract

The objective of the study was to compare the efficacy and compliance of disease-modifying therapies (DMTs) in patients with remitting-relapsing multiple sclerosis (RRMS) by performing a systematic review and network meta-analysis. They included 21 studies; the risk of relapses for most DMTs except Betaseron 50 µg was significantly lower comparing to placebo. Non-compliance in patients treated with DMTs was not significantly increased comparing to placebo. Dimethyl fumarate and ocrelizumab had superiority in improving magnetic resonance imaging (MRI) outcomes. Ocrelizumab and ofatumumab had the largest reduction of risk in disability progression at 3 months. Ofatumumab, alemtuzumab, and natalizumab showed the best efficacy and compliance. In conclusions, the present study demonstrated the hierarchy of DMTs treating RRMS. Ofatumumab, alemtuzumab, and natalizumab have superiority with respect to effectiveness and compliance. More studies are required to explore the long-term effect of DMTs. The findings could provide helpful information and contribute to clinical treatment decision-making.

COMMENT

This meta-analysis gives a clear information regarding the efficacy of various disease-modifying therapies (DMTs) especially in terms of their clinical and radiological effects. A DMT is deemed beneficial when it decreases the relapse rate, disability, disease progression, and also improves radiological outcome on magnetic resonance imaging (MRI). Hence, having a knowledge on the hierarchy of the DMTs gives a clear indication on the change of DMT a neurologist should undertake during multiple sclerosis (MS) treatment especially in deciding whether to escalate the therapy in cases of nonresponsiveness to the treatment. Among the available DMTs; ofatumumab, alemtuzumab, and natalizumab showed superiority with respect to effectiveness and compliance.

ARTICLE 2

Multiple Sclerosis, Disease-modifying Therapies and COVID-19: A Systematic Review on Immune Response and Vaccination Recommendations

Cabreira V, Abreu P, Soares-Dos-Reis R, Guimarães J, Sá MJ. Multiple sclerosis, disease-modifying therapies and COVID-19: A systematic review on immune response and vaccination recommendations.
Vaccines (Basel). 2021;9(7):773.

Abstract

This study analyses the risks of COVID-19 in patients with multiple sclerosis (MS) receiving disease-modifying therapies (DMTs) and their immune response to vaccination. A systematic review on COVID-19 course and outcomes in patients receiving different DMTs was conducted with data from 4,417 patients. Having MS per se does not carry a high risk of severe COVID-19; advanced age, comorbidities, and higher disability significantly impact COVID-19 outcomes. Most DMTs have a negligible influence on COVID-19 incidence and outcome, except for those causing severe lymphopenia and hypogammaglobulinemia, such as anti-CD20 therapies, there might be a tendency of increased hospitalization, worse outcomes, and a higher risk of reinfection. Blunted immune responses have been reported for many DMTs, with vaccination implications. Clinical evidence does not support an increased risk of MS relapse or vaccination failure, but vaccination timing needs to be individually tailored. For cladribine and alemtuzumab, it is recommended to wait 3–6 months after the last cycle until vaccination. For the general anti-CD20 therapies, vaccination must be deferred toward the end of the cycle and the next dose administered at least 4–6 weeks after completing vaccination. Serological status after vaccination is highly encouraged.

COMMENT

This article focuses on a very important topic of the risk of COVID-19 in a patient with multiple sclerosis (MS) especially in relation to the various disease-modifying therapies (DMTs) and the effect of vaccination when patients are on DMTs. The medications that cause lymphopenia and hypogammaglobulinemia (anti-CD20 therapy) may have higher risk of developing severe COVID-19 whereas MS per se does not cause increased risk of developing the infection. As there will be blunted immune response to the various DMTs, they have to be well-timed in relation to the infusion therapies so that there will be good adequate immunity following the COVID vaccination.

ARTICLE 3

Prodromal Emesis in Myelin Oligodendrocyte Glycoprotein-antibody-associated Disorder

Netravathi M, Holla VV, Saini J, Mahadevan A. Prodromal emesis in MOG-antibody associated disorder. *Mult Scler Relat Disord. 2022;58:103463.*

Abstract

This study aimed to evaluate the occurrence of emesis in patients of demyelinating disorders and determine their clinical and radiological features. Among 551 patients of central nervous system (CNS) demyelinating disorders; exclusive emesis without hiccups was observed in 1 (0.1%) patient of multiple sclerosis (MS), 17 (6.5%) patients of myelin oligodendrocyte glycoprotein-antibody-associated disorder (MOGAD) while none in aquaporin-4 (AQP4)-Ab-associated disorders ($p < 0.001$). There were 17 (M:F—8:9) patients with exclusive emesis in MOGAD with predominance seen in pediatric (58.8%) age group, followed by adults (35.3%) and late-onset (5.9%). ADEMON [acute demyelinating encephalomyelitis (ADEM) followed by optic neuritis] was observed in seven patients. Preceding clinical syndrome was optic neuritis (ON) (41.2%), brainstem syndrome (BS) (23.5%), involvement of both ON and BS in 23.5%, myelopathy (11.8%). Magnetic resonance imaging (MRI) analysis showed combination of lesions affecting the brainstem (11), ON (10), juxtacortical white matter (10), and periventricular lesions (3). Odds ratio for the presence of ADEM, lesions in medulla, pons, middle cerebellar peduncle (MCP), or any of the three areas was found to be significant. In conclusions, exclusive emesis without hiccups appears to be common in MOGAD and may occur as a prodromal illness or exclusive clinical episode. It is known to occur most commonly in association with ADEM and/or ON.

COMMENT

Area postrema syndrome is a core clinical feature very commonly observed in aquaporin-4 (AQP4)-related neuromyelitis optica (NMO) spectrum disorder. This study shows partial area postrema syndrome in the form of exclusive emesis to be more commonly seen in patients with myelin oligodendrocyte glycoprotein-antibody-associated disorder (MOGAD). They have also observed that among the different subtypes of MOGAD; exclusive emesis was most common feature in patients of acute demyelinating encephalomyelitis (ADEM) and/or optic neuritis.

ARTICLE 4

A Comparison of the Effects of Rituximab versus Other Immunotherapies for Myelin Oligodendrocyte Glycoprotein Immunoglobulin G-associated Central Nervous System Demyelination: A Meta-analysis

Bai P, Zhang M, Yuan J, Zhu R, Li N. A comparison of the effects of rituximab versus other immunotherapies for MOG-IgG-associated central nervous system demyelination: A meta-analysis.
Mult Scler Relat Disord. 2021;53:103044.

Abstract

Myelin oligodendrocyte glycoprotein-antibody-associated disorder (MOGAD) is now recognized as a nosological entity with specific clinical and paraclinical features. This study performed a meta-analysis to evaluate rituximab (RTX) efficacy and assessed the treatment efficacies based on relapse rates. A meta-analysis of five studies with 239 participants was conducted. Patients have received RTX in 82 of 239 (34.31%). The mean difference of annualized relapse rate (ARR) ratio of RTX therapy versus other immunotherapies was 0.16 [95% confidence interval (CI)–0.15 to 0.47]. No studies found to significantly affect heterogeneity. No major differences occurred in 9.2% of China patients (95% CI −0.20 to 1.86; $I^2 = 0$%) and 90.8% of non-China patients (95% CI −0.24 to 0.42; $I^2 = 0$%). Meanwhile there was no significant subgroup difference ($p = 0.18$) between them. In conclusion, RTX reduces the relapse frequency in most patients with MOGAD, but there is no differences between RTX and other immunotherapies in MOGAD.

COMMENT

Myelin oligodendrocyte glycoprotein-antibody-associated disorder (MOGAD) has been established to be a distinct entity from aquaporin-4 (AQP4)-neuromyelitis optica spectrum disorder (NMOSD). This study conducted a meta-analysis to study the difference in clinical response between rituximab and other immunotherapies.

There have been few case series that have showed rituximab to be less effective compared to other immunosuppressants especially in few subtypes of MOGAD. Hence, knowledge on the subtype of MOGAD and its management with rituximab or various immunosuppressants needs to be evaluated in future studies.

ARTICLE 5

Treatment of Myelin Oligodendrocyte Glycoprotein Immunoglobulin G-associated Disease in Paediatric Patients: A Systematic Review

da Costa BK, Banwell BL, Sato DK. Treatment of MOG-IgG associated disease in paediatric patients: A systematic review. *Mult Scler Relat Disord. 2021;56:103216.*

Abstract

This study aimed to perform a systematic review of the literature on treatment of pediatric patients (≤18 years) with MOG-IgG-antibody-associated disorder (MOGAD). They found 72 noncontrolled studies (observational studies, case reports, and expert recommendations). The most commonly reported acute phase treatment was intravenous methylprednisolone in 88% followed by oral steroids in 67%, intravenous human immunoglobulin (IVIG) in 66%, and plasma exchange in 33% of the studies. Long-term maintenance treatment was described by 53 studies mainly in relapsing disease course. The most frequently reported treatments were prolonged oral corticosteroids in 53% of the studies followed by azathioprine (51%), mycophenolate mofetil (45%), rituximab (41%), and periodic intravenous immunoglobulin (26%). In conclusions, long-term treatment in relapsing MOGAD pediatric patients are not those that have shown higher reduction in the annualized relapse rate in observational studies. Randomized controlled trials (RCTs) with standardized outcomes are needed to confirm the safety and efficacy of current and new treatments.

COMMENT

This meta-analysis aimed to study the efficacy of various medications in pediatric myelin oligodendrocyte glycoprotein-antibody-associated disorder (MOGAD). But there were no standard established clear treatment protocols followed and there were multiple various medications both in the acute as well as maintenance therapy.

ARTICLE 6

Distinct Patterns of Magnetic Resonance Imaging Lesions in Myelin Oligodendrocyte Glycoprotein-antibody Disease and Aquaporin-4 Neuromyelitis Optica Spectrum Disorder: A Systematic Review and Meta-analysis

Carandini T, Sacchi L, Bovis F, Azzimonti M, Bozzali M, Galimberti D, et al. Distinct patterns of MRI lesions in MOG antibody disease and AQP4 NMOSD: A systematic review and meta-analysis.
Mult Scler Relat Disord. 2021;54:103118.

Abstract

Distinct magnetic resonance imaging (MRI) features of myelin oligodendrocyte glycoprotein-antibody-associated disorder (MOGAD) and aquaporin-4 (AQP4)-neuromyelitis optica spectrum disorder (NMOSD) are still poorly defined. This study aimed to identify specific patterns of MRI abnormalities able to discriminate between MOGAD and AQP4-NMOSD. 14 case-series (1,028 patients) were included in the meta-analysis. MOGAD showed a higher number of MRI lesions than AQP4-NMOSD patients in the retrobulbar optic neuritis (ON) [odds ratio (OR) 5.67; 95% confidence interval (CI) 2.11–15.24; $p = 0.0006$] with ON head swelling (OR 8.20; 95% CI 4.13–16.28; $p < 0.00001$), corpus callosum (OR 2.30; 95% CI 1.11–4.76; $p = 0.02$), pons (OR 2.87; 95% CI 1.45–5.67; $p = 0.002$), and lumbar/conus spinal cord (SC) (OR 3.47; 95% CI 1.66–7.24; $p = 0.0009$). Conversely, lesions in the canalicular (OR 0.42; 95% CI 0.18–0.98; $p = 0.05$) and intracranial optic nerve (ON) (OR 0.30; 95% CI 0.11–0.84; $p = 0.02$), area postrema (OR 0.12; 95% CI 0.02–0.61; $p = 0.01$), medulla (OR 0.40; 95% CI 0.20–0.78; $p = 0.007$), and cervical SC (OR 0.29; 95% CI 0.09–0.92; $p = 0.04$) were prominent in patients with AQP4-NMOSD. In conclusions, this study provides further evidence that MOGAD and AQP4-NMOSD have distinct MRI features that may help clinicians for an early differential diagnosis.

COMMENT

Distinction between aquaporin-4 (AQP4) and myelin oligodendrocyte glycoprotein-antibody-associated disorder (MOGAD) is very important especially when the antibody reports are delayed or not available in view of financial constraints. Knowledge on the various areas of anatomical predilection helps in better understanding the disorder and initiating early adequate treatment.

ARTICLE 7

Brain Magnetic Resonance Imaging Activity during the Year before Pregnancy can Predict Postpartum Clinical Relapses

Lehmann H, Zveik O, Levin N, Brill L, Imbar T, Vaknin-Dembinsky A. Brain MRI activity during the year before pregnancy can predict post-partum clinical relapses.
Mult Scler. 2021;27(14):2232-9.

Abstract

There are fewer multiple sclerosis (MS) relapses during pregnancy, although relapse risk increases in the early postpartum period. The aim of this study was to evaluate the correlation between magnetic resonance imaging (MRI) changes in the year before pregnancy and the relapse rate in the year following postpartum. This was an observational retrospective case–control study that included 172 pregnancies in 118 females with MS. It was found a significant correlation for an active-MRI prepregnancy and relapses in the first 3 months postpartum ($p < 0.001$). Expanded disability status scale (EDSS) prepregnancy and relapses in the first 3 months postpartum were also significantly correlated ($p = 0.009$). In conclusions, an active-MRI in the prepregnancy period is a strong and sensitive predictor of early postpartum relapse, regardless of whether the woman had clinical evidence of disease activity prior to conception and delivery. This finding could provide clinicians with a strategy to minimize postpartum relapse risk in women with MS planning pregnancy.

COMMENT

Management of pregnancy is an important issue in people with multiple sclerosis (MS). It is very well known that there should not be clinical relapse and to have adequate control of MS symptoms prior to conception. This study also adds yet another magnetic resonance imaging (MRI) feature apart from clinical status so that postpartum relapse are prevented. Having absence of MRI disease activity prior to conception prevents postpartum relapse in patients of MS.

ARTICLE 8

A Randomized Study of Natalizumab Dosing Regimens for Relapsing-remitting Multiple Sclerosis

Trojano M, Ramió-Torrentà L, Grimaldi LME, Lubetzki C, Schippling S, Evans KC, et al. A randomized study of natalizumab dosing regimens for relapsing-remitting multiple sclerosis.
Mult Scler. 2021;27(14):2240-53.

Abstract

REFINE was an exploratory, dose- and frequency-blinded, prospective, randomized, study in relapsing-remitting multiple sclerosis (RRMS) patients. The objective was to examine the efficacy, safety, and tolerability of natalizumab administered via various regimens in RRMS patients. Clinically stable RRMS patients previously treated with 300 mg natalizumab intravenously for ≥12 months were randomized to one of six natalizumab regimens over 60 weeks: 300 mg administered intravenously or subcutaneously every 4 weeks (Q4W), 300 mg intravenously or subcutaneously every 12 weeks (Q12W), or 150 mg intravenously or subcutaneously Q12W. This study enrolled 290 patients. All Q12W dosing arms were associated with increased clinical and magnetic resonance imaging (MRI) disease activity and was closed early. In the 300 mg intravenous and subcutaneous Q4W arms, the mean cumulative number of combined unique active MRI lesions was 0.23 and 0.02, respectively; annualized relapse rates were 0.07 and 0.08, respectively; and trough natalizumab serum levels and α4-integrin saturation were comparable. Natalizumab 300 mg subcutaneous Q4W was comparable to 300 mg intravenous Q4W dosing with respect to efficacy, pharmacokinetics/pharmacodynamics, and safety.

COMMENT

This study is very important in studying the various natalizumab regimens. This is done basically to extend the dosing period so as to prevent the occurrence of progressive multifocal leukoencephalopathy (PML) as well as decrease the infusion dosage interval. This study found that: (i) Extending the dosage interval from 4 to 12 weeks was not helpful. (ii) Subcutaneous natalizumab was comparable to intravenous natalizumab thus it helps in decreasing the hospital visits, and may also improve adherence and compliance.

ARTICLE 9

Treatment Escalation versus Immediate Initiation of Highly Effective Treatment for Patients with Relapsing-remitting Multiple Sclerosis: Data from 2 Different National Strategies

Spelman T, Magyari M, Piehl F, Svenningsson A, Rasmussen PV, Kant M, et al. Treatment escalation vs immediate initiation of highly effective treatment for patients with relapsing-remitting multiple sclerosis: Data from 2 different National Strategies.
JAMA Neurol. 2021;78(10):1197-204.

Abstract

Treatment strategies for relapsing-remitting multiple sclerosis (RRMS) vary markedly between Denmark and Sweden. This study aimed to investigate the association of national differences in disease-modifying treatment (DMT) strategies for RRMS with disability outcomes. This cohort study used data on 4,861 patients from the Danish and Swedish national multiple sclerosis (MS) registries. A total of 2,700 patients from the Swedish MS registry [1,867 women (69.2%); mean standard deviation (SD) age, 36.1 (9.5) years] and 2,161 patients from the Danish MS registry [1,472 women (68.1%); mean (SD) age, 37.3 (9.4) years] started a first DMT between 2013 and 2016, were included in the analysis, and were observed for a mean (SD) of 4.1 (1.5) years. A total of 1,994 Danish patients (92.3%) initiated a low to moderately effective DMT [teriflunomide, 907 (42.0%)] and 165 (7.6%) initiated a highly effective DMT, whereas a total of 1,769 Swedish patients (65.5%) initiated a low to moderately effective DMT [teriflunomide, 64 (2.4%)] and 931 (34.5%) initiated a highly effective DMT. The Swedish treatment strategy was associated with a 29% reduction in the rate of postbaseline 24-week confirmed disability worsening relative to the Danish treatment strategy [hazard ratio (HR) 0.71; 95% confidence interval (CI) 0.57–0.90; $p = 0.004$]. The Swedish treatment strategy was also associated with a 24% reduction in the rate of reaching an expanded disability status scale score of 3 (HR 0.76; 95% CI 0.60–0.97; $p = 0.03$) and a 25% reduction in the rate of reaching an expanded disability status scale score of 4 (HR 0.75; 95% CI 0.61–0.96; $p = 0.01$) relative to Danish patients. The findings of this study suggest that there is an association between differences in treatment strategies for RRMS and disability outcomes at a national level. Escalation of treatment efficacy was inferior to using more efficacious DMT as initial treatment.

COMMENT

This study studied the disease-modifying treatment (DMT) usage pattern in two nations of Denmark and Sweden and found that escalation therapy was inferior to the usage of more efficacious DMTs in the treatment of relapsing-remitting multiple sclerosis (RRMS). Presently, it is a well-known fact that multiple sclerosis (MS) has both inflammatory phase in the initial period followed by degenerative phase. It is important to control the illness in the inflammatory phase by using more efficacious DMTs and prevent patients to progress to secondary progressive MS.

Section 16: Social Aspects of Neurology

Section Editor: Sudhir Shah

Associate Editors: Akanksha Jain, Zubin A Shah, Amey Bhise, Gaurav Shah, Umangkumar M Patel, Andelwar SL

ARTICLE 1

American Academy of Neurology Position Statement: Ethical Issues in Clinical Research in Neurology

Tolchin B, Conwit R, Epstein LG, Russell JA; Ethics, Law, and Humanities Committee, a joint committee of the American Academy of Neurology, American Neurological Association, and Child Neurology Society. AAN position statement: Ethical issues in clinical research in neurology.
Neurology. 2020;94(15):661-9.

Abstract

Aim: To provide guidance for ethical conduct in neurologic research involving human participants.

Clinical research involves work with human participants with the aim to develop or increase our knowledge about health and disease. It includes both interventional studies such as clinical trials and observational studies.

Seven principles should be fulfilled for clinical research to be considered ethically permissible.[1,2]

1. Social value—study must have the potential to benefit human health or increase society's knowledge of human biology.
2. Scientific validity—must use accepted scientific methods to produce valid and reproducible results.
3. Fair participant selection—study sites, populations, and participants must be selected based on scientific criteria.
4. Favorable risk–benefit—potential benefits to participants and society should be invariably greater than the risks to participants.
5. Independent review—studies should be reviewed and approved by individuals with appropriate knowledge of the research and are not associated with the research.
6. Informed consent
7. Respect for participants

Various ethical issues arise whenever a research study is planned.
- *Historical concerns institutional review board (IRB) review:* Many researchers believe that risks to participants in most clinical research is minimal, and that the overall costs versus benefits

analysis favors the removal of IRB review. However, eliminating IRBs can weaken the ethical foundation of clinical research and the safety of research participants.
- *Historical concerns: Equitable research participant inclusion*: Research should not exclude or restrict participants by sex, race, ethnicity, or age unless there is a scientific or ethical reason particular to that study.
- *Historical concerns: Cognitive impairment in research participants:* When participants are unable to make an informed consent like in participants with dementia or pediatric groups a legally appointed representative may make the decision on their behalf.[3]
- *Current controversies: International clinical research:* International clinical research in low- and middle-income countries (LMICs) has increased exponentially in the last two decades.[4] However, some companies conduct research in LMIC due to less rigid supervision (as well as lower study costs). Also, some individuals in LMICs who otherwise are not able to receive proper healthcare may get tempted to enlist in a clinical study to obtain otherwise unattainable healthcare. Besides there is also a concern that the interests of research participants in LMICs are not always reproduced in studies that are carried out in high-income country (HIC).
- *Current controversies: Replication crisis:* Replication crisis refers to the increasing phenomenon of peer reviewed and widely cited studies that show statistically significant results but the same cannot be replicated by other researchers.[5] It is mainly due to violations of the seven ethical principles mandatory in clinical research. Publication bias is one of the key contributors. To remove this all trials should be preregistered and reported in a timely manner.
- *Imminent ethical issues: Genetic research:* Genetic clinical research has its own ethical issues. There is likelihood of incidentally identifying unexpected genetic information, not related to the research but that is otherwise harmful for the participant. For instance, finding a disease-causing genetic mutation for which treatment is possible or revealing misattributed paternity.
- *Gene editing* that is insertion of self-propagating genetic sequences to modify the genetic makeup of a species has widespread ethical issues. It carries the risk of a new genetic sequence being accidently inserted in an incorrect location leading to undesired consequences.[6] Finally genetic editing of germ cells can even affect future generations.

In all the strict application of ethical principles leads to transparency, consistency, and fairness to ethical research and analysis.

COMMENT

Clinical research is fundamental for the progress of any scientific field. Properly guided research aimed for understanding the concepts of various pathological and physiological entities goes a long way in the advancement of science and development of newer treatment modalities for the benefit of human society. The seven principles of ethical research should be strictly followed. Before undertaking any research, institutional review board (IRB) review is mandatory. It seems to be a tedious process, but it is extremely necessary to see that the research is in the interest of patients and humanity. Steps can be taken to make this IRB approval less tedious and research friendly. Multisite studies can be taken under central IRBs, review of low-risk studies can be reduced, and research participants can be given options for broad consent to future studies. Researchers should disclose relevant conflicts of interest during the informed consent process. To safeguard the interests of participants both in low-income and high-income countries and for a nonbiased research unified guidelines should be made and followed and it should encompass the basic seven ethical principles. This ensures the research and the results of it to be unbiased and true. Also, clinical data, research protocols, statistical analyses, should be shared in open public platforms to remove any bias in the study. Other studies taken on further to check for replication of results as proposed by the original research should be funded and supported. Participants should be provided with an option to be informed—or not—of incidentally discovered results during genetic studies. The participants should be well-informed of the risks and benefits associated with research so as to allow for a free and informed consent without any persuasion or rewards attached.

Overall, ethically conducted clinical research is definitely a fundamental tool for the advancement of Science and society and for the progress of the nation and world as a whole.

ARTICLE 2

Ethical Issues in the Care of People with Dementia

Hughes J, Common J. Ethical issues in caring for patients with dementia.
Nurs Stand. 2015;29(49):42-7.

Abstract

Dementia causes many philosophical problems which add to the various ethical issues that clinicians have to face when caring for these patients.

The primary aim of this article is to focus on promoting autonomy and making best interests decisions. Every day, ethical issues including truth-telling, restriction, and limitations of freedom, exploitation, and liability are considered.[7]

Amnesia, poor attention-span, and reduced impulse control can create issues for general practitioners (GPs) treating people with dementia to acquire consent.

Family, caretakers, and close relatives can help establish the history of the patient and promote autonomy.[7]

Consideration of past and present desires can be a difficult process, and a patient's current best interests should not be ignored.

Rationalizing and reading about everyday ethical issues affecting people with dementia can help GP trainees identify and steer through them successfully when they are present.[8]

COMMENT

Factors to take into account when determining a person's best interests include:
- The person's past and present desires and opinions (in particular any relevant written statements made before the loss of capacity).
- The principles and morals that would have likely influenced the person's decision if they had the capacity.
- The views of others concerned with the person's well-being to determine what action would be in the person's best interests.
- Consider the underlying morals or principles on which the earlier choices were based. Have they honestly changed or can they be taken in a new light? Maybe the person is expressing "old" views or likings in a different way.
- How much suffering or gratification is it causing now? If maintaining a past faith is causing anguish, then it is likely that the person's existing welfare and not their previous independent interests should take preference.
- How important is the matter at stake? For example, maintaining a person's religious practice or moral beliefs are likely to have been much more important to them than issues of aesthetics, taste, or smartness of dress.
- Discover whether the apparent changes in preferences or values result from psychosocial factors or directly from dementia or whether on the other hand they are linked with a genuine gratification in doing things in a different way.

The nature of dementia raises many philosophical questions that may ultimately inform answers to various ethical questions that arise when caring for people with dementia. With so many elements to consider, clear and simple answers are not always easy to find.

ARTICLE 3

Disabling Stroke in Persons already with a Disability: Ethical Dimensions and Directives

Young MJ, Regenhardt RW, Leslie-Mazwi TM, Stein MA. Disabling stroke in persons already with a disability: Ethical dimensions and directives.
Neurology. 2020;94(7):306-10.

Abstract

Stroke is one of the leading cause of death and disability worldwide.[9] Currently mainstream management of acute stroke is intravenous (IV) thrombolysis and mechanical thrombectomy. The aim of these interventions is to restore perfusion and minimize neurological deficit and future disability. A disability is any physical or mental condition that substantially limits a major life activity such as walking, learning, or working. The Rehabilitation Act of 1973 and the Americans with Disabilities Act (ADA) provide official legal standards prohibiting limitation of healthcare services for people with disabilities relative to persons without a disability.[10]

The standard principles of bioethics are justice, respect for autonomy, beneficence, and nonmaleficence. Respect for patient autonomy, is a cornerstone of modern medicine, requires understanding patient preferences and values and allowing these ideals to inform care. When approaching stroke treatment decisions or undertaking advanced care planning, clinicians should understand patient or surrogate preferences, especially when it comes to potentially life-sustaining interventions. If an informed patient or surrogate chooses to forego a treatment, this should be respected and considered.

However, to limit this choice for patients with disabilities or to make the decision on their behalf assuming that such therapies would be undesirable simply because they are disabled is not only discriminatory but is also a total violation of their autonomy.[11] Ultimately the decision to opt in or out of any given treatment should always be in the hands of the patient regardless of disability.

COMMENT

Awareness of the cognitive vulnerabilities, social stigmas, and psychological factors associated with disability that may delay treatment decisions and trial design. The action that follows this awareness will ensure that these social and psychological forces do not magnify the impact of disability on this already vulnerable and growing population.

If reduction of long-term deficits from acute stroke is taken as a major factor deciding treatment course then this should be applied to all regardless of preexisting disabilities. Not providing equal standard of care for patient with disability is unethical and increase long-term costs and poor health outcomes in them.

ARTICLE 4

Driving and Epilepsy: Ethical, Legal, and Healthcare Policy Challenges

Kass JS, Rose RV. Driving and epilepsy: Ethical, legal, and health care policy challenges. *Continuum (Minneap Minn). 2019;25(2):537-42.*

Abstract

To drive a vehicle has become a basic human right of every individual. Driving by an epilepsy patient is a matter of social and legal importance as the patient may have a seizure while driving and cause harm to himself, others, and government property. In such cases, the victim of the accident can go to the court of law to file a case against the epilepsy patient who was driving and the treating neurologist might be made to appear in the court. The role of a neurologist in reporting his patient with epilepsy to the traffic department in view of his fitness to drive is different in different states in the USA.[12] There seems to be a lack of communication on the part of the treating neurologist while counseling the patient about his ability to drive and the risks associated with it.[13] However, state authorities while issuing driving licenses often rely on physicians' clinical assessment. The neurologist must think of counseling his patients with epilepsy about the risks of driving especially in drug resistance and poor compliance cases and if such a person insists upon driving despite proper counseling about the risks involved, neurologists should report such patients to the appropriate government authorities to avoid the imminent danger.

COMMENT

This article while giving examples of various lawsuits involving a doctor, his patient with epilepsy, and the accuser who suffered a road accident due to the patient having a seizure while driving, sheds light on the importance of the topic of epilepsy patients and driving and a neurologist's role in such cases. Although the example given is of the USA, this has worldwide implications as it is a common issue faced by neurologists worldwide. The neurologist tends to focus on treating epilepsy and does not give importance to other social aspects of patient's day-to-day life such as driving which should not be the case. The neurologist should stay up-to-date with his state's recent laws for driving for epilepsy patients and self-driving and act accordingly.

ARTICLE 5

Patients' Views on the Ethical Challenges of Early Parkinson Disease Detection

Schaeffer E, Rogge A, Nieding K, Helmker V, Letsch C, Hauptmann B, et al. Patients' views on the ethical challenges of early Parkinson disease detection.
Neurology. 2020;94(19):e2037-e2044.

Abstract

Early Parkinson's disease (PD) detection helps to decrease or stop degeneration in this disease.[14] The ethical challenges include: (1) the prodromal phase cannot be diagnosed with certainty,[15] (2) the duration between onset of the prodromal phase to motor manifestation is very prolonged—maybe decades, and (3) there is no treatment guidelines for the prodromal phase. In this study, 121 patients with PD according to UK brain bank criteria who could give written informed consent and understand the questionnaire were given 10 questions, and answers were analyzed. It was found that the median time for diagnosis was 1 year and the median of three consultations of general practitioner (GP) was followed by the neurologist was required, among whom 33% had another diagnosis. The most troublesome time was from motor manifestation to treatment initiation in 62%. 85% of patients would have liked to know the risk if they received instructions on lifestyle changes to alter disease. 39% of patients believed that if they would have known the risks they could have changed their lifestyle. 10% of patients thought that it would not be right to inform them about their disease, 23% said that information should be given, and 67% agreed to the risk disclosure under specific conditions. 54% of patients wanted discussion of the results with the family doctor or neurologist. 49% desired to have access to contact a person for regular follow-up.

Time from motor manifestation to final diagnosis, early risk announcement, personal right not to know[16-18] are some of the important aspects to be considered among individuals of this study.

COMMENT

The problem of innumerable consultations and inadequate or incorrect treatments can be reduced by increasing awareness among doctors.

Obtaining consent and risk disclosure among individuals can be critical given the uncertainty of progression of the disease and no disease modifying treatment option available during prodromal phase and it may lead to nervousness or fear. As the risk of disease has to be explained, the patient's right to not know the risk is not possible. So, to allow at-risk individuals to make an autonomous decision, risk disclosure should be merged with individual advice on lifestyle changes, exercise, and diet and appropriate consideration should be given to regular long-term follow-up and support.

ARTICLE 6

Ethical Considerations in Chronic Brain Injury

Hawley L, Hammond FM, Cogan AM, Juengst S, Mumbower R, Pappadis MR, et al. Ethical considerations in chronic brain injury.
J Head Trauma Rehabil. 2019;34(6):433-6.

Abstract

Chronic traumatic brain injury (TBI) varies in severity with the mortality going down due to the advent of new advancements in critical care but there are still long-standing sequelae in varying domains.[19] They carry a huge socioeconomic impact on the patient and their families. The outcome of TBI is heavily influenced by the services available which depends upon individual circumstances such as affordability and hence every patient might not get the best medical care possible. The challenge faced by clinicians working with cases whose outcomes can vary tremendously is ever-growing and needs a case-based approach with taking the relatives into confidence. The future trials regarding TBI should include outcomes that include qualities that are important for individuals with TBI and their families. Community training regarding the role of TBI patients in society is needed and TBI survivors should be a big part of such training activities.[20]

COMMENT

This article emphasizes the need to invest in the availability of affordable state of the art neurocritical care and rehabilitation facilities to the majority of the population. The counseling done by neurologists in cases of traumatic brain injury should not be too negative and too hurried as these patients may have delayed recovery. The patient's caretakers and patients' own thoughts should too be taken into account while prognosticating as the term good outcome can have different meanings for different people. Society's point of view toward patients with traumatic brain injury should change from being a burden on society to an active contributor.

ARTICLE 7

Ethical Principles in Patient-centered Medical Care to Support Quality of Life in Amyotrophic Lateral Sclerosis

Lulé D, Kübler A, Ludolph AC. Ethical principles in patient-centered medical care to support quality of life in amyotrophic lateral sclerosis.
Front Neurol. 2019;10:259.

Abstract

Quality of life (QoL) in amyotrophic lateral sclerosis (ALS) is the general well-being of a person and includes physical, psychological, and social dimensions. It is therefore, not simply a state of physical well-being.[21]

There are different intrinsic and extrinsic factors in medical care to assist QoL in ALS and the personal viewpoint in medical decision-making.

These factors may be included under the four ethical principles of good medical care namely, beneficence, nonmaleficence, autonomy, and justice.[22]

Beneficence: Therapeutic interventions are usually introduced by the physician to assist or increase QoL in ALS.[23]

Nonmaleficence: Maleficence in the sense of the emotional burden of diagnosis can be reduced by using a systematic approach for breaking the news as it may reduce the negative impact on QoL.[24]

Patient's Autonomy: Autonomy includes the sense of ability to make decisions and the feeling of being a creator of one's own action which is a key feature of self-efficacy and thus for QoL.[25]

Justice: This ethical principle of care requires that all patients are treated in an equal way without discrimination or social bias.[26]

COMMENT

Various intrinsic and extrinsic factors that can be used to increase quality of life (QoL) in amyotrophic lateral sclerosis (ALS) patients include:

- Permanent respiratory insufficiency causes disturbed sleep, lethargy, and reduced physical health, all these symptoms may be relieved by ventilation. Thus, ventilation may positively influence QoL. Fear of choking during meals is very common in patients with bulbar symptoms, so many patients fear to eat at all. Thus, insertion of percutaneous endoscopic gastrostomy (PEG) is a very useful approach to improve QoL. Other therapeutic interventions also help QoL such as the application of botox to stop drooling (sialorrhea).
- Aside from therapeutics, there is one key extrinsic factor that may significantly improve QoL which is social support. Family is the most important feature of individual QoL in ALS.
- Preferences regarding therapeutic procedures are highly determined by the patient's personal values, religious views, and cultural background.
- Patients can be included in family decisions and may participate in a daily routine if possible. This allows the patient to be an active part of the daily routine: to participate in decision-making, to be asked questions, to express concerns, address fears and anxieties, express wishes, and hopes.
- There is no justice in defining every person by the diagnosis with a nihilistic view of the disease which has to be prevented under all circumstances. Instead, to grant justice every patient has to be regarded as an individual with specific needs and the right to be treated the same according to his/her preferences, disregarding mental, societal, or financial status.

ARTICLE 8

Ethical, Palliative, and Policy Considerations in Disorders of Consciousness

Fins JJ, Bernat JL. Ethical, palliative, and policy considerations in disorders of consciousness.
Neurology. 2018;91(10):471-5.

Abstract

The American Academy of Neurology (AAN) guidelines for disorders of consciousness (DoC) replaced the term permanent vegetative state with the term chronic vegetative state.[27] The patients suffering from DoC include—first group misdiagnosed as DoC, second group patients who recovered after drugs or neuromodulation, the third group with cognitive-motor dissociation (CMD), and the fourth group who underwent late structural changes recreating network responses necessary for consciousness. Ancillary testing was suggested to avoid failing to identify consciousness when it is present. The guidelines advised reducing the threshold for clinical suspicion of pain suffering in individuals with DoC. Physicians should seek and discuss the patient's known preferences for living in vegetative state or minimally conscious state with the patient's lawful surrogate decision-maker.[28] Our healthcare system must provide the infrastructure and resources needed to offer quality care to patients with DoC.

COMMENT

This article reviews and critics the American Academy of Neurology (AAN) guidelines on disorders of consciousness. The newer terminologies chronic vegetative state and unresponsive wakefulness state are welcomed instead of the old term permanent vegetative state and vegetative state, respectively, this would help to avoid the stigma associated with the old terms and the propensity on part of the caretakers to take the decision to stop life support in view of likely poor outcome. The new terminologies would hopefully bring more enthusiasm in research in disorders of consciousness.

ARTICLE 9

Neuroethics of Neuromodulation: An Update

Zuk P, Torgerson L, Sierra-Mercado D, Lázaro-Muñoz G. Neuroethics of neuromodulation: An update.
Curr Opin Biomed Eng. 2018;8:45-50.

Abstract

During the past decade, there has been significant development in technologies for neuromodulation like deep brain stimulation (DBS), adaptive DBS (aDBS), transcranial magnetic stimulation (TMS), transcranial direct current stimulation (tDCS), and other such technologies. It has also created many ethical issues. Privacy of the patients can be unmasked due to development of detailed data registries.[29] Continued access to devices after the trial period is over can also be problematic due to cost-bearing responsibilities between patients and insurance companies.[30] Do-it-yourself neurostimulation has implications in its possible usage for cognitive enhancements.[31] Media coverage of latest technologies has important bearings on public perception of their possible benefits and disadvantages.[32] Neuromodulation in minors creates an ethical dilemma regarding responsibility for consent.[33] Research in these ethical issues is much needed because it affects the decisions regarding the development and public use of these technologies.

COMMENT

After any new technology has been rolled out for its general use, strict maintenance of registry and database is a must thing to facilitate clinical and research advancements, but with that, there is a risk of revelation of patients' identity. Another issue comes after the trial period is over for any new technology. If the patient has significantly benefited and wants to continue its further use, he might face significant difficulties for the same as insurance companies do not provide coverage for experimental therapies. Though trial conducting authority can offer removal after completion of the study period, the patient or his insurance company needs to bear its extra cost. Transcranial direct current stimulation (tDCS) can be used for cognitive enhancement of concentration and memory and for athletic reinforcement purposes. These may create ethical issues because of inequities they may create between those who have the resources to access these technologies and those who do not. Media plays an important part in creating a public mindset regarding any new technology and the trend has been favorable for most technologies especially for deep brain stimulation (DBS). An overly optimistic and simplified description of these new technologies may create exaggerated expectations for these technologies or create mistrust toward them when expectations are not met in reality. There have been concerns about changes in personality after these neuromodulation technologies. Neuromodulation has its role in refractory movement disorder treatment in minor patients also (< 18 years of age). In this patient population, the question arises of decision-making authority. Who determines what is in the best interest of the child, and who gets to make the final decision about whether neuromodulator interventions are used on children? Thus, the development of various neuromodulation tools also requires thoughtful reflection regarding their ethical aspects. They can be one of the most powerful means currently available for intervening on the human brain. Their refinement through further research promises to be a great contribution to the common good.

ARTICLE 10

The COVID-19 Pandemic and the Ethical Duties of the Neurologist

Rubin MA, Bonnie RJ, Epstein L, Hemphill C, Kirschen M, Lewis A, et al.; Ethics, Law, and Humanities Committee, a Joint Committee of the American Academy of Neurology, American Neurological Association, and Child Neurology Society; in collaboration with the Neurocritical Care Society Ethics Committee. AAN position statement: The COVID-19 pandemic and the ethical duties of the neurologist.
Neurology. 2020;95(4):167-72.

Abstract

The COVID-19 pandemic has made monumental changes in practice aspects of neurologists and also in the lives of their patients with non-COVID neurological diseases. Neurologists have to consider their fundamental obligations to their own individual patients with neurological disabilities as well as the greater community.[34] Deferring necessary but nonurgent investigations and selectively reallocating these available resources is very distasteful yet necessary during this pandemic times.[35] They may be asked to help with non-neurology patients from the surge. Apart from that, the education of next-generation neurologists might get affected during these days.[36] Neurologists need to adapt their daily clinical practice to recent needs and consider how they can care for their neurology patients while contributing to the care of all patients affected with COVID-19.[37]

COMMENT

With the expansion of the COVID-19 pandemic, every aspect of healthcare needs to undergo significant change. Inpatient admissions get restricted to those with medical necessity. Hospital spaces get reallocated to provide the highest quality of care for all COVID patients, especially for the most ill. Neurologists might need to defer planned interventions/investigations for their patients and reallocate medical resources to those who are in real need. For routine neurology patients, they can hold appointments via telehealth which is an evidence-based practice but it can be particularly problematic to neurologists because physical examination gets very limited with more emphasis on observation than their traditional "hands-on" approach. During this pandemic, neurologists may be called upon to help with nonneurology patients from the surge. Questions might get raised regarding the appropriateness of managing patients outside of one's primary skillset but if limited expertise is available and the neurologists being already trained to manage such patients, then the urgency of crisis makes it ethically permissible to offer the care which he or she is capable of. Apart from that, during routine days, many hospitals refer their patients to tertiary centers for specialty care. Tertiary centers, however, may be redirecting their neurology resources to confront the pandemic patient surge. But for the greater good of the community, referral centers should continue to provide urgent and emergent neurologic care. Education of the next generation of neurologists should continue during this pandemic. Neurology education is deeply rooted in the neurological examination and subsequent cognitive exercises of lesion localization and differential diagnosis. To replace this bedside teaching, they should practice remote-access-learning and perform video demonstrations of examination findings and facilitate interactive discussions. Despite these challenges, if neurologists fail to modify their practice, it would reduce our ability to control how many lives we can save with the equipment and staff that we have in this COVID-19 pandemic.

ARTICLE 11

The Ethics of Motivational Neuro-doping in Sport: Praiseworthiness and Prizeworthiness

Bowman-Smart, Hilary, Savulescu, Julian. The ethics of motivational neuro-doping in sport: Praiseworthiness and prizeworthiness.
Neuroethics. 2021;14(Suppl 2):205-15.

Abstract

Achievements in sports relies not only on the physical abilities of the athlete but also on "will" in achieving his goal.[38] The motivation of athletes leads to increasing the will to perform in sport. Motivation is of two types—intrinsic (where pursuing a task is enjoyable) and extrinsic (where task leads to the achievement of outcome-rewards).[39] Motivational enhancement impacts both kinds of motivation.[40] Motivational enhancement is the use of pharmaceuticals or technology to increase someone's motivation to complete a task or action. Motivational doping is an extreme form of motivation to enhance an athlete's performance.

Athletes gain achievements based on the amount of efforts undertaken, which leads to prizeworthiness (whether the athlete deserves prize)/praiseworthiness (whether the athlete deserves praise)/admiration (pure admiration of performance). The model proposed by Maslen et al.[40] suggests that praiseworthiness is dependent on the athlete's "costly commitment" to a particular valuable goal that is how much an athlete puts his physical efforts, mental efforts, time, money, and different opportunities missed during the time of training. According to this view, the morally relevant aspects of costly commitment are: (1) the voluntariness of the athlete, how desperate is the athlete to achieve the goal based on his personal, family, or national interest; (2) the costliness of effort that is physical efforts, mental efforts, time and money invested; (3) the value of the goal for the efforts applied by athlete–Olympic medal or prize at local community games; and (4) the strength of the athlete's commitment—will of the athlete.

Motivational doping reduces the effort to train, cost of training, decreases the time to train, increases voluntariness, and increases the strength to commitment.[41] However, praiseworthiness of the effort has to persist irrespective of prizeworthiness. On the other hand, it may lead to physiological as well as psychological side effects or may incur extreme life costs and decrease time in other tasks of priority.

COMMENT

Motivational doping is the enhancement of an athlete's will to engage in training efforts and take steps toward the goal, making it easier to take difficult tasks. According to the cost commitment model, performance can still be praiseworthy irrespective of prizeworthiness. However, extreme forms of motivation are not acceptable if they remove the voluntariness of the athlete, if the costs are reduced too greatly, if they reduce the strength of commitment required, or they remove the athlete's contribution to the sport.

ARTICLE 12

Challenges and Ethical Issues in the Course of Palliative Care Management for People Living with Advanced Neurologic Diseases

Sreenivasan V, Nobleza COS. Challenges and ethical issues in the course of palliative care management for people living with advanced neurologic diseases.
Ann Palliat Med. 2018;7(3):304-19.

Abstract

Aim: To discuss and summarize the challenges and ethical issues faced in the palliative care (PC) management of patients with advanced acute, rapidly progressive, slowly progressive or degenerative neurological conditions that are commonly seen in practice.

Palliative care is defined as care that provides relief from pain and other symptoms, that supports quality of life (QoL), and that is focused on patients with serious advanced illness and their families.[42] Various issues faced includes the following:

- *Timing of PC involvement:* There is currently no general guideline on the timing of PC for neurologic disease. "Simultaneous care"[43] wherein PC is incorporated early and throughout the disease process.
- *Surrogate decision-making:* Many patients have declined cognition or are not able to communicate properly. Both of these affect decision-making capacities (DMCs). Surrogates formally appointed by the patient may make decisions in his best interest. The surrogate should make their best judgement of what the patient may decide under the current situation and take decisions accordingly.[44]
- *Withholding and withdrawing treatment:* Prognostic tools can help with prognosis of the disease that may aid and guide this decision. Before withholding or withdrawing life-sustaining treatment (WLST) factors such as the patient and family's values, beliefs, and current emotional and psychological states should be taken into account.
- *Pain management, palliative sedation (PS):* Therapy to relieve pain and discomfort for patients currently in PC can also have several disadvantages like respiratory depression and further decrease in level of consciousness with the use of opioid or benzodiazepine use. Indications of PS include dyspnea, delirium,[45] pain, massive bleeding, or intractable vomiting.[46]
- *The use of neuromuscular blockade:* Patients who do not achieve regular respiration with adequate sedation are candidates for neuromuscular blockers. However, this may mask pain or other symptoms of discomfort. The use of neuromuscular blockers still continues to be debated and its use is very limited.
- *Initiating, withholding, or discontinuation of artificial nutrition and hydration:* Artificial nutrition includes oral nutritional supplements (ONSs), enteral nutrition (EN) delivered through nasogastric tube, percutaneous endoscopic gastrostomy (PEG), etc. Artificial hydration includes water or electrolyte solutions through feeding tubes or parenterally.[47] These pose an increased risk of infections, pressure sores, diarrhea, and fluid overload. The family should be made aware and educated about the goals, expectations, and possible outcomes of continuing oral intake. The surrogate has the right to refuse artificial hydration and nutrition (AHN).
- *Renal replacement therapy in acute brain injury:* Dialysis can be withdrawn in cases of severe neurologic impairment where the patient has no awareness, sensation, purposeful movement, or thought process.
- *Implantable cardiac devices:* Discontinuing a device like a pacemaker or an inotrope support is a major decision because stopping these may actually cause death. This should be made through informed consent where all the options and associated risk and benefits are considered. If the decision is made to deactivate the device, a do-not-resuscitate (DNR) status should also be signed simultaneously.[48]
- *Tracheostomy placement:* Tracheostomy prolong survival but has more expense and an increased caregiver burden. A balanced decision should be taken keeping in mind the prognosis of the underlying disease, patient's comorbidities, the risk and benefits of tracheostomy, and its effect on the patient's and caregiver's QoL.

Conclusion: There are many and variable challenges and ethical issues that are important to consider in the management of patients with advanced neurological disease. Further prospective studies are required to examine the effect of PC management and to improve PC utilization among patients with neurologic conditions.

COMMENT

Across the vast array of neurological diseases, a clinician as well as the family members are faced with a lot of ethical issues. Simultaneous care that includes palliative care early in the disease course with the aim of improving the quality of care, strengthening the support system to improve patient, and caregivers' quality of life should be done. Regarding surrogate decision-making there is an age-old debate among bioethicists because there is always a doubt into how reliable the surrogate can be in terms of knowing what the patient would have wanted. Whatsoever may be the case the nearest family member is the best person to take decisions on the patient's behalf if the need arises. On the part of the clinician, he/she should make sure that the surrogate decision maker is fully educated regarding all the alternatives and pros and cons of the various options available. Also, it is best to avoid early discontinuation of life sustaining therapy before 72 hours especially in patients with neurologic conditions with an unpredictable course. Terminally ill patients are in immense pain and discomfort. The clinician must decide and weigh carefully that palliative sedation does not cause more harm than good to the patient. Relieving a terminally ill patient of his pain either with sedation or with use of neuromuscular blockade is debatable but acceptable. In decisions pertaining to removal of life support devices like dialysis/cardiac pacemaker/tracheostomy a "time-limited trial" can be given wherein the support may be withdrawn if clinical improvement does not occur. The family members should be fully involved in these end-of-life care decisions. Palliative care should be individualized, and the best course of further treatment should be selected through a multidisciplinary approach along with open communication with the patient and family or caregiver.

ARTICLE 13

Reflections on Ethics and Humanity in Pediatric Neurology: The Value of Recognizing Ethical Issues in Common Clinical Practice

Ronen GM, Rosenbaum PL. Reflections on ethics and humanity in pediatric neurology: The value of recognizing ethical issues in common clinical practice.
Curr Neurol Neurosci Rep. 2017;17(5):39.

Abstract

The four principles of modern biomedical ethics are autonomy (each person is an individual worthy of respect), beneficence (doing good), nonmaleficence (doing no harm), and justice (fairness regardless of a person's circumstances).[49] Each of these principles is considered equally important.

The main elements namely, medical indications, quality of life, and patient's preferences decides the treatment course to be followed.

By sharpening our ability to recognize the ethical aspects of humanity relevant to daily healthcare issues experienced by patients, individual families, or specific populations (e.g., children with neurodevelopmental impairment), we will be able to improve our capacity and capability as a clinician to address and potentially resolve difficult situations.

Impairment and disability will always be a part of the human ailment despite remarkable technological progress. Given this reality, that despite great advancement in contemporary medicine we cannot cure all diseases. Thus, a major goal of healthcare would be to continue to focus on how to improve life quality and functioning of affected individuals.[50] In current situation, there is media hype about novel biomedical breakthroughs, offering complete cure to various neurological diseases, and giving false hope to the patients and their families despite lack of any proven evidence regarding the same.

Even if according to evidence-based medicine no beneficial treatment is currently available for the concerned neurological disease, a clinician could counsel the patients of possible treatment in near future and thus convey a sense of hopefulness that might help patient to lead a better life. This balanced approach could bridge the gap between evidence and humanity.

Screening of newborns for various neurological diseases like phenylketonuria (PKU), thyroid deficiency, galactosemia, etc., leads to early detection, management of these diseases which can be at times lifesaving for the child and prevent chronic disabilities.[51] However, it does not mean that screening tests should be applied irrationally without consideration of the prevalence of disease in community and its specificity and sensitivity.

COMMENT

Individual patients are not a singular population. Each patient has their own unique life situations, culture, goals, and expectations that need to be considered with humanity and humility. Despite remarkable technological progress in contemporary biomedicine, impairment, and disability will always be part of the human condition.

Ethics is one of the important pillars on which future medical education should focus on. It can be made a part of curriculum of medical training program. The objective is to identify the ethical issues inherent in any clinical scenario and to explore and learn from these ethical dilemmas.

ARTICLE 14

Drugs, Genes, and Screens: The Ethics of Preventing and Treating Spinal Muscular Atrophy

Gyngell C, Stark Z, Savulescu J. Drugs, genes and screens: The ethics of preventing and treating spinal muscular atrophy. *Bioethics. 2020;34(5):493-501.*

Abstract

Spinal muscular atrophy (SMA) affects approximately 1/12,000 live births, caused by deletion/mutation of *SMN-1* gene in an autosomal recessive manner.[52] Ex-ante approach includes preimplantation genetic diagnosis, prenatal testing, and termination of pregnancy. Gene editing technologies, such as the CRISPR-Cas9 system, can correct pathogenetic mutations at the embryonic stage.[53] Ex-post (post birth) treatment includes antisense oligonucleotide-Nusinersen which has an estimated cost of US$750,000 initially, then US$3,750,000/year.[54] Gene therapy includes AVSX-101, which is a genetically modified virus, costs around US$2.125 million dollars. The aspects which could be considered in decision-making are:

- *Autonomy:* Means ability to take independent decision without external influence and should own full responsibility of the decision taken by the individual.[55] The availability of carrier screening enables a greater range of reproductive choices for parents. Ex-post therapies technically give parents a little choice for effective therapy.
- *Beneficence*: Means improvement of individual with the treatment given.[56] Using ex-ante approach individual would not have survived as pregnancy would be terminated, while the next child born after ruling out SMA on screening would have normal life expectancy. Until we have more empirical data about these treatments, it is difficult to compare these two approaches.
- *Justice:* Deals with equitable distribution of medical service and cost-effectiveness of treatment. In the public health system, with limited resources, cost plays an important part. Ex-ante intervention ensures healthy individual, while ex-post interventions only increase life by few years. The screening of the population may be expensive, thus if individuals know they are carriers, then prenatal screening is to be considered and should be promoted on justice grounds.[57]

COMMENT

For the couples using the ex-ante approach, the chance of the next child having spinal muscular atrophy (SMA) is greatly reduced and using the ex-ante approach is much cheaper and helps to prioritize carrier screening for SMA enabling couples to make an informed decision. Thus, couples who are known carriers, should use ex-ante methods, like preimplantation genetic diagnosis, prenatal testing, and termination, and based on the moral principles of autonomy, beneficence, and justice to reduce the burden of SMA.

ARTICLE 15

Understanding and Addressing Gender Equity for Women in Neurology

Silver JK. Understanding and addressing gender equity for women in neurology.
Neurology. 2019;93(12):538-49.

Abstract

Gender bias and disparities provide fertile ground for sexual harassment, and medical profession is not an exclusion. Whatever form they take, the evidence demands that both gender discrimination and sexual harassment, which are overwhelmingly directed at women, must be recognized by the medical and scientific community as morally unjustifiable and unethical.[58] Gender bias must be eliminated as discrimination is stigma to the healthcare professionals. Gender discrimination itself harms women and supports organizational environments in which sexual harassment is more prone.[58] Sexual harassment is the result of gender discrimination that is highly prevalent in academic institutions. This can also limit the capable women to rise as a leader and to obtain grant of funds to advance their research work and careers. Physician burnout is a common issue among all specialties. Neurology has been ranked among the top specialties at risk for burnout, and risk is likely more pronounced in women.[59] Therefore, we must conclude that leaders of all healthcare-related organizations have a moral and ethical imperative to genuinely address both gender discrimination and sexual harassment of women in medicine.[60]

COMMENT

Gender bias and sexual harassments are common problems for medical profession. It is our moral responsibility to contain it. At this unique time in history, there is an opportunity for leaders in neurology to strategically address its workforce gender disparities. Leaders will have to plan a path to overcome barriers and to create an equitable and safe work environment for women. Leaders in all organizations must take responsibility for gender equity. The aim is to focus on ethical principles and behavior to address gender disparities for women in medicine.

REFERENCES (Social Aspects of Neurology)

1. Emanuel EJ, Crouch RA, Arras JD, Moreno JD, Grady C (Eds). Ethical and Regulatory Aspects of Clinical Research: Readings and Commentary, 1st edition. Baltimore: Johns Hopkins University Press; 2004.
2. Emanuel EJ, Abdoler E, Stunkel L. Research ethics: how to treat people who participate in research. Bethesda: National Institutes of Health; 2010.
3. US Department of Health and Human Services. Federal policy for the protection of human subjects. Final rule. Fed Regist. 2017;82(12):7149-274.
4. George M, Selvarajan S, Dkhar SA, Chandrasekaran A. Globalization of clinical trials: where are we heading? Curr Clin Pharmacol. 2013;8:115-23.
5. Schmidt S. Shall we really do it again? The powerful concept of replication is neglected in the social sciences. Rev Gen Psychol. 2009;13:90-100.
6. Zhang XH, Tee LY, Wang XG, Huang QS, Yang SH. Off-target effects in CRISPR/Cas9-mediated genome engineering. Mol Ther Nucleic Acids. 2015;4(11):e264.
7. Hughes JC, Baldwin C (Eds). Ethical Issues in Dementia Care: Making Difficult Decisions, 1st edition. London: Jessica Kingsley Publishers; 2006.
8. Strech D, Mertz M, Knüppel H, Neitzke G, Schmidhuber M. The full spectrum of ethical issues in dementia care: systematic qualitative review. Br J Psychiatry. 2013;202:400-6.
9. Gorelick PB. The global burden of stroke: persistent and disabling. Lancet Neurol. 2019;18(5):417-8.
10. Gostin LO. The Americans with Disabilities Act at 25: the highest expression of American values. JAMA. 2015;313(22):2231-5.
11. American Stroke Association, Regenhardt RW. (2018). Acute stroke treatments for patients with pre-stroke disability: are we discriminating against the disabled? [online] Available from https://journals.heart.org/bloggingstroke/2018/11/13/acute-stroke-treatments-for-patients-with-pre-stroke-disability-are-we-discriminating-against-the-disabled/ [Last Accessed September, 2022].
12. Epilepsy Foundation. State driving laws database. www.epilepsy.com/driving-laws/ 2008691. Accessed January 31, 2019.
13. Noe K. Counseling and management of the risks of living with epilepsy. Continuum (Minneap Minn). 2019;25(2):477-91.
14. Salat D, Noyce AJ, Schrag A, Tolosa E. Challenges of modifying disease progression in prediagnostic Parkinson's disease. Lancet Neurol. 2016;15(6):637-48.
15. Berg D, Postuma RB, Adler CH, Bloem BR, Chan P, Dubois B, et al. MDS research criteria for prodromal Parkinson's disease. Mov Disord. 2015;30(12):1600-11.
16. Hunter DJ. Uncertainty in the era of precision medicine. N Engl J Med. 2016;375(8):711-3.
17. Simpkin AL, Armstrong KA. Communicating uncertainty: a narrative review and framework for future research. J Gen Intern Med. 2019;34(11):2586-91.
18. Andorno R. The right not to know: an autonomy based approach. J Med Ethics. 2004;30(5):435-9.
19. Corrigan JD, Hammond FM. Traumatic brain injury as a chronic health condition. Arch Phys Med Rehabil. 2013;94(6):1199-201.
20. Kim H, Colantonio A. Effectiveness of rehabilitation in enhancing community integration after acute traumatic brain injury: a systematic review. Am J Occup Ther. 2010;64(5):709-19.
21. The World Health Organization quality of life assessment (WHOQOL): position paper from the World Health Organization. Soc Sci Med. 1995;41(10):1403-9.
22. Beauchamp TL, Childress JF (Eds). Principles of Biomedical Ethics, 6th edition. Oxford: Oxford University Press; 2009.
23. Bourke SC, Bullock RE, Williams TL, Shaw PJ, Gibson GJ. Noninvasive ventilation in ALS: indications and effect on quality of life. Neurology. 2003;61(2):171-7.
24. Creemers H, de Morée S, Veldink JH, Nollet F, van den Berg LH, Beelen A. Factors related to caregiver strain in ALS: a longitudinal study. J Neurol Neurosurg Psychiatry. 2016;87(7):775-81.
25. Galin S, Heruti I, Barak N, Gotkine M. Hope and self-efficacy are associated with better satisfaction with life in people with ALS. Amyotroph Lateral Scler Frontotemporal Degener. 2018;19(7-8):611-8.
26. Bede P, Oliver D, Stodart J, van den Berg L, Simmons Z, Brannagáin DO, et al. Palliative care in amyotrophic lateral sclerosis: a review of current international guidelines and initiatives. J Neurol Neurosurg Psychiatry. 2011;82(4):413-8.
27. Giacino JT, Katz DI, Schiff ND, Whyte J, Ashman EJ, Ashwal S, et al. Practice guideline update recommendations summary: disorders of consciousness: report of the guideline development, dissemination, and implementation subcommittee of the American Academy of Neurology; the American Congress of Rehabilitation Medicine; and the National Institute on Disability, Independent Living, and Rehabilitation Research. Neurology. 2018;91(10):450-60.
28. Bernat JL. Nosologic considerations in disorders of consciousness. Ann Neurol. 2017;82(6):863-5.
29. D'Haese PF, Konrad PE, Dawant BM. Big data and deep brain stimulation. In: Krames E, Peckham PH, Rezai A (Eds). Neuromodulation: Comprehensive Textbook of Principles, Technologies, and Therapies, 2nd edition. Cambridge: Academic Press; 2018. pp. 137-45.
30. Lázaro-Muñoz G, Yoshor D, Beauchamp MS, Goodman WK, McGuire AL. Continued access to investigational brain implants. Nat Rev Neurosci. 2018;19(6):317-8.

31. Dubljević V, Racine E. Moral enhancement meets normative and empirical reality: assessing the practical feasibility of moral enhancement neurotechnologies. Bioethics. 2017;31(5):338-48.
32. Gilbert F, Ovadia D. Deep brain stimulation in the media: over-optimistic portrayals call for a new strategy involving journalists and scientists in ethical debates. Front Integr Neurosci. 2011;5:16.
33. Smeets AYJM, Duits AA, Horstkötter D, Verdellen C, de Wert G, Temel Y, et al. Ethics of deep brain stimulation in adolescent patients with refractory Tourette syndrome: a systematic review and two case discussions. Neuroethics. 2018;11(2):143-55.
34. National Public Radio, Breslow J. (2020). NYC could need up to 45,000 additional medical workers this month, Mayor says. [online] Available from https://www.npr.org/sections/coronavirus-live-updates/2020/04/09/830973097/nyc-could-need-up-to-45-000-additional-medical-workers-this-month-mayor-says [Last Accessed September, 2022].
35. AMA code of medical ethics' opinion on allocating medical resources. Virtual Mentor. 2011;13(4):228-9.
36. Gallagher TH, Schleyer AM. "We Signed Up for This!" - student and trainee responses to the Covid-19 pandemic. N Engl J Med. 2020;382(25):e96.
37. Hatcher-Martin JM, Adams JL, Anderson ER, Bove R, Burrus TM, Chehrenama M, et al. Telemedicine in neurology: Telemedicine Work Group of the American Academy of Neurology Update. Neurology. 2000;94(1):30-8.
38. Ilieva IP, Farah MJ. Enhancement stimulants: perceived motivational and cognitive advantages. Front Neurosci. 2013;7:198.
39. Ryan RM, Deci EL. Intrinsic and extrinsic motivations: Classic definitions and new directions. Contemp Educ Psychol. 2000;25(1):54-67.
40. Maslen H, Savulescu J, Hunt C. Praiseworthiness and motivational enhancement: 'No pain, no praise'? Australas J Philos. 2019;98(2):304-18.
41. Faber NS, Savulescu J, Douglas T. Why is cognitive enhancement deemed unacceptable? The role of fairness, deservingness, and hollow achievements. Front Psychol. 2016;7:232.
42. Dying in America: improving quality and honoring individual preferences near the end of life. Mil Med. 2015;180(4):365-7.
43. Meyers FJ, Linder J. Simultaneous care: disease treatment and palliative care throughout illness. J Clin Oncol. 2003;21(7):1412-5.
44. Johansson M, Brostrom L. Empirical fallacies in the debate on substituted judgment. Health Care Anal. 2014;22(1):73-81.
45. Chiu TY, Hu WY, Lue BH, Cheng SY, Chen CY, et al. Sedation for refractory symptoms of terminal cancer patients in Taiwan. J Pain Symptom Manage. 2001;21(6):467-72.
46. Rady MY, Verheijde JL. Sedation for the imminently dying: survey results from the AAN ethics section. Neurology. 2010;75(19):1753.
47. Druml C, Ballmer PE, Druml W, Oehmichen F, Shenkin A, Singer P, et al. ESPEN guideline on ethical aspects of artificial nutrition and hydration. Clin Nutr. 2016;35(3):545-56.
48. Ayach B, Malik A, Seifer C, Zieroth S. End of life decisions in heart failure: to turn off the intracardiac device or not? Curr Opin Cardiol. 2017;32(2):224-8.
49. Beauchamp TL, Childress JF (Eds). Principles of Biomedical Ethics, 6th edition. Oxford: Oxford University Press; 2009.
50. Ronen GM, Rosenbaum PL (Eds). Life quality outcomes in children and young people with neurological and developmental conditions: concepts, evidence and practice, 1st edition. London: Mac Keith Press; 2013.
51. Al-Qabandi M, Gorter JW, Rosenbaum P. Early autism detection: are we ready for routine screening? Pediatrics. 2011;128(1):e211-7.
52. Verhaart IEC, Robertson A, Wilson IJ, Aartsma-Rus A, Cameron S, Jones CC, et al. Prevalence, incidence and carrier frequency of 5q-linked spinal muscular atrophy - a literature review. Orphanet J Rare Dis.2017;12(1):124.
53. Ma H, Marti-Gutierrez N, Park SW, Wu J, Lee Y, Suzuki K, et al. Correction of a pathogenic gene mutation in human embryos. Nature. 2017;548(7668):413-9.
54. Institute for Clinical and Economic Review. (2018). Spinraza® and Zolgensma® for spinal muscular atrophy: Effectiveness and value. Retrieved from https://icer-review.org/wp-content/uploads/2018/07/ICER_SMA_Draft_Evidence_Report_122018-1.pdf
55. Coggon J, Miola J. Autonomy, liberty, and medical decision-making. Camb Law J. 2011;70(3):523-47.
56. Callahan D. Managed care and the goals of medicine. J Am Geriatr Soc. 1998;46(3):385-8.
57. Boardman FK, Sadler C, Young PJ. Newborn genetic screening for spinal muscular atrophy in the UK: The views of the general population. Mol Genet Genomic Med. 2018;6(1):99-108.
58. National Academies of Sciences, Engineering, and Medicine. Sexual Harassment of Women: Climate, Culture, and Consequences in Academic Sciences, Engineering, and Medicine. Washington, DC: The National Academies Press; 2018.
59. Dyrbye LN, Burke SE, Hardeman RR, Herrin J, Wittlin NM, Yeazel M, et al. Association of clinical specialty with symptoms of burnout and career choice regret among US resident physicians. JAMA. 2018;320(11):1114-30.
60. Silver JK. #BeEthical: a call to healthcare leaders: ending gender workforce disparities is an ethical imperative. Available at: sheleadshealthcare.com/wp-content/uploads/2018/10/Be_Ethical_Campaign_101418.pdf. Published September 17, 2018. Accessed March 13, 2019

INDEX

Page numbers followed by *t* refer to table.

A

Acetazolamide 102
Acetyl-l-carnitine 123, 124
Acid alpha-glucosidase 281
Activated protein C 54
Acute disseminated
    encephalomyelitis
    syndrome 204, 207, 208
Acute stroke 49
    registry 176
Acute STroke Registry and
    Analysis of Lausanne 176
Acute vestibular syndrome 1, 2
Adeno-associated virus 137,
    142, 150
Adiponectin 137
Adiporon 137
Adrenal insufficiency,
    management of 136
Adrenocorticotropic hormone
    62, 64
    stimulation test 137
Adult cerebral malaria 32
Advanced neurologic diseases
    306
Aerobic exercise, effects of 228
Alzheimer's disease 81, 108-
    110, 112-115, 118-120, 248,
    255, 256, 258
Amino acid decarboxylase 87
Amyloid-β precursor protein
    264, 265
Amyotrophic lateral sclerosis
    300
Angiotensin receptor blockers
    146
Angiotensin-converting enzyme
    127, 146
Antecedent infections 127
Antiaquaporin-4-
    immunoglobulin G 198

Anti-connective tissue growth
    factor 143
Anti-gamma-aminobutyric acid
    201
Anti-N-methyl-D-aspartate 57,
    201, 206
Antiseizure medication 63, 73
Antitubercular drugs 39
Apolipoprotein E 262
Aquaporin-4 286
    neuromyelitis optica
        spectrum disorder 289
Argyll robertson pupils 26
Arrhythmias 146
Artificial intelligence 279
Artificial nutrition and
    hydration 307
Ashworth scale, modified 231
Aspiration thrombectomy 45
Aspirin 47, 49
Ataxia 90, 99
    rating of 93, 94, 96
    telangiectasia 96
Atrial fibrillation 53
Attention deficit hyperactivity
    disorder 254, 255
Autism spectrum disorders 66
Autoimmune
    disorders 197
    encephalitis 199, 201, 202,
        206
Autosomal dominant 100, 101

B

Bacterial neuroinfections,
    acute 37
Barthel index, modified 231
Basic human right 297
Basilar artery
    acute 44
    occlusion 44

Beck's depression index 129
Berg balance scale 217, 218, 226
Best-corrected visual acuity 275
Biallelic trinucleotide 238
Bladder dysfunction,
    management of 218
Botulinum neurotoxin 212
    injection 88
Botulinum toxin 88, 212
Brain 28
    injury, acute 307
    magnetic resonance imaging
        11, 185, 265
    swelling, determinants of 32
Breathing, sleep disordered 177

C

Calcitonin gene-related peptide
    12
Calcium-binding protein
    calprotectin 130
Calpainopathy 151
Calprotectin 129
Campylobacter jejuni 125, 127,
    128
Cannabidiol 63, 253
Cardiorespiratory fitness 113,
    114
Cardiovascular disease 6, 161,
    173
Cardiovascular health study 111
Caregiver stress 117
Casimersen 144*t*
Cataplexy, number of 170
Catechol-o-methyltransferase
    254, 255
Central nervous system 10, 37,
    199, 204
Central sleep apnea 169
    moderate-to-severe 169
    treatment of 169

Centronuclear myopathies 270
Cerebellar artery, posterior inferior 206, 207
Cerebellar ataxia 25
  types of 97
Cerebellar function 95
Cerebellar inhibition 95
Cerebellar tonsillar ectopia 185
Cerebellar transcranial direct current stimulation 94
Cerebellospinal stimulation 94
Cerebral amyloid angiopathy 265
Cerebral malaria 32, 33
Cerebral small vessel disease 167, 168
Cerebral venous
  sinus thrombosis 9, 10
  thrombosis 10
Cerebrospinal fluid 11, 26, 31, 32, 37-39, 85, 119, 127, 185-187, 193-195, 198, 202, 263, 264
  classical 37
  mutant huntingtin 87
  spontaneous spinal 12, 14
Cerebrovascular disease 160
Charcot-Marie-Tooth disease 263, 264
Chikungunya 127
Cholesterol 79
Chronic inflammatory demyelinating polyneuropathy 129, 130
Chronic migraine, prevention of 2
Classic infantile pompe disease 249
Clinical dementia rating 109, 117
Cochin hand functional disability 124
Cognition 105
Cognitive deficiency 215
Cognitive impairment 91, 92, 294
  mild 108, 109
Completing vaccination 285
Compound muscle action potentials 201
Consciousness, disorders of 302

Continuous positive airway pressure 160, 161, 166, 177, 178
Corneal nerve
  fiber length 127
  fractal dimension 127
Coronary artery disease 160
Coronary heart diseases 163
Corticosteroids 134
COVID-19 30, 76, 116, 165, 285
  cornea of 126
  diagnosis 29
  infection 26, 27, 117, 126, 131
  isolation 118
  pandemic 3, 14, 15, 76, 117, 118, 165, 166, 304
  risk of 285
  severe 122
  vaccination 27
Cranial nerve, branches of 17
Cycloserine 38
Cytokine
  release syndrome 32
  storm 131
    syndrome 31

D

Daily living, activities of 209, 260
Deep brain stimulation 66, 86, 303
Deflazacort 246
  therapy 135
Dementia 25, 105, 108, 117, 202, 295
  risk factors 113
  with lewy bodies 171
Demyelination 284
Dengue 127
Derived neurotrophic factor 83
Dermatomyositis 157
Dichlorphenamide 154
Diplopia 189, 190
Direct oral anticoagulant 10
Disability 34
Disabling stroke 296
Disease-modifying therapies 284, 285
  compliance of 284
Disease-modifying treatment 292

Divergent pallidal pathways 84
Domagrozumab 144t
Dopamine
  agonists 86
  loss, effects of statins on 79
  transporter 79
Dravet syndrome 63, 73, 75
Drisapersen 144t
Drug-resistant epilepsy 164
Dual sensory impairment 110, 111
Duchenne muscular dystrophy 134, 136-139, 141-143, 145, 146, 150, 276
  treatment of 142
    strategies of 144t
Dysferlinopathy 151
Dystonic tremor 88

E

Edasalonexent 144t
Efficacy 284
Electrocardiogram 53
Electrochemiluminescence 101
Electroencephalography 71, 205, 252
Electronic health records 29
Emotion regulation index 74
Encephalitis 31
Encephaloceles 185
Endovascular stroke treatment 47
Endovascular therapy 44
Endovascular treatment 44, 46-48
  assessment of 44
Enzyme 273
  replacement therapy 249, 250
Enzyme-linked immunosorbent assay 37, 127
Epidermal neurite density 132
Epidural blood patch 12
Epilepsy 61, 65, 252, 297
  prevention of 70, 252
  thalamus for 66
  treatment-resistant 254
Epileptic encephalopathy 63, 256, 257
Episodic ataxia 102
Episodic migraine 19, 21, 22

Episodic positional vertigo 2
Episodic spontaneous vertigo 1, 2
Epworth sleepiness scale 170, 180
Erythrocyte sedimentation rate 206, 207
Eteplirsen 144*t*
Excessive day time sleepiness 171, 180, 181
Eye movement sleep behavior disorder 85
Ezutromid 144*t*

F

Facial pain 17
Facioscapulohumeral dystrophy 152, 267, 268
Fampridine 102
Fatigue severity scale 98, 129
Fibromyalgia 132
Fluorescent in situ hybridization 264, 265
Fluoxetine 234
  effects of 58, 233
Food and drug administration 144*t*
Friedreich's ataxia 237, 238, 271, 272
  natural history of 272
  rating scale, modified 238
Frontotemporal dementia 109, 110
Fugl-Meyer scale 216
Fukuyama congenital muscular dystrophy 246
Functional gait assessment 217, 218
Functional oral intake scale 228
Functional reach test 226

G

Gait freezing 218
Gastrointestinal infection 136
Gender bias 311
Gene
  editing 294
  therapy 87
General practitioner 299
Genetic determinants 153

Genetic frontotemporal dementia 109
Genetic markers 256
Genetic screening 279
Giant cell arteritis 206, 207
  extracranial 206
Givinostat 144*t*
Glial fibrillary acidic protein 263
Glucocerebrosidase gene 260
Glucocorticoids 136, 139
  tapering 155
Glucosamine 273
Glycosaminoglycan 239
Glycosylphosphatidylinositol deficiencies 245
Golodirsen 144*t*
Gross motor function measure 246
Guillain-Barré syndrome 125, 127, 128, 130, 131

H

Hank's balanced salt solution 149
Headache 1
  attributed restriction 5
  disorders 5
    classification of 19
Healthcare policy challenges 297
Hematopoietic stem 239
Histone deacetylase 144*t*
Hospital anxiety and depression scale 161, 215
Human T-lymphotropic virus 35, 36
Humphrey visual field 275
Huntington disease 278
Hurler's disease 240
Hyperglycemia 57
Hypertension 5
Hypogammaglobulinemia 285

I

Idebenone 144*t*
Idiopathic intracranial hypertension 14, 186-188, 192
Imminent ethical issues 294

Immune thrombotic thrombocytopenia 10
Immunoglobulin 96, 144*t*
Immunosuppressive therapy 203
Immunotherapeutic management 205
Immunotherapies 287
Impaired nonmotor symptoms 86
Implantable cardiac devices 307
Impulse control disorders 86
Impulsive-compulsive disorders 86
Infantile spasms 64
  steroids for 64
Inflammatory myopathies 156
Infliximab 157
Inherited glycosylphosphatidylinositol deficiencies 245
Innumerable consultations 299
Insomnia 172
  behavioral therapy for 166
  chronic 175
Intensive blood pressure 48
Intensive care unit 206
Intensive caregiver education program 214, 215
Intensive systolic blood pressure 48
Internal carotid artery 46, 48
International League against Epilepsy 72
Intracranial hypertension 187, 193, 194
Intracranial pressure 185, 186, 195
Intravenous immunoglobulin 131
  high-dose 10
Intravenous pulse methylprednisolone 65
Ischemic stroke 51, 176
  acute 56, 214

J

Japanese encephalitis 127, 128
Juvenile
  dermatomyositis 155
  fibromyalgia 132

K

Karolinska sleepiness scale 180

L

Lasmiditan 8
Lateral cutaneous nerve 121
Leber hereditary optic neuropathy 275
Lecanemab 118
Left ventricular ejection fraction 145
Lennox–Gastaut syndrome 63
Leprosy 34
  management information system 33
  presenting symptoms of 33
Leukocyte telomere length 261
Leukoencephalopathy 282
Levetiracetam 68, 70
Levodopa 79
Lewy body 171
  dementia 81
Limb-girdle muscular dystrophies 147, 148, 148t, 149, 150
Lower urinary tract symptoms 219
Lumbar puncture 194
Lymphopenia 285

M

Major histocompatibility complex 242
Manual muscle test 157, 158
Maximal expiratory pressure 147
Maximal inspiratory pressure 147
Maximally tolerated dose 54
Maximum voluntary contraction 152
Mayo sleep questionnaires 171
Meckel's caves 185
Memory enhancement training 114
Meningitis 25, 32, 39
Mental distress 181
Methylation 254
Methylphenidate 254
Middle cerebral artery 46, 48

Migraine 12, 14, 15
  attacks 7
  chronic 2, 3, 19, 21, 22
  disability assessment 22
  physical function impact diary 22
  treatment of 19
Mini mental state examination score 224
  test 215
Minute walk
  distance 135
  test 136, 140
Mirror therapy 231
Mitogen-activated protein kinase inhibitor 252
Mobile stroke units 59, 60
Moderate-intensity aerobic exercise 229
Modern biomedical ethics 309
Monoclonal antibodies 4, 13
Mononeuritis multiplex 122, 123
Mononeuropathy, characterization of 121
Montreal cognitive evaluation 215, 233
Motivational doping 306
Motor axonal neuropathy, acute 125
Motor relearning program 224
  effects of 224
Movement disorders 79
  behavior 85
Mucopolysaccharidosis 240, 249
Multibacillary 34
Multifocal motoric neuropathy 129
Multiple sclerosis 228, 229, 284-286, 291, 292
  relapsing-remitting 284, 292
Multiple sleep latency test 181
Multiple system atrophy 95, 100, 219
  diagnosis of 96
Muscle cells, denaturation of 246
Muscle disorders 134
Muscle-specific tyrosine kinase activation 201

Muscular dystrophies, management of 152
Mutated isocitrate dehydrogenase 1 242
Myasthenia gravis 200
Myelin oligodendrocyte glycoprotein 199, 204, 208
  antibody 286, 289
  immunoglobulin G, treatment of 288
Myelitis 25
  asymptomatic neurosyphilis 25
Myeloradiculopathy 204
Myocyte membranes 246
Myopathy-functional activity scale 273
Myotonic dystrophy 153

N

Natalizumab 291
National Cholesterol Education Program 6
National Institute of Health Stroke Scale 41, 42, 58, 234
Nerve conduction study 122
Neurocysticercosis 28
Neurodegenerative
  ataxia 94
  dementia syndromes 201
Neurogenetics 236
Neurogenic detrusor overactivity 219
Neuroinfections 25
Neurological disorders 26, 27
Neurological symptoms 31
Neurology 84, 311
  clinical research in 293
  social aspects of 293
Neuromodulation
  devices 19
  neuroethics of 303
Neuromuscular blockade, use of 307
Neuromuscular junction 201
Neuromuscular transcutaneous electrical stimulation 227
Neuromyelitis optica
  associated optic neuritis 191, 192
  spectrum disorder 190, 191, 198, 199, 203

Neuro-ophthalmology 185
Neuropathic facial pain 16
Neuropathy, treatment of 123
Neuroprotection 53
Neuropsychiatric inventory 117
Neurosyphilis 25, 26
Newborns, screening of 309
Next-generation sequencing 266
Nicotinamide riboside 96
N-methyl-D-aspartate agonists 256
N-methyl-D-aspartate receptor 201
  antibody encephalitis 205
Noncardioembolic ischemic stroke 49
Nondisabling neurologic deficits, minor 41
Noninvasive neuromuscular electrical stimulation 227, 228
Noninvasive vagus nerve stimulation 83
Nonmotor symptoms 81
Nonsteroidal anti-inflammatory drugs 124
Nuclear factor-kappa B 140, 144t
Nucleus, anterior 66

O

Obstructive sleep apnea 160, 161, 162, 167, 168, 177, 178
Ocular surface disease 126
  index 126
Omaveloxolone 236-238
Optic nerve drusen 195
Optical coherence tomography 188, 189, 194
Oral anticoagulation 53
Oral prednisolone 246
Oropharyngeal dysphagia 227, 228

P

Pain
  chronic 174
  management 307
Palliative care management 306

Palliative sedation 307
Palmitoylethanolamide 123, 124
Pamrevlumab 144t
Papilledema 188
Paraneoplastic neurologic syndromes 197
Parkinson's disease 79-82, 84-87, 180, 218, 247, 260, 262, 263, 298
  dementia 79
  detection 298
  pathophysiology of 84
  prevalence of 217
Parkinsonian behavioral deficits 84
Paucibacillary 34
Peak cough flow 147
Pediatric neurology 308
Percutaneous endoscopic gastrostomy 301
Periodic paralysis, primary 154
Perioptic subarachnoid space 186
Peripheral nervous system 204
  syndromes 203
Peripheral neuropathy 121
Permanent respiratory insufficiency 301
Persistent idiopathic facial pain 16
Pharmacology 32
Phrenic nerve stimulation 169
Pittsburgh sleep quality index 171, 229
Placebo-controlled trial 81
Plaque reduction neutralization test 128
Plasmodium falciparum 32
Pluripotent stem cells 142
Polymerase chain reaction 37, 264, 279, 280
Polymyositis 157
Polysomnography 167, 173, 178
Pompe disease 280
Positron emission tomography 119
Postvaccinal neurological disorders 27
Praiseworthiness 305
Prednisolone 156t, 246
Pregnancy, management of 290

Prizeworthiness 305, 306
Prodromal emesis 286
Progenitor cells 239
Progressive myoclonus epilepsy 266
Proprioceptive neuromuscular facilitation 224
Pseudodeficiency alleles 280
Pseudotumor cerebri syndrome 195
Pyridoxine, high-dose 244

Q

Quality of life 300, 301
Quantitative polymerase chain reaction 35

R

Raised intracranial pressure, syndrome of 187
Randomized clinical trial 43
Randomized controlled trial 2, 3, 50, 69-71, 75, 82, 170, 179, 180, 253
Rankin scale, modified 44, 55, 56
Rapid eye movement 164, 171, 172, 180
  sleep-onset 181
Recurrent neurocysticercosis 28
Refractory epilepsy 66
Refractory movement 303
Rehabilitation 209
Relapsing-remitting multiple sclerosis, treatment strategies for 292
Renal replacement therapy 307
Respiratory management 146
Restore brain study 58
Retinal nerve fiber layer 188, 189, 194
Reverse transcription-polymerase chain reaction 27
Rheumatic diseases 123
  neurological complications of 123
Rheumatoid arthritis 123, 124
Rituximab 199, 287

S

Sarcoglycanopathy 151
SARS-COV-2 infection 26, 126, 128
Schirmer tests 126, 127
Self-rating anxiety scale score 215
Self-rating depression scale 215
Serum
 calprotectin 129
 C-reactive protein 37
 neurofilament light chain 100, 129, 130
Severe acute respiratory syndrome coronavirus 2 31 infection 130
Sex differences 112
Sexual harassment 311
Sialorrhea 301
Silent brain infarction 168
Sleep
 behavior disorder 171, 172
 disorders 174
 duration 162
 heart health study 173
 medicine 160
Sleep apnea 161
 cardiovascular endpoints 160
 treatment of 176
Sleep disturbances 172, 174, 181
 spectrum of 181
 square 228
Small fiber neuropathy 126, 132
Social handicap 5
Solitary cysticercus granuloma 28
Spinal muscular atrophy 237, 240, 241, 243, 278, 280, 310
Spinocerebellar ataxia 90-92, 98, 100, 101
Spontaneous intracranial hypotension 11, 12
Spontaneous microembolic signals 52
Standard prophylactic drugs 12
Stroke 41, 163, 209-211, 233, 296
 and death, prevention of 49
 chronic 216
 recovery 56

Subcutaneous natalizumab 291
Subjective cognitive decline 108, 114, 115
Subthalamic nucleus-deep brain stimulation 86
Sudden unexpected death 65
Surrogate decision-making 307
Survival motor neuron 236, 237
Symptomatic intracerebral hemorrhage 42
Symptomatic spinal muscular atrophy 244
Symptomatic therapy 252

T

Talditercept alfa 144*t*
Task-based mirror therapy 230, 231
Telomere length 261
Thrombolysis 41
Thrombotic thrombocytopenic syndrome 9, 10
Ticagrelor 49
Tissue plasminogen activator 46
Tracheostomy placement 307
Transcranial direct current stimulation 303
Transcranial magnetic stimulation 95
Transdermal cannabidiol gel 62
Transient ischemic attack 49, 163
Traumatic brain injury, chronic 299
Treatment disability score 129
Treatment-emergent adverse events 8
Treponema pallidum hemagglutination assay 26
Trigeminal autonomic cephalalgia 19
Trigeminal neuralgia 16
Tuberculosis 32, 39
 meningitis 38
Tuberous sclerosis 252
 complex 70, 71, 252
Tumor necrosis factor alpha 31, 83

U

Ultrasound 267
Unfractionated heparin 47
Unified Huntington's disease rating scale 87
Unified Parkinson's disease rating scale 180, 217, 248, 260
Unpleasant soft symptoms 267
Upper limb motor function 230
Urinary symptoms 218

V

Vaccination implications 285
Vagus nerve stimulation 65, 66, 84
Vamorolone 144*t*
Vestibular disorders activities 102
Vestibular migraine 1
Vestibular rehabilitation 220, 221
Vestibular test 1
Video electroencephalography 253
Video head impulse tests 1
Video oculography 1
Virtual epilepsy clinics 75
Virtual reality 218, 232
Vision and hearing impairment 111

W

Wakefulness test 170
West syndrome 61, 64
White matter hyperintensities 168
Whole-exome sequencing 266
Withholding and withdrawing treatment 307
Writer's cramp 213
 disability scale 212, 213
 impairment scale 212, 213
 occupational therapy for 212
 rating scale 212, 213

X

X-linked recessive disorder 141

Y

Yoga 114